Springer

Berlin
Heidelberg
New York
Barcelona
Budapest
Hong Kong
London
Milan
Paris
Santa Clara
Singapore
Tokyo

Manual of Internal Fixation in the Cranio-Facial Skeleton

Techniques Recommended by the AO/ASIF Maxillofacial Group

Editor: Joachim Prein

Chapter Authors:
Leon A. Assael · Douglas W. Klotch · Paul N. Manson
Joachim Prein · Berton A. Rahn · Wilfried Schilli

With 190 Figures in 565 Separate Illustrations

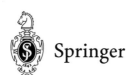 Springer

Joachim Prein, M.D., D.M.D.
Professor of Maxillofacial Surgery
Chairman of Clinic for Reconstructive Surgery
Unit for Maxillofacial Surgery
University Clinics of Basel, Kantonsspital
4031 Basel, Switzerland

ISBN 3-540-61810-4
Springer-Verlag Berlin Heidelberg New York

Library of Congress Cataloging-in-Publication Data
Manual of internal fixation in the cranio-facial skeleton: techniques recommended by the AO/ASIF-Maxillofacial Group / J. Prein ... [et al.]. p. cm. Includes bibliographical references. ISBN 3-540-61810-4 (alk. paper) 1. Facial bones – Surgery – Handbooks, manuals, etc. 2. Cranium – Surgery – Handbooks, manuals, etc. 3. Internal fixation in fractures – Handbooks, manuals, etc. 4. Surgery, Plastic – Handbooks, manuals, etc. I. Prein, J. (Joachim), 1938– . II. Arbeitsgemeinschaft für Osteosynthesefragen. [DNLM: 1. Skull – surgery. 2. Fracture Fixation, Internal – methods. 3. Facial Bones – surgery. 4. Surgery, Plastic – methods. WE 705 M294 1998] RD763.M336 1998 617.5`2059 – dc21 DNLM/DLC for Library of Congress 97-35559 CIP

Springer-Verlag Berlin Heidelberg New York a member of BertelsmannSpringer Science+Business Media GmbH
© Springer-Verlag Berlin Heidelberg 1998
Printed in Germany

The use of general descriptive names, registered names, trademarks, etc. in this publication does not imply, even in the absence of a specific statement, that such names are exempt from the relevant protective laws and regulations and therefore free for general use.

Product liability: The publisher cannot guarantee the accuracy of any information about dosage and application contained in this book. In every individual case the user must check such information by consulting the relevant literature.

Drawings: Kaspar Hiltbrand, Basel
Cover design: design & production, Heidelberg
Typesetting: Data conversion by B. Wieland, Heidelberg
Printing and bookbinding: Konrad Triltsch, Print und digitale Medien GmbH, 97199 Ochsenfurt-Hohestadt, Germany
SPIN: 10879710   24/3111 – 5 4 3
Printed on acid-free paper

Chapter Authors and Contributors

Leon A. Assael, D.M.D.
Professor of Oral and Maxillofacial Surgery
Chairman of Department Oral
and Maxillofacial Surgery
The School of Medicine of the
University of Connecticut Health Center
Farmington, CT 06030, USA

Wolfgang Bähr, M.D., D.M.D.
Ass. Professor of Maxillofacial Surgery
University Clinic for Maxillofacial Surgery
79106 Freiburg i. B., Germany

Benjamin Carson, Professor
Department of Neurosurgery
Johns Hopkins University
Baltimore, MD 21205, USA

Christopher R. Forrest, M.D., M.Sc., F.R.C.S.(C)
Ass. Professor, Craniofacial Program
Division of Plastic Surgery
The Hospital for Sick Children
Toronto, Ontario M5G 1X8, Canada

Beat Hammer, M.D., D.M.D.
Ass. Professor of Maxillofacial Surgery
Clinic for Reconstructive Surgery
Unit for Maxillofacial Surgery
University Clinics of Basel, Kantonsspital
4031 Basel, Switzerland

Douglas W. Klotch, M.D., F.A.C.S.
Associate Professor of Surgery
Director of Division of Otolaryngology
Department of Surgery, College of Medicine
University of South Florida
Tampa, FLA 33606, USA
Chairman of Maxillofacial Technical Commission

Christian Lindqvist, M.D., D.D.S., Ph.D.
Professor of Oral and Maxillofacial Surgery
Head of Department of Oral and Maxillofacial Surgery
University of Helsinki
00130 Helsinki, Finland

Nicolas J. Lüscher, M.D.
Professor of Plastic Surgery
Head of Plastic Surgery Unit
Clinic for Reconstructive Surgery
University Clinics of Basel, Kantonsspital
4031 Basel, Switzerland

Paul N. Manson, M.D.
Professor of Plastic Surgery
Chief of Division of Plastic, Reconstructive
and Maxillofacial Surgery
Johns Hopkins University
Baltimore, MD 21287–0981, USA

Bernard L. Markowitz, M.D., F.A.C.S.
Ass. Professor of Plastic Surgery
Division of Plastic Surgery
University of California
Los Angeles, CA 90095, USA

Stephan M. Perren, M.D., Dr. sc. (h.c.)
Professor of Surgery
AO Development
7270 Davos, Switzerland
Chairman of AO/ASIF Technical Commission

John H. Phillips, M.D., F.R.C.S. (C)
Professor of Plastic Surgery
Medical Director, Craniofacial Program
Division of Plastic Surgery
The Hospital for Sick Children
Toronto, Ontario M5G 1X8, Canada

Carolyn Plappert
Product Manager Maxillofacial
STRATEC Medical
4437 Oberdorf, Switzerland

Joachim Prein, M.D., D.M.D.
Professor of Maxillofacial Surgery
Chairman of Clinic for Reconstructive Surgery
Unit for Maxillofacial Surgery
University Clinics of Basel, Kantonsspital
4031 Basel, Switzerland
Chairman of European Maxillofacial
Educational Committee

Berton A. Rahn, M.D., D.M.D.
Professor of Maxillofacial Surgery
AO Research Institute
7270 Davos, Switzerland

Wilfried Schilli, M.D., D.M.D.
Professor emeritus of Maxillofacial Surgery
Director emeritus of University Clinic
for Maxillofacial Surgery
79106 Freiburg i.B., Germany

Mark A. Schusterman, M.D.
Ass. Professor of Plastic Surgery
Chairman of Department of Plastic Surgery
University of Texas
M.D. Anderson Cancer Center
Houston, TX 77030, USA

Peter Stoll, M.D., D.M.D.
Ass. Professor of Maxillofacial Surgery
University Clinic for Maxillofacial Surgery
79106 Freiburg i.B., Germany

Patrick K.Sullivan, M.D.
Associate Professor of Plastic Surgery
Brown University
Providence, R.I. 02905, USA

Craig A. Vander Kolk, M.D.
Associate Professor
Director of Cleft and Craniofacial Center
The Johns Hopkins Outpatient Center
8152D, Baltimore, MD 21287–0981, USA

Foreword

Clinical research continues to confirm that no truth is more transitory than that in the sphere of scientific knowledge. Developments in the field of traumatology at the end of this century provide a striking example of this. As early as 1890 Lambotte carried out osteosyntheses with plates and screws. These remained a mere episode, however, until Danis renewed the idea of internal fixation 50 years later. Danis combined internal fixation with the new technique of interfragmentary compression, which led to primary bone healing that allowed full function at the same time. Reacting to disconcerting statistics about the results of conservative fracture treatment, Mueller then applied interfragmentary compression to 80 patients in Switzerland and confirmed its usefulness.

Mueller, recognizing the need for further developments in clinical application, and scientific analysis, assembled a group of friends consisting of general and orthopedic surgeons in 1958 with the aim of creating the necessary armamentarium for internal fixation and to form a study group for clinical trials. This group came to be known as the *Arbeitsgemeinschaft für Osteosynthesefragen* (AO), and later in English-speaking countries as the "Association for the Study of Internal Fixation" (ASIF). Building on the conviction that the objectivity of nature is not merely an illusion, the initiators of AO/ASIF – Müller, Allgöwer, Willenegger, Schneider, and Bandi – transformed the pragmatically oriented concept into a scientific method of applied physics, mathematics, and biology. In combination with systematic teaching of specialists in AO/ASIF courses, subjectivity was thus excluded as much as possible from the choice of means. The goals and principles of AO/ASIF are built on this basis and are summarized in the AO/ASIF philosophy.

Convinced of its benefit by this approach, the maxillofacial unit of the Department of Surgery at the University of Basel adopted the AO/ASIF philosophy in 1966. The consistent application of the two principles of anatomical reduction of fracture fragments and stable internal fixation guaranteed the immediate, active, and pain-free opening and closing of the lower jaw. The results were also considerably improved by the early total care of the severely traumatized patient in the first hours following the accident.

The further development of the AO/ASIF concept led to today's comprehensive craniofacial surgery in the fields of traumatology, orthognatics, tumor, and reconstructive surgery.

AO/ASIF courses contributed fundamentally to the development of these fields. In the course of its worldwide response, the AO/ASIF philosophy has been able to attract distinguished authors to join the faculty of AO/ASIF courses. By sharing their clinical, experimental, and theoretical experience, they take part in shaping a special internal fixation technique in the craniofacial skeleton. The philosophical aspect of AO/ASIF courses in theory and practice assures high standards of quality. After all, the enormous progress in metal implantology should not hide the fact that lack of knowledge and experience, on the one hand, and false compromises, on the other, can cause much greater damage than with conservative methods.

Thus this interdisciplinary manual provides standards for the application of the AO/ASIF principles. The scientific and technological background is based on the laws of nature. Resulting from the interaction between pure research and clinical practice, it comprises in the widest sense the fields of organization, biomechanics, anatomy, and osteology as well as metallurgy and the application of tools.

The accumulated knowledge is integrated in topographically defined surgery of the skull (splanchnocranium), including the walls of the upper respiratory and digestive tracts.

The bottom line of this surgery is internal fixation. The differences in its application are dictated by the variety of craniofacial bones with respect to their function and structure. On the one hand, we are dealing with a motional apparatus in the area of the mandible; on the other, the maxilla represents a supportive frame of lamellas, among others for nose and eyes, and the cranial vault a supportive frame of diploë for the brain. Correspondingly, two qualities of stability are being distinguished in practice: *functionally stable and locally stable fixation.*

In the past 10 years there has been a rapid increase in the degree of perfection in treating most complicated fractures, disturbances of growth in the regio masticatoria and facialis, and malformations in the areas of the nose, eyes, and skull. These operations are further improved by preoperative planning with spiral 3 DCT, 3D laser stereolithography, and virtual-reality prosthetic design. These techniques still depend highly on international cooperation. Initial experiences have shown how complex craniofacial injuries, including the loss of functionally and anatomically important bone parts, can be simulated ad hoc and immediately treated with adequate autologous bone, if necessary in combination with hydroxyapatites.

Looking back to the beginnings in the 1970s and 1980s, one can observe with great satisfaction that this progress has been the work of distinguished representatives of the disciplines involved. I am most thankful for the honor of their personal friendship and acquaintance.

This manual will be a safe standard for teaching and applying internal fixation in AO/ASIF courses as well as in the operating room.

Great acknowledgement is due to the editor and the authors.

Prof. Dr. Dr. Bernd Spiessl

Preface

This *Manual of Internal Fixation in the Craniofacial Skeleton* is the result of fascinating developments in internal fixation techniques for the facial skeleton over the past 30–40 years. These techniques are based on the AO/ASIF philosophy for fracture care in the general skeleton – ensuring early pain-free movement, precise anatomical reduction, and adequate fixation according to the various functional forces. The principles and techniques described here have grown out of continuous international cooperation involving a great number of specialists working in the craniofacial area. It also continues the ideas originally developed by pioneers in the field who carried out important clinical and experimental research. In this context we should mention particularly Champy, Michelet, Luhr, Spiessl, and Tessier.

In its early days in the 1950s and 1960s this approach to internal fixation of facial bones found application principally in the treatment of trauma patients. The favorable experiences gathered in the meantime, however, have led to many of the advantages of internal fixation being extended to the reconstruction of tumor defects and the stabilization of major osteotomies in orthognathics and craniofacial surgery.

Today we also appreciate the important role that facial trauma plays in the early definitive treatment of polytraumatized patients, particularly in reducing adult respiratory distress syndrome and multiple organ failure. Close cooperation among all those working in the various related disciplines and specialties for the craniomaxillofacial area is essential to ensure optimal results for patients. This is especially so regarding the participation of the neurosurgeon in cases of traumatology and craniofacial surgery. The concept of early definitive treatment sometimes means many hours of surgery, and therefore another crucial participant in the treatment team is the anesthesist, and important progress has also been made in this area over recent years.

Four major advances underlie the great progress in craniofacial surgery in recent decades: (a) the technique of approach, (b) the technique of internal fixation with plates and screws, (c) the development of optimal materials such as titanium, and (d) modern imaging techniques like CT and MRI.

This first AO/ASIF *Manual on Internal Fixation Techniques in the Craniofacial Skeleton* is the product of collaborative work on the part of many cranio-maxillofacial specialists worldwide. Since the first maxillofacial course in Davos in 1974 and the first AO/ASIF course in the United States in 1984, 20 courses have been conducted in Davos and 109 worldwide, with several thousand persons participating. In addition to these courses, numerous international workshops have been organized to deal with specialized topics. The principles presented in this *Manual* have developed out of both the good and the disappointing experiences during this experimental, educational, and practical work. An important feature of all the courses on internal fixation in cranio-maxillofacial surgery is that they were organized by and for *oral* and *maxillofacial surgeons*, *plastic surgeons*, and *ENT surgeons*. In this Manual we try to demonstrate the results of this close international cooperation, including the substantial clinical experience and research carried out principally in the AO/ASIF Research Institute in Davos.

The fact that this *Manual* deals only with techniques for open internal fixation does not reflect an opinion on our part that every fracture should be operated on. However, it is our opinion that internal fixation – employing the appropriate technique for the correct indication – entails substantial safety and diminishes morbidity for patients. One could even maintain that adequate and safe internal fixation provides the best protection against infection and is of even greater importance than antibiotics. Internal fixation, especially in traumatology, can also have a very considerable socioeconomic impact when one considers the various factors that affect treatment costs – including the duration of surgery, cost of materials, training of the surgeon, as well as the patients' absence from work.

This *Manual* is divided into seven chapters, with a single author responsible for each; only the first chapter on research and instruments has two authors. International contributors, who are mentioned before each respective chapter, have put in their knowledge and have made significant contributions.

The material presented here reflects our present knowledge of the subject, and its correct application can surely mean comfort and benefits to our patients. On the other hand, however, it represents only the latest milestone on the way to further progress. We hope that this *Manual* proves an important help both during courses and during surgery.

In the name of all the coauthors and contributors who have invested a tremendous amount of time, knowledge, and work, I wish to thank especially Mrs. Helga Reichel-Kessler, whose continuous and never-ending encouragement was essential in finalizing the manuscript and thus in completing the whole project.

I want to thank especially Mr. Kaspar Hiltbrant for his very clear and precise drawings, which are a particular feature of this *Manual*. I am also grateful to Mrs. Ruth Rahn, who provided very important prestudies for these drawings.

Finally, I thank the staff of Springer-Verlag for their excellent help in preparing this *Manual* for publication.

Prof. Dr. Joachim Prein

Contents

CHAPTER 1

Scientific and Technical Background

1

Chapter Authors: Joachim Prein
Berton A. Rahn
Contributors: Joachim Prein
Berton A. Rahn
Carolyn Plappert
Stephan M. Perren

1.1 Introduction

1.1.1 The AO/ASIF Foundation

The Association for the Study of Internal Fixation (ASIF) was founded in 1958 in Switzerland under its original German name "Arbeitsgemeinschaft für Osteosynthesefragen (AO)," a working group to deal with questions on internal fixation of fractures. This group in the meantime has become an international organization dedicated to improving the care of patients with musculoskeletal injuries and their sequelae through research and education in the principles, practice, and quality control of the results of treatment. In 1984 this study group was transformed into a nonprofit foundation providing an umbrella structure for its activities in the fields of research, development, education, and documentation. New technologies and products developing from ideas and from research and development activities are licensed to the three Synthes producers, Mathys AG Bettlach, Stratec Medical Oberdorf, both in Switzerland, and Synthes USA, Paoli. The royalties which they pay finance the activities of the AO/ASIF Foundation.

The activities of the Foundation are supervised by an international Board of Trustees, comprising 90 leading surgeons in various specialities in orthopedics and trauma, including cranio-maxillo-facial surgery. The Academic Council establishes the basic medical and scientific goals of the foundation, taking specific regional needs and socioeconomic aspects into account. It provides input to research and development and suggests new therapeutic recommendations and teaching methods to be associated with them. The Academic Council is responsible, on behalf of the Board of Trustees, for the strategic and middle-range planning, and a Board of Directors ensures that the goals of the Academic Council can be implemented.

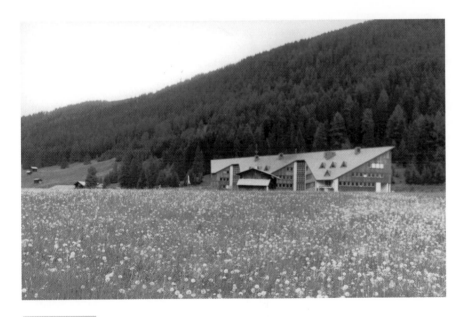

Fig. 1.1

The AO/ASIF Center. This institution serves as an international service center, coordinating the various worldwide activities of the foundation and providing support in research, development, education, and documentation relevant to trauma care. It is located in an attractive Alpine environment in Davos, Switzerland

Products before they are adopted by the AO/ASIF are submitted to a Technical Commission, with representatives from both the medical and the manufacturing sides. Speciality Technical Commissions exist for various fields of surgery, including a Maxillofacial Technical Commission. Although it is not possible to incorporate into this commission every single speciality group performing surgery in the cranio-maxillo-facial region, this Technical Commission tries to cover, across the speciality borders, the medical needs in a most comprehensive way. In the Maxillofacial Technical Commission, as within all Technical Commissions, the medical side outweighs the manufacturing side by a five to three majority. This principle ensures that professional decisions regarding medical concepts and ideas are not dominated by commercial issues. On the other hand, this structure allows for direct input from the medical market place reflecting the needs of the surgeons in the field.

The AO/ASIF Center (Fig. 1.1), located in Davos, Switzerland, is conceived as an international service center, providing worldwide support in research, development, education, and documentation.

1.1.2 Research

To promote the AO/ASIF Foundation as a clinical and scientific research organization several mechanisms have been set up to encourage research relevant to trauma care. The AO/ASIF Research Institute (ARI) in Davos is a nonprofit institution dedicated to basic and applied research in the treatment of trauma of the skeletal system and in related topics. Its scientific independence is maintained by an international scientific Board of Trustees. A multidisciplinary team of some 60 coworkers includes specialists in surgery, dentistry, biology, materials science, biomechanics, and biomedical engineering. The Research Institute works with clinical and basic scientists and with manufacturers in addressing topics relevant to the understanding and treatment of musculoskeletal injuries and their sequelae. A number of other institutions are included in the worldwide network of common interests and receive support from the foundation. The AO/ASIF Research Commission provides grants to support research projects dealing with trauma, surgery of the skeletal system, and related basic and clinical topics. Its aim is to provide "seed money" intended especially to fund work on novel concepts and work by young researchers.

1.1.3 Development

The goal of development activities at the AO/ASIF is to support the AO/ASIF Foundation in attaining its medical objectives by providing new techniques and safe equipment for treating injuries to the skeletal and locomotor system. Such development should be as universal as possible and of high quality and safety standards. In combination with the appropriate theoretical and practical teaching these methods should be simple enough for general use.

AO/ASIF development comprises the Development Coordination Group, the AO/ASIF Development Institute (ADI), the development groups of each of the three manufacturers, and the AO/ASIF Technical Commission, the only organization authorized to approve a device. The ADI involves 30 collaborators, mainly technically and application oriented. It functions in close collaboration between clinicians, research, and the three manufacturers and is guided and supervised by its own Steering Committee, consisting of three medical persons and one representative from each of the three manufacturers. Documentation and decisions in all phases conform to ISO 9001, EN 46001, MDD 93/42 EEC, FDA, and Japanese Standards.

1.1.4 Education

AO International (AOI) is the educational link, within the foundation, between national and regional AO/ASIF sections, surgeons, operating room staff, hospitals, and working groups involved in trauma and orthopedic-surgery throughout the world. This body coordinates courses worldwide, selects from an extensive faculty pool to assign speciality-specific and region-specific course faculty, and supports these teaching efforts with appropriate educational material. In these courses the scientific background is presented, the principles developed from this basic knowledge, and the way in which these principles are to be applied in a practical situation. Bone models presenting the most important fracture patterns are used for practical training, and videotapes show the appropriate procedures in a step-by-step approach.

Fellowships and scholarships are available in many countries in approved AO/ASIF teaching clinics for surgeons and for operating room personnel. Membership in the AO/ASIF Alumni Association is open to AO/ASIF faculty members, former scholarship fellows, and participants of advanced AO/ASIF courses. This Association promotes communication between surgeons and the AO/ASIF bodies and supports symposia and meetings to alumni up to date on current trends and activities in the fields of research, development, education, and documentation.

1.1.5 Documentation and Clinical Investigations

In its early days the AO/ASIF Documentation Center sought to collect information on all cases treated within the group. This offered an enormous help during the pioneering phase in assessing the efficiency and the risks of approaches which at the time often seemed very aggressive methods of treatment. Today the emphasis is more on prospective studies. A decentralized documentation system has been developed. This system uses a uniform design that permits local documentation but the possibility of pooling data between different centers. The documentation department provides guidelines and assistance in coordinating such multicenter studies, from the planning phase to the final evaluation.

1.1.6 Fracture Classification

A comprehensive classification has been developed by the AO/ASIF group that includes the site of the fracture, its degree of severity, and the approach to treatment. This classification (Fig. 1.2) is based on the differentiation of bone segment fractures into three types, their further division into three groups and their subgroups, and the arrangement of these in an ascending order of severity according to the morphological complexities of the fracture, the difficulties in their treatment, and their prognosis. In graphic representations the colors green, orange, and red and darkened arrows indicate the increasing severity. A1 indicates the simplest fracture with the best prognosis, and C3 the most difficult frac-

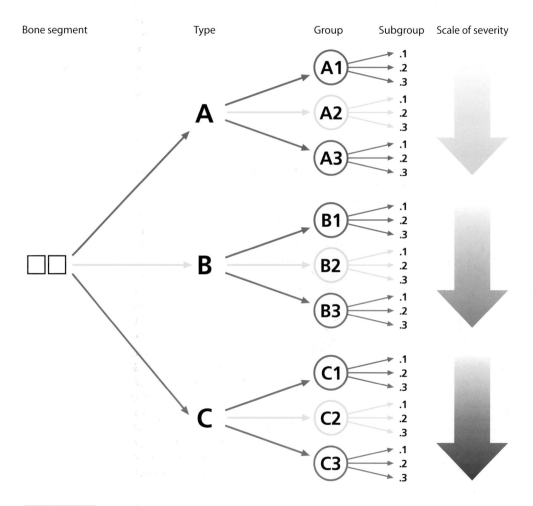

Fig. 1.2

The principle of the comprehensive AO/ASIF classification. In ascending severity the fractures are subdivided into three major types: A, B, and C. Within each type a further tripartition into groups (A1, A2, A3, etc.) and subgroups (A1.1, A1.2, etc.) is performed, again ranked in order of increasing severity.

Darkening arrows, increasing severity in terms of both potential difficulties in treatment and the expected prognosis of outcome. *Green*, lowest severity; *yellow*, intermediate severity; *red*, highest severity. (From Müller et al. 1991)

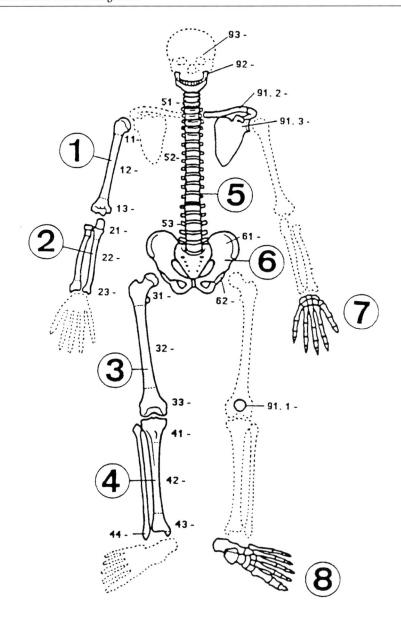

Fig. 1.3

The anatomic location in the AO/ASIF classification. In developing this comprehensive classification system the authors focused primarily on long bones.

An adaptation to the specific needs of cranio-maxillo-facial surgery has not yet been performed, but it appears feasible to subdivide this area into mandible, facial, and cranial regions. The mandible could then further be subdivided into collum, ramus, and corpus; the facial area into lateral, central caudal, and central cranial; and the cranial area into a frontal region, cranial vault, and skull base. (From Müller et al. 1991)

ture with the worst prognosis. Classifying a fracture thus establishes its severity and provides a guide to its treatment.

The AO/ASIF classification system was developed based particularly on fractures of long bones (Fig. 1.3).

In this classification the cranio-maxillo-facial area is not considered as a single entity; only the mandible is included, listed among varia together with the patella, clavicle, and scapula. The anatomical relationships and patterns are more complex in cranio-maxillo-facial fractures than in long bones, and typical fracture planes frequently involve more than one bone. Therefore a comprehensive fracture classification, although offering certain interesting features, would require major modifications to become suitable for cranio-maxillo-facial surgery.

Classifications of cranio-maxillo-facial fractures began with the classical Le Fort types, an approach which is simple and practicable but not sufficient for fractures of a higher degree of complexity. In the case of the mandible the early descriptive types of fracture classification were gradually replaced or supplemented by an approach concentrating on the number of fragments, the site, displacement and occlusion, soft tissue involvement, and accompanying fractures in the upper jaw (see Spiessl 1986).

Classifications in the cranio-maxillo-facial region hitherto were limited to specific functional areas, such as the mandible or the midface, and attempts were made to differentiate and to regionally expand the classifications taking into account the increasing complexity and severity of fracture patterns caused by the increasing influences of high-velocity injury. These efforts led to a subdivision into comminuted fractures of the upper midface, lower midface, with or without concomitant mandibular fractures, central midface, and craniofacial and panfacial fractures. It is now accepted that only imaging in three dimensions can identify and encompass the complex fracture patterns observed in the cranio-maxillo-facial area, and it is this three-dimensional approach that will provide the basis for any future comprehensive classification system.

Developing a comprehensive approach for a cranio-maxillo-facial fracture classification comparable to that described for long bones requires that the specific needs of this specific region are addressed. When the entire cranio-maxillo-facial area is to be classified at the same hierarchical level as a single long bone, a further subdivision of the anatomical site is absolutely necessary. Describing the anatomic location with sufficient precision requires subdivisons at least to segment and subsegment levels. If the principle of tripartition as described in the original AO/ASIF classification is to be maintained, an adaptation for the cranio-maxillo-facial region could consist of a subdivision into mandible, facial region, and cranial regions. The mandible could then further be subdivided into collum, ramus, and corpus; the facial area into lateral, central caudal, and central cranial region; and the cranial area into frontal area, cranial vault, and skull base. The original idea of further classification according to complexity and severity could then follow the suggested pattern depicted in Fig. 1.2, using the types A, B, C, the groups A1, A2, A3, B1, B2, etc., and then further subgroups.

1.2 Bone as a Material

1.2.1 Structure

In the gross aspect, cancellous bone is distinguished from compact and from cortical bone. These terms describe the arrangement of the bony substance but provide no information on its origin or composition. In cancellous bone a contiguous system of trabeculae is visible, whose dimensions, volume density, and arrangement vary with site, loading conditions, and age. Grad-

ual transitions may occur between cortical and cancellous structures. By eroding new cavities inside the compact structure osteoclasts carve cancellous bone out of the cortical bone, or osteoblasts fill the spaces in the cancellous network to transform it into compact bone. During growth-related remodeling processes no net bone loss should occur; under pathological conditions, such as osteoporosis, the balance between osteoblastic and osteoclastic activities is disturbed, resulting in a weakening of skeletal structures.

On a microscopic level the arrangement of the organic fibers is used to discriminate between different forms of organization. Woven bone contains bundles of collagen fibers arranged as in connective tissue and connected to the neighboring connective tissue, for instance, the periosteum. This type of tissue can be interpreted as connective tissue stiffened by the incorporation of mineral to become bone. In the embryonic skeleton woven bone is almost ubiquitous. In adults ossified collagen bundles are still found at the insertion sites of tendons and ligaments. The mechanism of woven bone formation is encountered in situations requiring rapid bone repair processes since this mechanism allows ossification of relatively large areas in a short period of time. Usually the quality of such rapidly formed woven bone structures is inferior to a slowly developing compact bone, and after its rapid formation it frequently undergoes further remodeling to result in a structure adapted to the local requirements.

In the adult the major portion of both cortical and cancellous bone consists of lamellar bone. Lamellar bone appears to be on a more specific level of differentiation. The arrangement of its collagen fiber bundles seems to follow certain functional criteria. Comparable to technical composite structures, such as steel-reinforced concrete or fiber-glass, the orientation of these collagen bundles presents a relationship to the mechanical function of the corresponding bone site. The formation of these highly differentiated lamellar bone structures, deposited layer after layer, proceeds much more slowly than the formation of woven bone. Osteoblasts usually are able to form approximately 1–2 µm lamellar bone per day. These layers are deposited superficially on the surfaces of compact bone or on cancellous bone trabeculae. Remodeling processes, a concerted action between resorption and formation, take place on both the outer surface and in the interior of compact bone. During internal remodeling osteoclasts drill tunnels into the compact bone; osteoblasts follow and deposit new bone concentrically on the walls of the tunnel until the lumen is narrowed to the dimension of the central capillary. Such newly formed structures are called secondary osteons or Haversian systems. The result of this remodeling is a gradual internal renovation of an existing structure while it permanently continues to fulfill its function. This internal remodeling mechanism allows adaptation of the bony structure to a changing environment.

The blood supply to the bone in the cranio-maxillo-facial region is abundant, with many collaterals found at most sites. Inside the bony structures the nutritional pathways follow the Haversian systems, and these canals are cross-connected by the Volkmann canals. Each system usually contains a single vessel of the capillary type. There is evidence that inside these intracortical low-pressure systems the flow direction alternates depending on the current conditions. Peripheral to these capillaries the perfusion pathways follow the canalicular system related to the osteocytes. These canaliculi allow perfusion over a distance of a few tenths of a millimeter beyond the capillaries.

The blood supply of compact bone, especially in a thick cortex, requires correspondingly long low-pressure connections inside the bone and makes the compact structure more susceptible to disturbing influences. Once the intracortical circulation is interrupted, a long remodeling process is required to reattach the intracortical vessels to circulation. In cancellous structures the vascular supply reaches the bone surfaces directly, and there are only few and short intraosseous vessels. All the biological reactions – resorption, remodeling, healing – may thus take place more rapidly and more intensely. In the mandible the structure conforms more to the type found in long bones; in the craniofacial region the bones often consist of thin sheets, which although compact in their design still have the nutritional characteristics of cancellous bone, a high surface to volume ratio, and thus probably are less prone to disturbance of circulation. As a result the susceptibility to infection is low, and the healing times are short.

1.2.2 Chemical Composition

Bone matrix is a composite of organic and inorganic constituents. The inorganic portion comprises approximately 65% and consists principally of hydroxyapatite $[Ca_{10}(PO_4)_6(OH)_2]$, in addition to magnesium, potassium, chlorine, iron, and carbonate in significant amounts. Of the organic constituents 90% are collagen, predominantly of type I, and the remaining 10% are noncollagen proteins, including approximately 23% osteonectin, 15% osteocalcin, 9% sialoproteins, 9% phosphoproteins, 5% α2-HS glycoproteins, 3% albumin, and further proteins in smaller amounts.

1.2.3 Mechanical Properties

The material "bone" is a composite consisting of mineral components, which are primarily responsible for its compressive characteristics, and organic components,

primarily the collagen structures, which determine the tensile behavior. This composite structure is comparable to structures designed for technical applications, such as steel-reinforced concrete or fiber-glass. Compact bone is a highly anisotropic material, i.e., its mechanical properties differ along different axes. The orientation of its internal components is believed to be related to the functional requirements and the loading history of the corresponding region. The inhomogeneous appearance that bone sometimes presents on a microscopic level may be due to its modeling and remodeling history. Anisotropy does not seem to play a major role in internal fixation.

Even during normal daily activities bone must resist large forces. The ultimate strength of bone is approximately 1 MPa, about one-tenth that of steel. The dimensions of bony structures are oversized in relation to the requirements of normal use, and the strength of a bone therefore retains reserves for the requirements of heavy physical activity. Compression applied to bone can be maintained due to the springlike compressibility of the material. Young's modulus of axial stiffness of cortical bone is about 20 GPa. By way of illustration, a human tibia loaded axially with 1 000 N would undergo a shortening by 10 μm. The reserves of this spring effect are thus limited, and minimal bone resorption, for example, at an implant-bone interface or between fragment ends, would immediately lead to a loss of preload. The comparably small loss (10%–20%) observed without resorption is explained by the time-dependent deformation under load ("creep," or, vice versa, "stress relaxation"). A special characteristic of bone is its brittleness. When deformed, for example, in elongation, it tolerates a deformation of only 2% before it breaks, resulting in characteristics which are closer to the behavior of glass than of rubber.

Bone is found in a compact form in the skeleton, and in a more or less loose arrangement, as cancellous bone. The strength of cancellous bone varies but is typically less than 10% of cortical bone. The mechanical properties of cancellous bone depend on the amount of "bone" material that it contains, the design, orientation, and connections of trabeculae in relation to the direction of load, and the microstructure inside the trabeculae.

1.2.4 Mechanical Glossary

A force (expressed in newtons, N) acting upon a material results in a state of internal stress. A force acting with a lever arm is called a moment; this is expressed in newton meters (Nm). The unit of stress (σ), force/area, is N/m^2. Force deforms a material. The deformation ratio, strain ($\varepsilon = \delta L/L$), is unitless and is reported as percentage change of the original dimension. The relationship between the acting force and the resulting deformation is called stiffness: the less the stiffness the larger the deformation. The term rigidity is often used synonymously with stiffness in the medical literature. All three elements – force, stress, strain – may be split into static (constant) and dynamic (changing over time) components.

A load may consist of up to three components of force and three components of moment. Load acts upon a material or device. It may or may not change with time. A load which does not change with time is called static, while a periodically or intermittently changing load is dynamic in nature. The compression exerted by an implant applied under tension is static, the forces generated by the function (e.g., mastication) are dynamic or functional forces.

No component under consideration neither the static force generated by the implant, the dynamic force resulting from function, nor the amount of surface area upon which the forces act – is distributed evenly over a fracture area. Therefore at different sites different mechanical conditions may exist at different times.

1.3 Fractures in the Cranio-Maxillo-Facial Skeleton

1.3.1 Origin of Skull Bones

Two different mechanisms of bone formation are observed during embryogenesis: membranous and endochondral bone formation. In membranous bone formation the ossification process takes place by direct mineral deposition into the organic matrix of mesenchymal or connective tissue. In the skull this is the major mechanism observed. The frontal, parietal, and nasal bone, the maxilla, zygoma, and the mandible are all of membranous origin.

In endochondral bone formation primarily a cartilaginous template is formed. This cartilage is gradually transformed; it becomes mineralized and is then replaced by bone. While this mechanism is the main process of formation for long bones, in the skull the cartilaginous origin is restricted to the nasal septum and to internal bony components of the nose, occipital bone, and cranial base. Appositional growth in all bones, whether of membranous or endochondral origin, proceeds via membranous bone formation. Due to the ongoing modeling and remodeling processes scarcely any original bony material is left in the skull after growth is completed, and no remainders of calcified cartilage are detected. It is often discussed whether the origin of the bone plays a significant role in later repair processes. This question has not yet been addressed in a comprehensive manner, but there is no evidence that possible differences in repair processes observed in long bones are actually due to the embryological origin

rather than to local or regional boundary conditions, such as dimensions of the bony structures, blood supply, and loading history.

1.3.2 Load-Bearing Structures in the Cranio-Maxillo-Facial Skeleton

The anatomy of the cranio-maxillo-facial skeleton is designed to provide protection for soft structures of vital importance and to permit mastication. Important protective functions include encasement of the central nervous system, eyes, and respiratory pathways. The shell of the cranial vault consists of a composite structure, including an outer and inner compact layer connected by a cancellous intermediate. The hemispherical design, together with the layered structure, makes it specially suited to protect against direct impact. In the midface the cellular structure, reenforced by the orbito-zygomatic frame, is able to act as a shock-absorbing structure.

During mastication the mandible moves relative to the rest of the skull. Forces act at the attachment sites of the masticatory musculature and in the occlusal plane. These forces are transmitted from the teeth to the alveolar bone, and from there to the bony structures of mandible and maxilla. The maxilla is connected by four main trajectories to the orbito-zygomatic frame, which is then connected to the neurocranium.

These structures are of paramount importance in the repair of facial fractures, and they are addressed specifically in the respective chapters. The mandible has a shape which is closer to the shape of a tubular bone. The major muscle forces meet the mandible in the area of the angle and in the ascending ramus. Reactive forces in the occlusal plane are generated during mastication. This tends to bend the anterior portion of the mandible caudally. Thus an important tensile component is created in the alveolar portion of the mandible. In the case of an interrupted mechanical integrity of the mandible the repair must concentrate primarily on these tension zones, and the correct placement of the implants is determined by the location and type of fracture and its relationship to the tension zones. However, it cannot be assumed that placement of an implant on the presumable tension side immobilizes a fracture under all possible physiological loading conditions. The corresponding chapter on the treatment of mandibular fractures expands on these aspects and indicates the preferred sites of implant placement for the specific types of fractures.

Loading of the occlusal plane may reach quite high values. Maximum bite forces in an average population are found in an order of magnitude of 200–300 N in the incisor area, 300–500 N in the premolar region, and 500–700 N in the molar area. Electromyographic investigations have shown that the masticatory musculature is activated in a more or less symmetric fashion, even when the load in the occlusal plane acts asymmetrically. The values found during normal mastication are usually much smaller, amounting to only a fraction of the maximum biting force.

In the case of a fracture in the angle of the mandible, 70 mm distant to the incisors, and a biting force in the incisor area of 300 N, a moment (force times lever arm) of approximately 20 Nm would result. The higher loads in the premolar or molar region, combined with the correspondingly shorter lever arms, result in similar values for the moment. Additional torsional components must be considered the greater the load deviates from the midline.

Assuming the mandibular body to have a height of 30 mm, and muscle forces to act symmetrically, a unilateral fracture must still bear 10 Nm of this moment. This means that under maximum loading conditions, and provided that the fragment ends are in contact, an implant placed at the cranial border of the mandible and its anchoring devices must still be able to resist a load of more than 300 N.

1.3.3 The Fracture

The skeleton provides a rigid frame for physical activity and for the protection of soft organs. The basic requirement for optimal function is adequate anatomic shape and stiffness (i.e., resistance to deformation under load). Fractures are the result of mechanical overload. Within a fraction of a millisecond the structural integrity and thus the stiffness of the bone can be interrupted. The shape of the fracture depends mainly upon the type of load exerted and upon the energy released. Torque results in spiral fractures, avulsion in transverse fractures, bending in short oblique fractures, and compression in impaction and in higher comminution. The latter mechanisms are encountered principally in cancellous areas and in shell-like structures as they are found in the cranio-facial area, where the honeycomb design acts as a shock absorber.

The degree of fragmentation depends upon the energy stored prior to the process of fracturing; thus wedge fractures and multifragmentary fractures are associated with high energy release. In this context the rate of loading plays a role.

A special phenomenon is the implosion which occurs immediately after disruption. Such an implosion is followed by marked soft tissue damage due to cavitation, comparable to the damaging mechanism in a gunshot wound. Thus in addition to the disruption of the intracortical blood vessels, the vascular damage is extended into the neighboring soft tissue regions. This damage is then superimposed to the direct action of the trauma, including vascular and nerve damage, soft tissue contusion, and other injuries.

Concomitant injuries may include nerve damage (mandibular, infraorbital, optical, facial nerves), and vessels. Due to a rich network of collaterals, however, the latter does not pose severe problems to the blood supply of the region. Even lethal complications may result from dramatic blood loss through an injured maxillary artery. Penetration of the skin or the mucosa, in contrast to the situation in long bones, is unproblematic in the cranio-maxillo-facial area.

The vascular situation in the mandible is to some extent comparable to the situation in a long bone. The cortex reaches a certain thickness, and if the intracortical circulation is interrupted, a corresponding delay must be expected until the blood supply has been reestablished. In contrast to long bones, however, closed muscle compartments do not pose a problem in the skull. In the midfacial and cranial region the bony walls are thin; they frequently remain attached to the surrounding soft tissues. Experience in cranio-facial surgery reveals that even if the soft tissues are stripped, the connection to circulation recovers rapidly. Thus the susceptibility to infection is minimal, and the tendency for healing is good.

In summary, the fracture event leaves us with an interrupted force transmission in the involved skeletal parts, with an interrupted blood supply inside the bone, and with a more or less disturbed circulatory situation in the environment of the injured bone, whereby the nutritional problem is by far not as severe as in a long bone.

1.3.4 Biological Reaction and Healing of Bone

Healing is defined as restoration of original integrity. Clinically this goal is reached when the bony structures can resume their full function, even if on a microscopic level the structure of the bone has not yet reached the appearance of an unaltered bone. For successful healing minimal requirements of both a mechanical and a biological nature must be met. Biologically the healing process depends on the presence and appropriate functioning of cells that are able to participate in the various phases of the healing process. These cells must reach the site of repair, and their activities must be supported by adequate nutritional supply. A sufficient blood supply is therefore a primary prerequisite. Biological events in fracture healing at any time are strongly affected by the mechanical boundary conditions. Biological reactions in turn may affect the mechanical environment.

The situation at the onset of fracture healing is characterized by the intracortical blood supply to the fragment ends being interrupted by the fracture trauma, by an injured soft tissue bed, and possibly by damage to major afferent or efferent vessels. Depending on the local situation and the fracture pattern, intracortical perfusion of the fragment ends is interrupted over a distance of several millimeters. Surgery then may produce additional trauma.

As a reaction to disturbed blood supply, a process of internal and surface remodeling of the affected bone begins; the first traces of resorptive activity may become visible 2–3 weeks after injury. During this remodeling process nonperfused bone is replaced by new vital bone. In parallel, beginning as early as the end of the first week, new bone formation is observed predominantly in the subperiosteal region. The further course of the entire healing process is then determined by an interrelationship between mechanics and biology.

Simplistically, only the healing patterns under the two mechanical extremes are described, namely absolute immobilization of the fracture and full range of interfragmentary motion, ignoring that the situation may be different at different sites and may change with time.

Under interfragmentary motion the tissues are continuously torn and squeezed. The tolerance of various types of tissues to deformation differs, being high (up to 100%) for connective tissue, much lower for cartilage (10%–15%), and lower still for bone (2%). Tissue can be assumed not to form under circumstances that would not allow its existence. If minimal deformation exists from the start, the conditions are met for the formation of bone. These are the conditions which allow the osteoclasts, as a cutter head, to drill their canal across the immobilized contact zone, and the newly formed osteons to link the two fragments together. This process is called direct or primary bone union. Smaller gap areas, when immobilized by neighboring contact zones, still permit direct lamellar ossification inside the gap. In larger but still immobilized gaps woven bone formation in a first step subdivides the space; the smaller compartments produced by this subdivision are filled by lamellar bone in a second step.

In the case of high interfragmentary motion, the strain in the fracture gap exceeds the level tolerated by bone, and ossification is not possible. Here one observes a tissue differentiation cascade from granulation tissue to connective tissue, fibrocartilage, mineralized cartilage, woven, and finally compact bone. Along this differentiation cascade there is a gradual increase in strength and in stiffness of these tissues, while at the same time the tolerance for strain is reduced. This brings about a gradual reduction of motion and thus a reduction of interfragmentary strain. This differentiation cascade permits a consecutive tissue always to be formed under the protection of its precursor.

There are clearly various degrees of immobilization of a fracture. Even in the same fracture plane a certain part may present the pattern of direct healing which is characteristic for minimal strain, or the healing via a cascade of tissue differentiation which is observed under interfragmentary motion. This can be attributed to the fact that the degree of immobilization changes with time, and that even in the same fracture different strain conditions may be present (Fig. 1.4). At one site the conditions for direct remodeling across the fracture plane could be met primarily, produced by full immobilization of the fracture by the implant, or secondarily when callus has bridged at other sites which would then provide the conditions for remodeling across the fracture only at a later stage. The simultaneous occurrence of both patterns is also possible when the mechanical conditions within the same fracture vary. Then at one site immobilization is sufficient for direct union while at other sites interfragmentary motion determines a healing pattern with resorption of the fragment ends and a union via a differentiation cascade.

After complete immobilization of the fracture plane the radiological aspect of a healing fracture differs from the conventional appearance in which the progress of healing can be judged by the amount of callus formed. The fracture is barely visible after a perfect alignment. After internal remodeling has begun, there is a gradual reduction of radiological density in the fracture area which is due to the internal remodeling activities. With time the fracture site appears increasingly diffuse in the radiogram and gradually disappears. It is difficult to determine from the radiological appearance when function can be allowed again. Experience shows that the remodeling of a mandible to full load bearing and plate removal requires 4–6 months, a shorter period than in long bones, with a recommended period to implant removal of 1.5 years in the tibia and 2 years in the femur. In the midfacial and cranial regions the healing process is even faster. Here bony fixation of fragments may be observed even after 1 month. This is due to the excellent circulatory conditions in this region of the body and to the thin dimensions and the cancellous character of bone, allowing a more rapid recovery of interrupted blood supply. The healing of grafted bone follows the same rules, with accessibility to circulation of the bony structures of the graft and the mechanical relationship at the graft-host interface playing an important role.

The current preference is to reduce the iatrogenic disturbance of blood supply to bone by designing implants that interfere less with blood supply and by introducing more biology-friendly fixation techniques. These so-called "bio-logical" plating techniques offer advantages especially in comminuted fractures, where additional exposure would result in the production of dead bone, and in condylar fractures. For this type of treatment it is hoped that a certain compromise on the mechanical side is compensated by the clear gain on the biological side by preserving vascular connection to the bony fragments.

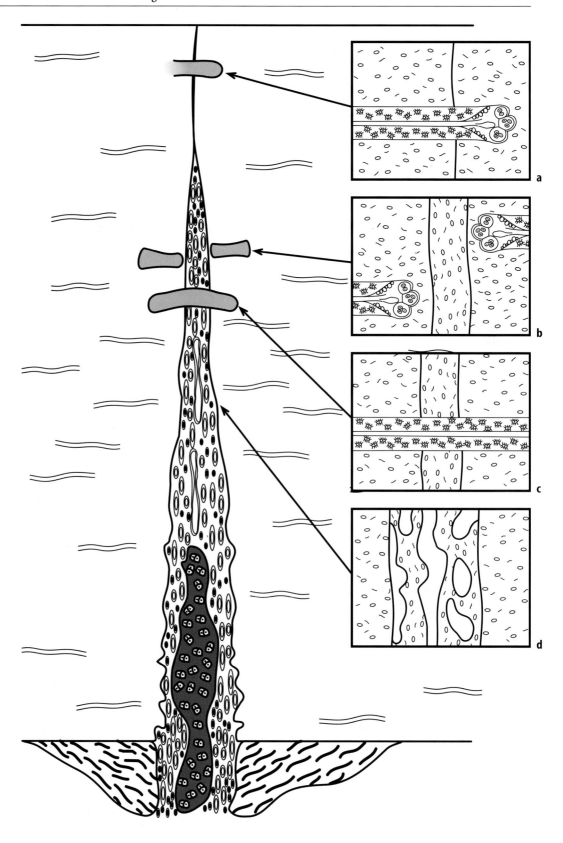

Fig. 1.4

◀ Patterns of fracture healing. The appearance of a healing fracture is determined by the geometry of the fracture zone, the
degree of immobilization at various sites, and their changes
occurring over time.

An absolutely perfect alignment of the entire fracture is not
possible; direct contact between the fragment ends is restricted
to only small portions. The remainder consists of a gap of varying width. Complete absence of interfragmentary motion is
possible only in contact areas and in gap zones in their close
vicinity. If this zone is completely immobilized, whether from
the beginning or as a sequel to bony bridging at other sites,
direct intracortical remodeling across the fracture plane may
take place at contact sites (**a**). In a first step small immobilized
gaps are filled directly with lamellar bone (**b**). Then secondary
remodeling (**c**) in the axis of the bone gradually leads to reconstruction of the original integrity. This phenomenon of fracture healing without intermediate steps of tissue differentiation is called direct, or primary, bone healing. Pure direct healing, an extreme healing pattern on the one side of the scale,
seems to be relatively rare.

The further away from the contact areas, the higher is the
chance of interfragmentary motion of various degrees, and the
gap is usually wider. The healing pattern in these zones is characterized by resorption of the fragment ends, callus formation,
and interfragmentary ossification via a cascade of tissue differentiation. This leads to a gradual immobilization during the
healing process. This pattern, found on the other extreme of
the scale, is frequent. Intermediate stages, for instance, the subdivision of a wide gap by the formation of woven bone (**d**), may
be observed between the two extremes.

At a specific phase during the healing process it may happen
that some sites of the same fracture are under relative motion
while others become immobilized. Thus in a single fracture it
is possible to observe a broad spectrum of different healing
patterns. As a routine, however, only a narrow band from the
full range of healing patterns reflects the situation of that specific fracture.

Over the past decade distraction osteogenesis has
been very popular for lengthening procedures in long
bones and in bone segment transfer, and it is now gaining increasing importance in the cranio-maxillo-facial
field. During distraction woven bone forms in the distraction gap. The speed of distraction must be high
enough to prevent bony bridging, and slow enough to
permit the differentiation to bone. A total amount of
1 mm per day, in one to four steps, has been found to be
adequate. Under continuous distraction the daily distraction distance can be approximately doubled, which
means that the overall treatment time can be correspondingly reduced.

Efforts at pharmacological enhancement of healing
by systemic or regionally applied substances, osteodynamic agents, cytokines, hyperbaric oxygen, or physical
stimulation, for example, by electric, magnetic, or ultrasound effects have shown varying degrees of success in
experimental settings. These methods have not yet
matured to a stage at which they can be considered for
general clinical application.

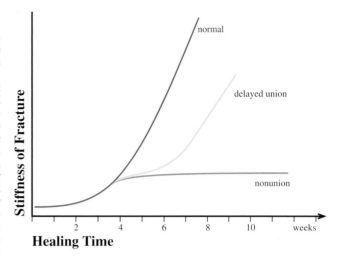

Healing Time

Fig. 1.5

Fracture healing: recovery of mechanical function. Initially a
healing fracture presents low strength and low stiffness. During approximately the fourth to sixth weeks a dramatic change
in mechanical properties occurs towards the properties of normal bone. In an undisturbed situation mineralization across
the fracture plane takes place at this time. If the loading of the
mineralizing fracture does not exceed certain limits, healing
proceeds normally. Undue loading of such a uniting fracture at
a critical moment may disturb the mineralization process and
lead to a delay in bony union, or, if compensatory healing
mechanisms fail, to a nonunion.

Potential complications in fracture healing include
infection, refracture, delayed healing, nonunion, implant
failure, and implant loosening. Some of these complications are related to the use of implants, and some are
more general phenomena in fracture healing.

Due to the rapid healing in the cranio-maxillo-facial
region the bone regains sufficient strength very early. In
contrast to the situation in long bones, in the cranio-
maxillo-facial area a refracture does not occur without
adequate trauma.

The flora in infection may include both aerobic and
anaerobic germs, and *Aspergillus* and *Actinomyces*.
Infection generally begins when the soft tissues are
severely damaged, and perfusion to the bone and its surrounding tissues is interrupted. An open wound alone,
in the skin or in the oral cavity, with implant exposure,
does not necessarily mean that a deep infection will
ensue.

Nerve injury may be due to the original trauma, for
instance, in mandibular fractures. Since it cannot be
excluded that surgical procedures further compromise
nerves, it is very important that the neurological situation be described prior to surgery in order to avoid nonjustified claims.

Healing is considered to be delayed when the union
takes clearly longer than the expected duration, for the

midface more than 4–6 weeks (Fig. 1.5). With the mandible, if little occurs within 12 weeks, one can expect there to be a problem and must take some action. Discovering a delayed union in conventional radiograms is difficult, and not reproducible. Standardized, soft radiograms repeated at intervals can sometimes be investigated for changes. Once a nonunion or pseudarthrosis has developed, it does not require resection since the tissue in a nonunion represents only an early stage of tissue differentiation, and the only problem is too excessive a strain to permit mineralization of the moving fracture gap. The use of a stiffer and stronger implant, for example, a reconstruction plate of any type, would allow the further progress of the differentiation process.

Screw loosening, with subsequent loss of stability, may be a source of complications. Monocortical screws lacking angular stability in the plate are especially prone to such complications. Other possible causes include insufficient numbers of screws, their inappropriate placement, and undue functional loading. Inadvertent stripping of screws during insertion, perhaps hidden behind a higher moment with self-tapping screws, may be problematic in a thick cortex; direct mechanical bone damage can be induced by the insertion of non-self-tapping screws into a pilot hole that is too narrow.

1.4 Indications for Operative Treatment of Fractures

Modern bone surgery aims at rapid recovery of form and function. This must be the goal of every surgeon treating craniofacial fractures and tumors with consecutive bone defects or performing osteotomies for the correction of craniofacial deformities. The degree of stability required in each situation depends on the fracture pattern. Optimal, not maximal, stability is required. Under these conditions undisturbed healing takes place, and the fixation is optimal or adequate. Absolute and relative indications can be defined for internal fixation in patients with facial fractures. The decision for conservative or surgical treatment depends on the type and condition of fracture and on the patient's condition and situation. It is an absolute precondition for surgeons using internal fixation for fractures to understand conservative treatment first.

Closed and simple fractures can well be treated with conservative methods, the simplest method being intermaxillary fixation for several weeks.

Functionally stable internal fixation is indicated for:

- Multiple or comminuted fractures of mandible and maxilla
- Panfacial fractures
- Defect fractures
- Wide open fractures
- Dislocated midface fractures

- Fractures of the atrophic mandible in geriatric patients
- Infected fractures of the mandible.

Another absolute indication for internal fixation which affects even the type of fixation is the patient's inability or unwillingness to cooperate. This is sometimes the case with elderly, mentally retarded patients, alcoholics, and drug addicts. The first and most important reason for adequate internal fixation must be the immediate restoration of form and function, the relief of pain, and the avoidance of late sequelae. Socioeconomic factors such as short hospitalization time and early return to work are of secondary concern but do play a role depending on the economic situation, which may vary in different parts of the world.

Especially in polytrauma patients there is an absolute and principal indication for early definitive care. In these patients surgery should be performed for all fractures simultaneously. Swelling is not a reason for delayed treatment of facial fractures.

Sufficient (adequate) stability is the safest protection against infection and is more important than antibiotics. Furthermore, stability prevents the collapse of the reconstruction in traumatology and tumor surgery. In orthognathic surgery internal surgery together with precise planning helps to predict the result, but it cannot prohibit relapse if the planning is not well coordinated with pre- and postoperative orthognathic treatment.

1.5 Operative Reduction and Internal Fixation

1.5.1 Reestablishing Stability

Fracture treatment in general strives for complete and early recovery of skeletal function. Therefore solid, complication-free union in appropriate anatomical shape is the basic goal. The appropriate anatomical shape varies depending on site and character of the fracture. In an intra-articular fracture precise reconstruction of the articular surfaces is a goal in its own right. Any incongruity of the articulating surfaces gives rise to areas of high stress and thus promotes posttraumatic arthrosis. Fractures through the dentate regions require a precise realignment, as occlusion may otherwise be endangered, and fractures involving the orbit demand perfect reconstruction to avoid problems with vision. In addition, the esthetic appearance of the face, which is determined largely by its underlying skeletal parts, deserves special attention. Early reconstruction of the normal anatomy generally offers the best prospects for optimal recovery of function and esthetics and is preferred to "tolerable malalignment" which requires corrective surgery at a later stage.

The general goals of operative treatment include the early anatomical reduction of fracture fragments, maintaining their position after reduction, and guaranteeing union in the desired position. Completely immobilizing the fracture requires that the means of fixation act directly at the fracture site. These fixation devices must neutralize the loads occurring under everyday functional requirements in a specific situation. To obtain appropriate stability one must therefore consider the personality of the patient, type and site of the fracture, soft tissue conditions, and many other boundary conditions which can affect the outcome. In selecting an appropriate implant it is necessary to estimate the expected magnitude and duration of load for each specific case. A special danger is underestimation of loading conditions, for instance, in collum fractures and fractures in an atrophic mandible. While miniplates in the horizontal ramus of the mandible can perform perfectly when they are loaded in tension, their stabilizing function may be insufficient when they are placed at a site subjected to varying types of load. In addition, the requirements for a fixation device change over time. During a normal healing process bone takes over gradually, and the implant is unloaded. If the healing process is delayed, the implant must take care of additional load, and it may then undergo fatigue failure.

After a fracture the transmission of compressive forces can still take place across a fracture plane. The bone remains able to take over the compressive tasks, and the implant must substitute for the lost tensile properties. This load sharing between the bone and the implant allows implant dimensions to be used that are much smaller than those necessary for the full loading spectrum. In the case of a bony defect and in comminuted zones a plate is loaded in bending. Sooner or later even a strong plate will fail in fatigue, since plates are not designed to cover a prosthesis function permanently. Under such conditions the bone regeneration must be monitored carefully, and active intervention is required if the healing process does not proceed in the expected way.

1.5.2 Implant Materials

An implant material for fracture fixation must be strong and ductile, adaptable to fit the bone surface, and biocompatible. Today one uses principally metals such as stainless steel, chromium-molybdenum alloys, or commercially pure titanium. Except for a short period in the early 1970s when soft titanium was used, the metal of choice of cranio-maxillo-facial surgery was stainless steel until approximately 1986. For the maxillo-facial field, however, titanium is now almost exclusively the material of choice.

1.5.2.1 Stainless Steel

Stainless steel consists mainly of iron (62.5%), chromium (17.6%), nickel (14.5%), and molybdenum (2.8%) and further components in minor amounts. The implant quality of 316L stainless steel meets the metallurgical requirements established by the American Society of Testing and Materials (ASTM) and the International Organization for Standardization (ISO). Two grades of carbon contents and four grades of cold work are defined from annealed to extra hard. For AO/ASIF maxillo-facial implants steel was the metal of choice until 1986. Corrosion resistance and compatibility are fair. Implant metals are protected from corroding by a passive layer consisting of nonsoluble corrosion products. Corrosion is observed principally when one metal component frets against another metal component (fretting corrosion, Steinemann 1977).

Surgeons in many countries prefer not to remove implant material. One of the reasons may be that the removal of up to 10 plates and 50–60 screws used in fixing facial fractures often means an additional major surgical intervention. For this reason the Maxillofacial Technical Commission has decided to ask for implants made of commercially pure titanium. Although titanium is more expensive than steel, it may be more cost effective in the long run because of its favourable characteristics (no known allergies, no second intervention).

1.5.2.2 Titanium

Commercially pure titanium consists of titanium and oxygen. It is extremely insoluble and consequently is inert and biocompatible. Today it is available in grades I–IV, combining high strength and ductility. The basic differences in grades lie in their oxygen content. All cranio-maxillo-facial implants are available in titanium. Only the 2.7 line (screws and implants) is still available in steel.

Severe trauma of the facial skeleton may require a great number of screws and plates, and titanium implants are therefore preferable because they can be left in place. According to Steinemann (1988) the body is saturated with titanium, and no additional soluble titanium can thus become active. In contrast to steel and its components, pure titanium is physiologically inert, and its unmatched tissue tolerance has been scientifically and clinically proven. Titanium has a high corrosion resistance due to the spontaneously forming thin oxyde layers on the surface which guarantees that the material behaves passively.

The golden color of AO/ASIF titanium implants is due to the anodizing process. A variety of colors can be produced, depending on the thickness of the oxyde film. No accompanying corrosion is observed even in cases of unstable internal fixation with tissue stained dark by pure titanium abrasion particles (O. Pohler, personal communication, 1988). Pure titanium and its wear products behave passively and provoke neither toxic nor allergic reactions. AO choose not to add alloys to pure titanium in order to preserve its excellent biocompatibility. Implants of titanium alloys are available only for special high-strength indications outside the maxillofacial area.

1.5.2.3 Biodegradable Polymeric Materials

Since it is generally desirable for no foreign body material to remain, efforts are being made to develop biodegradable materials. However, biodegradable polymeric materials are not yet available for use with conventional techniques of internal fixation which dissolve after a certain period in the body, and which combine adequate strength, ductility, maintenance of compression and degradability, and lack of tissue reaction. A search has been going on for biodegradables and ceramic material especially for surgery of the facial bones. A decade ago we expected to be using mainly biodegradable material by now. For many reasons, however, including stiffness of the material, bending characteristics, and especially the unfavorable characteristics of late resorption this has not come true. While adequate biodegradable implants are not yet available for fracture fixation in highly loaded areas or defect reconstruction, it seems that for the fixation and reconstruction of midfacial walls (especially orbital walls) resorbable implants will be available in the near future. Resorbable implants are especially desirable for bone surgery in children because of the danger of implants being displaced through the growth and bone apposition of the growing facial skeleton. On the other hand, one must be sure that the process of resorption does not disturb the growth process.

1.5.3 Implant Removal

In treating fractures the function of the implant extends only so long as is required for the affected bone to acquire enough strength to resist the corresponding functional loads. Thereafter, in the case of nonresorbable materials, the options exist of removing the implants or leaving them without function. No general recommendations can be given for implant removal, and the pro's and con's must be balanced in each individual case.

An argument against removal is that this would mean an additional surgical intervention, with additional costs, a risk of damaging important structures (e.g., nerves) during the procedure, an additional, but minor, risk of infection, and the hazards of anesthesia. These criteria are less important at sites of easy access in outpatients in whom the procedure can be performed under local anesthesia.

There are a whole series of criteria which favor implant removal, related to both the patient's concerns and medical considerations. Patients may request that the implant be removed for cosmetic reasons when it is shining through thin skin. A general feeling of disturbance may be caused by subacute complications including chronic infection, compatibility problems, and allergic reactions. If the implant is at a prominent location, such as the eyebrow region, it may lead to mechanical problems, for instance, in impact sports, and in cold climates an implant immediately underneath the skin can increase sensitivity to coldness. Problems with dentures in the upper and lower jaws may also encourage implant removal.

Complications such as screw loosening, implant failure, and infection very often require surgery. If screws loosen before the fracture unites, restabilization is needed. An argument for removing loose screws is the chance of their migration to undesired sites. Infection in the presence of an implant is not necessarily a reason for removing the implant. If the fixation is considered to be stable, an implant can be left until the fracture is completely united since controlling an infection is easier under conditions of stability; the implant can be removed later when the bone has united. Wound contamination is not a contraindication for the placement of an implant since stability helps in fighting infection. If an infected internal fixation is unstable, implant removal and restabilization are mandatory.

The materials used in implants for fracture fixation have proven their biocompatibility. Stainless steel, however, contains components that may be problematic if released from the alloy. This can happen when implants fret against each other, which leads to destruction of the oxide layer on the surface of the implants. In this context allergic reactions deserve special attention. It has been shown that up to 20 % of certain populations are sensitive to nickel, a major constituent of stainless steel. The occurrence of severe allergic reactions is an indication for replacing the steel implants with their titanium equivalents.

In children implant removal is advocated not primarily for growth disturbance but rather for their possible translation by drift phenomena. As long as major growth must take place, there is a chance that these growth mechanisms can lead to an intracranial displacement of the implants. Plate removal remains an issue in pediatrics in view of the long life expectancy of very young patients, and the lack of knowledge about the very long term outcome.

The major function of an implant during the healing process is the mechanical protection of the fracture site. A frequently mentioned indication for implant removal is their adverse stress protection effect. Experience with heavily loaded long bones of the lower extremity shows that this aspect is of only minor concern unless extreme amounts of hardware are used. It cannot be denied that a fractured bone treated by implants placed directly on the bone surface undergoes a remodeling in the vicinity of the implants, and that a first step in this remodeling process consists of temporary porosis. This process takes place during the first few postoperative months, and it is located in the zone where blood supply to the bone was disturbed. A remodeling of bone underneath the plates and around the screws soon leads to an adaptation of the bone structure to the new loading conditions. This porosis is completely absent when intracortical circulation is preserved by using circulation-friendly implants and implantation techniques.

1.5.4 Principles of Stabilization

1.5.4.1 Splinting

Splinting consists of connecting a more or less stiff device to the fractured bone. This device reduces the mobility of the fracture in proportion to the stiffness of the splint-bone composite but does not aim at completely abolishing fracture mobility.

External splinting seeks to reduce the fracture fragments without surgical intervention. Such external splints may be fixed to the teeth or applied to mucosal or skin covered surfaces. Under these conditions there is always a soft intermediate structure, either periodontium or soft tissues, and forces are not directly transmitted from the splint to the bone. As a consequence a certain mobility at the fracture site remains. Under most circumstances this mobility does not interfere with the healing process, but it cannot be guaranteed that the initial alignment of the fragments will be maintained to its full extent until the bone has united.

In internal splinting the stabilizing devices are fixed directly to the fracture fragments, with the bone-implant complex still allowing for some interfragmentary motion. Internal splints usually lead to more reduction in interfragmentary motion than external splints. Wire sutures or flexible plates are among the devices that are considered to act as internal splints. External fixators, having internal and external components, belong to the same category of fixation devices in terms of their functional effect.

1.5.4.2 Compression

The use of compression is an elegant method to exclude interfragmentary motion. Compression fixation consists in pressing together two surfaces, either bone to bone or implant to bone. The effect of compression is twofold: it produces preload in the fracture plane, and it acts by increasing interfragmentary friction. Thus the fracture remains immobilized as long as the axial preload is higher than the tensile loads produced by function, and as long as the interfragmentary friction prevents displacement by shear forces. In bone the compression may be maintained over a period of several weeks to several months, usually long enough to allow for a bony connection between the fragment ends.

Compression is no absolute precondition for undisturbed healing, but in specific applications it means more safety and includes a biological and mechanical advantage. Biologically compression means undisturbed healing because it guarantees absolute stability even under the condition of function. Mechanically it allows load sharing between bone and implant. Under these conditions the implants for the osteosynthesis can be smaller than in load-bearing osteosynthesis where larger and thicker plates are necessary. Compression provides a maximum strength with a minimum of fixation material. In the facial skeleton compression for fracture fixation is applicable only in noncomminuted, simple fractures of the mandible; occasionally it may be useful at other locations.

When resorption at the fragment end has taken place (late surgery, infection) compression cannot be used.

In the maxillary area, because of the thin bones, compression can rarely be applied. On the other hand, because of the different type of functional load (static) there is almost no need for compression in the midface area.

In some areas, such as the zygomatico-frontal suture, the root of the zygomatic arch, and sagittal fractures of the palate, compression with lag screws may guarantee the repositioned position of the fracture with small and few implants only. Compression osteosynthesis can be performed either with compression plates or with lag screws.

Compression with a Plate. The special geometry of the plate hole (Fig. 1.6a–c) together with eccentric placement of the screw (Fig. 1.6d) allows interfragmentary compression in an axial direction when the screw is driven fully into the screw hole (Fig. 1.6e,f). The screw hole is a section of an inclined and horizontal cylinder that permits the downward and horizontal movement of a sphere, the screwhead (Fig. 1.6c). As soon as the screw head arrives at the outer rim of the plate hole, it meets the intersection of the inclined and horizontal cylinder. The screw head then makes the spherical contact in the plate hole and glides horizontally towards the opposite (inner aspect) of the plate hole. Since the screws also engage the bone, they move the bone inwards towards the fracture line. Only one screw on each side of the fracture line should be placed eccentrically (Fig. 1.7a–c).

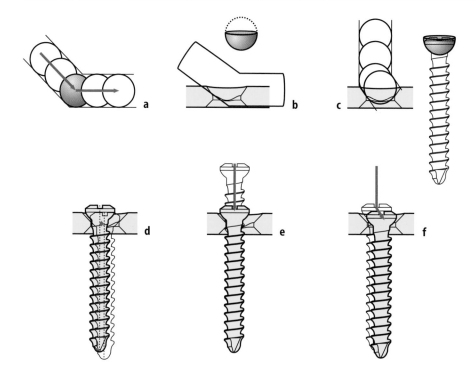

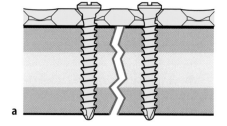

Fig. 1.6 a–f

a The screw head moves in the oval-shaped plate hole like a ball in an angled cylinder.
b The screw hole is a section from of an inclined and a horizontal cylinder.
c Movement of the screw head with its spherical undersurface in the DC hole of the plate.
d The eccentrically placed screw arrives at the rim of the platehole.
e As the screw is driven in, it glides within the platehole to its final position (**f**).

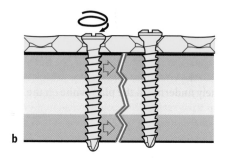

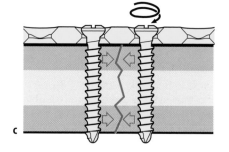

Fig. 1.7 a–c

Compression with a plate.
a The two innermost screws should be placed eccentrically ▶ within the DC holes.
b As these screws are driven in, they approximate the fragments.
c With final tightening of the screws compression is achieved.

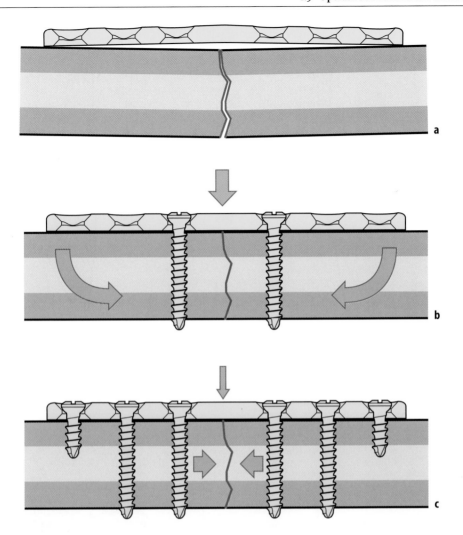

Fig. 1.8 a–c

If a plate is correctly overbent (**a**), the inner screws should be placed first (**b**). If the outer screws are placed first, the fracture in the cortex near to the plate may be opened because then the plate may be too long in relation to the bone spanned between the outer screw holes. Depending on the strength needed, the additional screws are placed mono- or bicortically.

If the fracture was preloaded before the first two screws were placed, tightening of the screws causes axial compression. The other holes of a plate should then be loaded with screws in a centric (neutral) position. It should always be kept in mind that a plate acts eccentrically, and complete closure of a fracture results only immediately underneath the plate while on the opposite side a gap may result. Overcoming this tendency may require a plate or splint to be used as a tension band, or slight overbending of the plate, as indicated in Fig. 1.8 a–c, or combining the plate with an additional lag screw across the fracture plane.

Compression with a Lag Screw. Any screw from the maxillo-facial set can be used as a lag screw. In most instances 2.4 or 2.0 screws are used as lag screws. The lag screw technique is used either for fracture fixation or for the fixation of bone grafts. Ideally a lag screw should cross the fracture plane at a perpendicular angle. Use of the lag screw technique in the mandible is ideal after a sagittal split osteotomy, in oblique fractures of the body

of the mandible (Fig. 1.9 a), in chin fractures (see also Fig. 3.4 a, b), and in more complicated applications such as the mandibular angle (see Fig. 3.20 a).

Since all screws of the maxillo-facial set are fully threaded, a so-called "gliding hole" must be drilled into the first (near) cortex and a threaded hole into the second (far) cortex. The first hole is overdrilled so that the hole in the cortex has at least the size of the outer diameter of the screw thread. A special drill guide is placed into the first hole to locate the second hole centrally in the far cortex. Thereafter the hole in the far cortex is drilled to the diameter of the pilot hole. lts size is determined by the size of the core of the screw. lf used with-

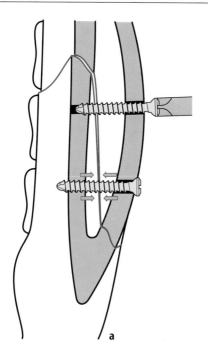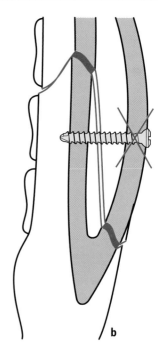

Fig. 1.9 a, b

a Oblique fractures can be fixed very efficiently with lag screws. A gliding hole (same size as the diameter of the thread) must be drilled into the outer cortex. A thread hole is made in the far cortex. As the screw is tightened (lower screw) the fracture is closed and compressed.

b If no gliding hole is placed, and both holes are threaded, the fracture can be neither closed nor be compressed.

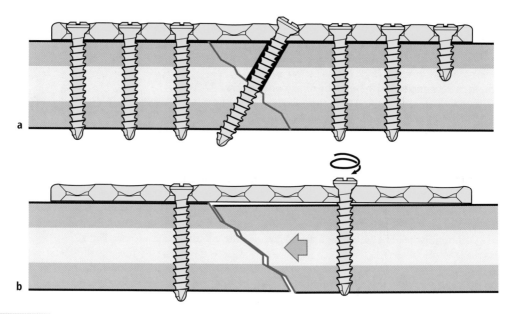

Fig. 1.10 a, b

Compression with a lag screw and plate.
a If a lag screw in combination with a DC plate is used for fixation, the lag screw should be placed first. Thereafter the remaining screws must be placed in a neutral position.

b If no lag screw is used above an oblique fracture line, the plate must be fixed first to the fragment which forms an obtuse angle with the fracture; then as the screw in the opposite fragment is activated (*right*) the spike of the opposite fragment is driven against the plate.

out a plate, a countersink for the screw head is cut into the bone before placement of the screw. Self-cutting screws can then be placed immediately; for non-self-cutting screws a thread corresponding exactly to the thread of the screw is cut into the far cortex with a tap. The use of self-cutting screws as lag screws may be hazardous, however, since the holding capacity of their tip is diminished due to the flutes.

If the gliding hole is in one fragment and the threaded hole in the other as the screw is tightened, the fragments are squeezed together, and interfragmental compression is generated (Fig. 1.9a). The type of compression generated by a lag screw is referred to as static interfragmental compression. It is static because it does not change significantly with load. A lag screw is the most efficient way of achieving interfragmental compression and therefore stability, but it does not provide a great deal of strength. Therefore rarely only a single lag screw is applied. At least three lag screws are generally placed in fractures of the mandible or sagittal split osteotomies, or a lag screw is used in combination with a plate. Whenever a lag screw is used through a plate hole in the case of a dynamic compression (DC) plate (Fig. 1.10a), all the other screws must be placed in a neutral position, or the fragments may shift.

To achieve maximal interfragmentary compression the lag screw must be inserted into the middle of the fragment equidistant from the fracture edges and directed at a right angle to the fracture line. If the screw is not inserted perpendicularly to the fracture plane, a shearing force is introduced as it is tightened, and the fragments may dislocate. Similarly, insertion of a screw at an acute angle to the fracture plane introduces a shearing moment as it is tightened, and the fragment tend to displace. These fundamental errors in screw insertion are often responsible for a loss in reduction. With loss in reduction, decreased structural continuity and stability are inevitable. If the oblique plane is too short or the opposite cortex has been damaged so that a lag screw cannot be applied, the plate must be fixed first to the fragment which forms an obtuse angle with the fracture (Fig. 1.10b).

1.6 Design and Function of Implants and Instruments

AO/ASIF implants and instruments are highly standardized and meet with special technical specifications of material and dimension. Their continuous evaluation by the Technical Commission guarantees a high standard of quality and technical development and especially the maintenance of tolerances within the system. Combining instruments and implants from different manufacturers may lead to complications such as broken drills and taps, broken screws, and damaged implants.

Although a clinical study conducted by Rüedi (1975) showed no negative clinical effect, mixing of implants and screws made of different materials (titanium and steel) should be avoided. A mixed metal system increases the risks inherent in product liability, a major concern of clinical complications.

Systems of different dimensions designated by numbers are used at various areas of the facial skull. The smallest system is the 1.0 system. The designation of the system indicates the screw size (diameter of the thread).

1.6.1 Screws

1.6.1.1 Function of Screws

Screws are the basic element for the fixation of plates or similar devices onto bone or as lag screws to hold fragments together. The correct selection and placement of screws are the key to successful stabilization of fractures or osteotomies. The best plate is useless if it is not fixed correctly with screws. Screws are designated according to the outer diameter of their thread (Fig. 1.11).

1.6.1.2 Types of Screws

In cranio-maxillo-facial surgery all screws are fully threaded and have an asymmetrical buttress thread profile (Fig. 1.11) This type of a thread is a cortical thread. Only the 1.0 standard and the 1.2 emergency screws have a metric thread due to their size.

Screws used in cranio-maxillo-facial surgery are between 1.0 and 2.7 mm in size. Only for the special reconstruction plates (UniLOCK and titanium hollow reconstruction plate, THORP) special screws are used. For each screw there is an emergency screw which is slightly larger in size and must be used in case the regular screw strips.

All screw heads to date have a cruciform recess except the 2.7 screw and its emergency screw, 3.2 mm, which have a hexagonal recess (Fig. 1.11). Another exception is the 4.0 mm THORP screw head which due to its locking

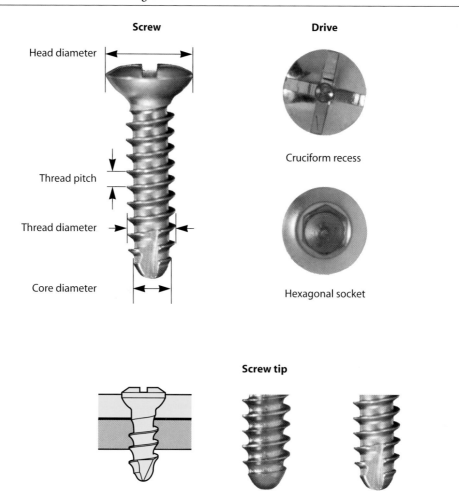

Fig. 1.11

Cranio-maxillo-facial screws are fully threaded. Except for 1.0 and 1.2 emergency screws, they have an asymmetrical buttress thread profile. Screw tips are either blunt or fluted. Nonfluted screws are thread forming and have a higher torque whereas fluted screws are thread cutting and therefore self-tapping.

Inset: In thin bone one must ensure that at least two threads engage within the bone. Screws should have a small pitch in these instances.

device, which uses an additional locking screw, has a special recess. In the future a star drive may gain increasing importance.

Screws are also differentiated by the manner in which they are inserted in the bone (pretapped or self-tapping), their function, and their size, according to the thickness of bone for which they are intended.

While pretapped or non-self-tapping screws have blunt tips, most self-tapping screws have two or three flutes at the tip to facilitate penetrating the pilot hole and cutting their thread simultaneously (Fig. 1.11). While fluted screws are thread cutting, nonfluted screws are thread forming. In thick and solid bone it is advisable to place a thread with a tap before inserting the screw because otherwise the torque during insertion may become too high, and the screw may break. On the other hand, 2.7 screws and the 4.0 screw for the THORP system are blunt screws that require a pretapped hole. All the other screws from 1.0 to 3.0 can be used in a self-tapping manner, and most have flutes.

Another major difference between screws is the manner in which they couple with the screwdriver. Two types of screwdrivers are available, those with a screw-holding device (holding sleeve) and those which are self-retaining. These screws couple securely with the screwdriver, which completely obviates any screw-holding device on the screwdriver (see Fig. 1.18a–f).

Craniofacial Screws

Screw	Thread (Ø in mm)	Core (Ø in mm)	Pitch (Ø in mm)	Head (Ø in mm)	Drive
Standard screw	1.0	0.7	0.25	1.6	
Emergency screw	1.2	0.9	0.25	1.6	
Standard screw	1.3	0.9	0.5	2.4	
Emergency screw	1.7	1.1	0.6	1.6	
Standard screw	1.5	1.1	0.5	3.0	
Emergency screw	2.0	1.4	0.6	3.5	
Standard screw	2.0	1.4	0.6	3.5	
Emergency screw	2.4	1.7	1.0	3.5	

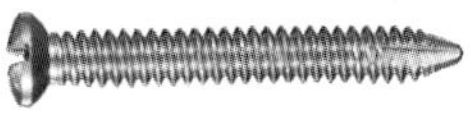

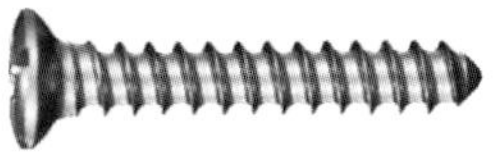

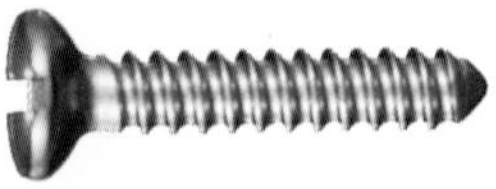

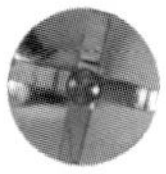

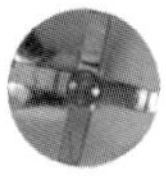

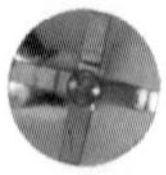

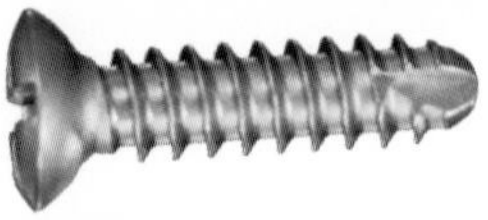

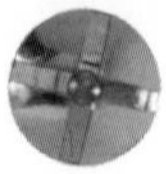

1.6.1.3 List of Screws

Craniofacial Screws 1.0–2.0 (Fig. 1.12). The size of screws generally used in the cranial and midfacial areas is between 1.0 and 2.0 mm. From January 1998 on all these screws will have fluted tips. The pitch in small screws is smaller than in larger screws. All screw heads have a cruciform recess.

Fig. 1.12

List of cranio-facial screws.

Mandible Screws

Screw	Thread (Ø in mm)	Core (Ø in mm)	Pitch (Ø in mm)	Head (Ø in mm)	Drive
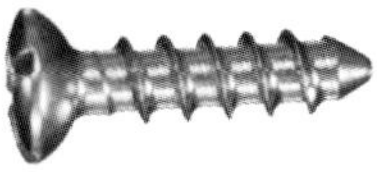					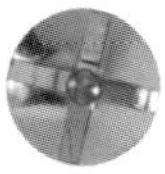
Standard screw	2.0	1.4	1.0	3.5	
Emergency screw	2.4	1.7	1.0	3.5	
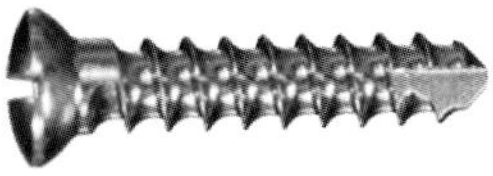					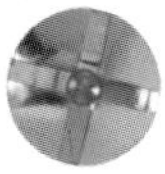
Standard screw	2.4	1.7	1.0	4.0	
Emergency screw	2.7	1.9	1.0	4.0	
UniLOCK screw 2.4	2.4	1.7	1.0	4.0	
UniLOCK screw 3.0	3.0	2.4	1.0	4.0	
Emergency screw	Not existing				
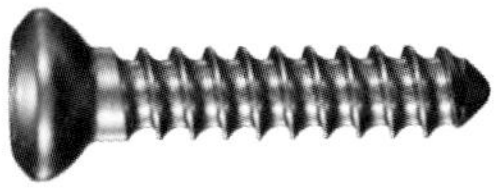					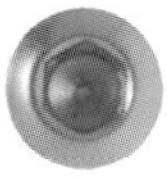
Standard screw	2.7	1.9	1.0	5.0	
Emergency screw	3.2	2.1	1.25	5.0	
THORP screw	4.0	3.0	1.25	4.5	
Emergency screw	Not existing				

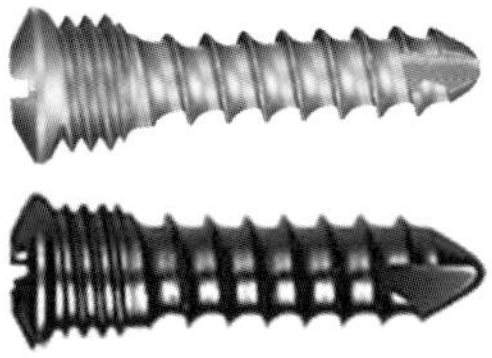

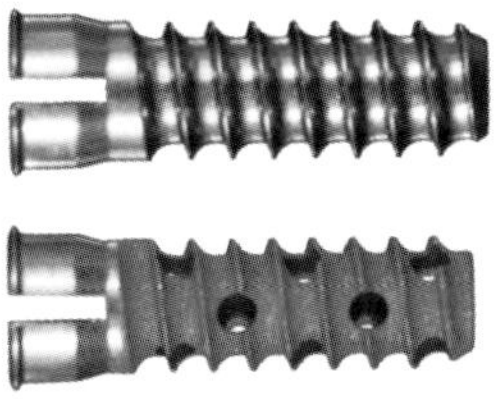

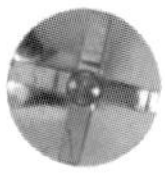

Mandible Screws 2.0–4.0 (Fig. 1.13). Screw sizes for the mandible vary between 2.0 and 4.0 mm. The pitch of the 2.0 screw for the mandible is 1.0 mm, in contrast to the 2.0 screw for midface application with a pitch of 0.6 mm. The 2.0 and 2.4 screws have a cruciform drive, while the 2.7 screw has a hexagonal drive, and the THORP screw has a special configuration for the application of the locking screw.

Fig. 1.13

List of mandible screws.

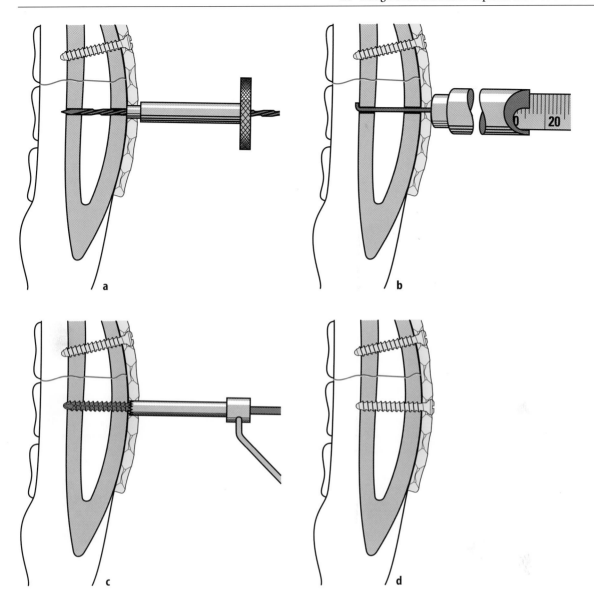

Technique of screw insertion.
a Drilling of the pilot hole with a drill corresponding to the core diameter of the screw.
b The length of the hole in the bone is measured with a depth gauge either through the plate hole or after countersinking. Note: Measure before tapping if tapping is necessary.
c Tapping through a tissue protector.
d Placement of the screw thereafter.

1.6.1.4 Technique of Screw Insertion

Correct and precise placement of the screw is one of the most important steps in plate fixation and, as a consequence, fracture and osteotomy fixation. It must be well understood that the stability of the fixation depends on the rigidity of the plate but, most importantly, on the holding capacity of the screws. Incorrect handling of the screw hole in the bone either when drilling or at the time of the placement of the screw may cause failure due to early mechanical overload of the system.

It is very important to use the various instruments for placement of the screws in the correct sequence. The correct drill bit should correspond to the core diameter of the screw. Cooling of the drill during drilling is very important to prevent overheating the bone. The length of the screw hole depends on whether self-tapping or pretapped screws are used. Thread tapping with the tap is followed by placement of the screw (Fig. 1.14).

Self-tapping screws with flutes at their tips are designed in a way that once a pilot hole is drilled, and the length of the screw is measured, they can be inserted by simply screwing them in. The pilot hole is somewhat larger than the core of the screw. Because the screw must cut its own thread when it is inserted, it may encounter considerable resistance, particularly in thick cortical bone. In these instances, even if a self-cutting screw is used, it is better to use a tap before the torque resistance becomes greater than the strength of the screw, which then causes a fracture of the screw. In addition, resistance to screw insertion may interfere with the accuracy of insertion, particularly when the surgeon is trying to insert the screw obliquely into bone to lag fragments together. It may be problematic to go in and out with self-tapping screws several times. At reinsertion it may happen that a second thread is cut accidentally on top of the first thread in the bone. This new path which destroys the earlier cut thread is disadvantageous and may considerably lower the holding capacity of the screw or lead to stripping of the screw.

The flutes in the tip areas of the screw reduce the holding capacity of the screw in this area. This is especially disadvantageous when the screw is used in a lag manner. Lag screws should either be blunt or their tip 2 mm longer than the depth gauge indicates

Studies show that in extremely thin cortical bone, such as midfacial bones, self-tapping screws hold better than non-self-tapping screws of corresponding size. Non-self-tapping screws are clearly superior in cancellous bone and in flat bones such as those of the mandible, skeleton, and pelvis.

Non-self-tapping screws with a blunt tip require pre-drilled pilot holes and then a careful cutting of their thread into the bone with a tap that corresponds exactly to the profile of the screw thread. Because the thread is cut with a tap, the size of the pilot hole corresponds almost to that of the core of the screw, and the screw thread has a much deeper bite into the adjacent bone. Much less heat is generated when the screw is inserted because there is less resistance. The tap is designed in such a way that it is not only much sharper than the thread of the screw, but it also has a more efficient mechanism of clearing the bone debris which therefore does not accumulate and clog its threads to obstruct its insertion. This allows the surgeon to work with much greater precision, particularly in thick cortical bone. The screws can easily be removed and reinserted without the fear of inadvertantly cutting a new channel as the screw alone is not able to cut a channel in cortical bone. The screws are spun, and therefore their core is perfectly straight and their surface is polished. Thus at the time of removal fully threaded screws are easily removed. Depending on the pitch of the screw, in very thin bone only few threads can gain a hold in the bone (see inset in Fig. 1.11). It is therefore important that these delicate thin bones are not partially destroyed when inserting screws.

1.6.1.5 Instruments for Screw Insertion

The instruments for screw insertion include drill bits (Figs. 1.15, 1.16), drill sleeves (Fig. 1.17a,b), depth gauges (Fig. 1.17d), taps (whenever necessary; Fig. 1.17e,f), and screwdrivers (Fig. 1.17g–i, 1.18).

Drill Bits (Fig. 1.15). Various drill bits are available for the different types of screws in different lengths, with and without stop, and with various couplings (corresponding to different power tools). Drill bits correspond to the core diameter of each screw for which they should be used to place the pilot hole. They have either two or three

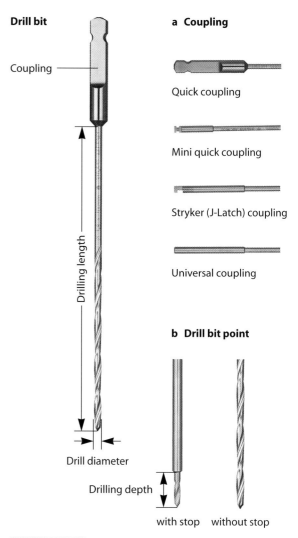

Fig. 1.15 a, b

Drill bit consisting out of shaft with coupling, drilling length, and drill diameter, which corresponds to the core of the screw and cuts the pilot hole.
a The various couplings for the drill bits.
b The tips of the drills may be either with or without stops.

Screw	Drill bit		Tap

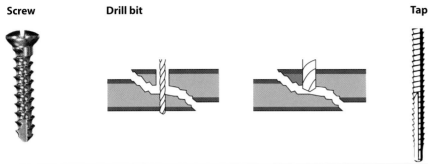

Thread Ø in mm	Threaded hole Ø in mm	Gliding hole Ø in mm	Ø in mm
1.0	0.76	–	–
1.3	1.0	–	–
1.5	1.1	1.5	Optional
2.0	1.5	2.0	Optional
2.4	1.8	2.4	Optional
2.7	2.0	2.7	Standard
4.0	3.0	–	Standard

Fig. 1.16

List of screws with corresponding drill bits for either threaded holes or gliding holes. Taps are either not necessary, optional, or indicated as for 2.7 or 4.0 screws.

flutes. They should be used with drill guides of corresponding size.

Care must be taken not to damage drill bits by contact with metal or to use unnecessary bending forces during drilling. Irrigation is mandatory during drilling to prevent heat damage to the bone.

Drill Sleeves (Fig. 1.17a). Drill sleeves are available in short and long dimensions for the various drill bits. There are special drill guides (Fig. 1.17b, c) for centric or eccentric placement of the screw hole for plates with DC holes.

Drill guides for transbuccal usage are shown with the transbuccal instrumentation (see Fig. 1.33).

Depth Gauges (Fig. 1.17d). The purpose is the placement of correct screw length which guarantees good screw hold in opposite cortex. The screw tip should exit slightly the cortex to guarantee optimal holding capacity. The gradation of screws and depth gauges is generally every 2 mm. If the measurement indicates placement between the calibration points, the longer screw should be chosen.

Depth measurement is not necessary when using a drill with stop. Depth must be measured before tapping when using pretapped screws.

Taps (Fig. 1.17e, f). Although most of the screws are self-tapping and have fluted tips, taps are available for all of them (except 1.0 and 1.3 screws). When screws are used in hard cancellous bone with a considerable thickness (4–8 mm), it is recommended to use a tap in order not to break the screw.

Instruments for Screw Insertion

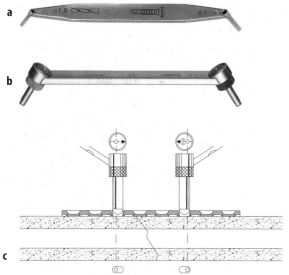

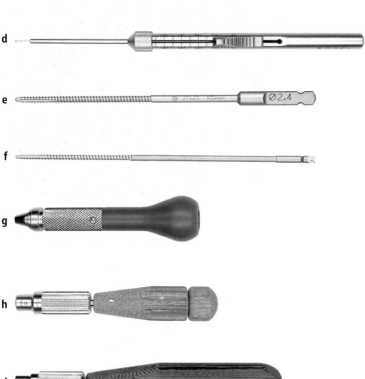

Fig. 1.17 a–i

a Drill sleeves for precise placement of screw holes and for protection of soft tissues. Double sleeves for various screw sizes offer the appropriate diameters (pilot hole and gliding hole) for the drill bits.

b Double drill guide for centric or eccentric placement of screw holes for plates with dynamic compression holes.

c Eccentric placement of the first two screws.

d Depth gauge measures the length of the hole in the bone and allows correct selection of the screw length.

e Tap for 2.4 screw with quick coupling.

f Tap for 2.0 screw with mini-quick coupling.

g Handle with mini-quick coupling.

h Short handle with quick coupling.

i Long handle with quick coupling.

Instruments for Screw Insertion

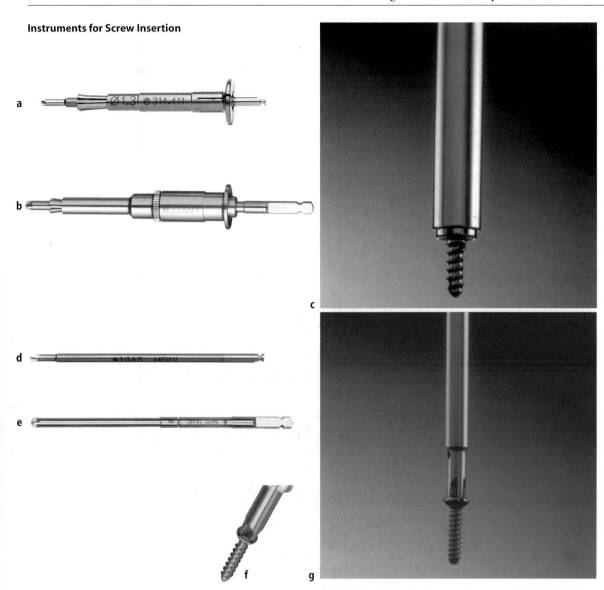

The thread diameter marked on the tap corresponds to the screw size. Taps for 1.5 and 2.0 screws are used with handle with mini-quick coupling whereas for 2.4, 2.7, and 4.0 screws they match with those with quick couplings.

Screwdrivers (Fig. 1.18). Screwdrivers with holding sleeves and with self-retaining tips are available. For transbuccal application they are used without a holding sleeve (see Fig. 1.34c). Screwdrivers for 1.0–2.0 screws are provided with mini-quick couplings; for 2.4 and 2.7 screws they have quick couplings.

Fig. 1.18 a–g

a Screwdriver with cruciform tip with holding sleeve and mini-quick coupling.
b Screwdriver with cruciform tip for 2.4 screws with holding sleeve and quick coupling.
c Screw attachment to tip of screwdriver with holding sleeve.
d Screwdriver with self-holding tip cruciform and mini-quick coupling.
e Screwdriver with self-retaining tip and quick coupling.
f,g Screw attached to tip of screwdriver via self-holding tip.

Craniofacial Plates

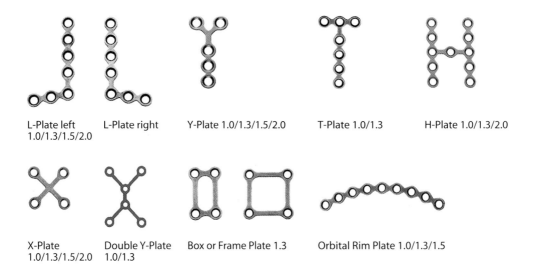

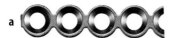

Adaption plate 1.0/1.3/1.5/2.0

L-Plate left L-Plate right   Y-Plate 1.0/1.3/1.5/2.0   T-Plate 1.0/1.3   H-Plate 1.0/1.3/2.0
1.0/1.3/1.5/2.0

X-Plate   Double Y-Plate   Box or Frame Plate 1.3   Orbital Rim Plate 1.0/1.3/1.5
1.0/1.3/1.5/2.0   1.0/1.3

1.6.2 Plates

1.6.2.1 Craniofacial Plates (Figs. 1.19, 1.20)

The shape of plates for midfacial and cranial applications corresponds generally to adaption plates. They have the form of X, Y, double-Y, H, T, L (left- and right-curved for orbital rim), and straight plates. Their thickness varies in between 0.5 mm (for the 1.0 system) and 0.9 mm (for the 2.0 system).

For special indications orbital floor plates, burr hole covers or screen as a cover for cranial or other bone defects are available.

Another special plate for the 2.0 system is the DC plate which can be used at the lateral orbital rim area and occasionally for pediatric mandibular fractures, as a tension band plate for mandibular fractures, and for fixing subcondylar fractures.

Fig. 1.19 a, b

a Magnified view of round plate holes for cranio-facial plates.
b Cranio-facial plates are designed for the various screw sizes in between 1.0 and 2.0. These are used mainly for the mid-face and cranial areas. Their thickness varies in between 0.5 and 0.9 mm.

Craniofacial Plates

Orbital floor plate universal
1.0/1.5

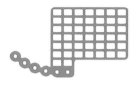

Orbital wall plate right
1.0/1.3/1.5

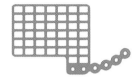

Orbital wall plate left
1.0/1.3/1.5

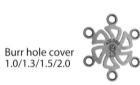

Burr hole cover
1.0/1.3/1.5/2.0

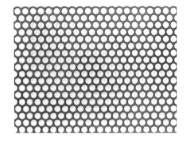

Screen 1.0/1.3

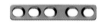

Zygomatic DCP® 2.0

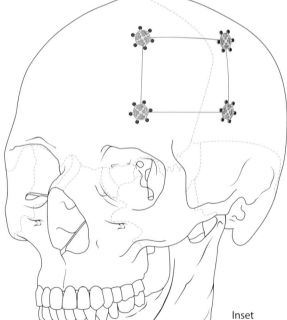

Inset

Fig. 1.20

Special plate configurations (orbital floor plates, burr hole covers, screen, zygomatic DC plate).

Inset: Application of burr hole covers for fixation of cranial bone after osteotomies or fractures.

Mandible Plates 2.0

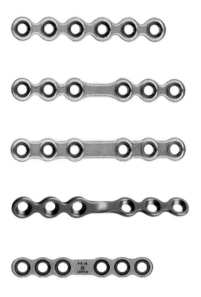

Small 2.0 plates for noncomminuted mandibular fractures. These are thicker (1.0 mm) and therefore stronger than 2.0 miniplates for the midface.

LC-DCP® Plates 2.4

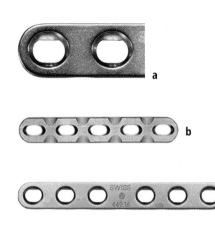
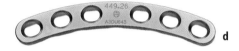

Fig. 1.22 a–d

a 2.4 plates with bidirectional DC holes. Thickness 1.65 mm.
b Limited contact design for minimal contact with the bone without impairing the implant strength.
c Straight six-hole 2.4 LC-DC-plate.
d Crescent six-hole 2.4 LC-DC-plate for chin and angular area of the mandible. (Thickness 2.0 mm).

1.6.2.2 Mandible and Reconstruction Plates
(Figs. 1.21–1.28)

Plates for mandibular fractures or defect reconstruction vary in thickness from 1.0 mm (2.0 system) to 3.0 mm (THORP system). The mini-mandible plates (2.0 system) have round holes while the straight or crescent plates for the 2.4 system have a bidirectional dynamic compression unit (DCU) screw hole. The 2.4 fracture plates have a limited contact design (undercuts) to reduce interference with the vascular supply of the bone when pressed against the surface of the bone (LC-DC plates).

Other special plates have notches at the edges. These notches allow bending in all three dimensions; especially bending edgewise and twisting is possible. The thinner and smaller variety is for special fracture situations (universal fracture plate; Fig. 1.24) while the stronger reconstruction plate is used to stabilize defect situations or comminuted zones (Fig. 1.25). Care must be taken not to overload these implants as this entails the danger of fatigue fractures. While universal fracture plates can be used only in load-sharing situations where the bone protects the plate, reconstruction plates can act temporarily as load-bearing implants.

If the plate holes of the reconstruction plates are supplied with a thread, special 2.4 screws (UniLOCK screw) with a second thread below their head can be locked in these holes.

The same is possible with the specially designed but technically more demanding THORP system (Fig. 1.27). Both plates, THORP and UniLOCK, are fixed to the bone in a manner similar to an external fixator but much closer to the bone surface. Since these plates need not be pressed against the bone surface, they are more circulation friendly, while the angular stability of the screw in the plate still guarantees sufficient stability.

Orthognathic Plate for Sagittal Split Osteotomy

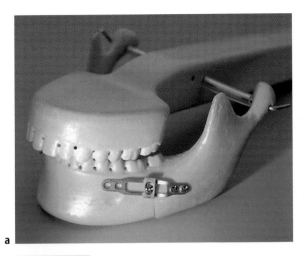 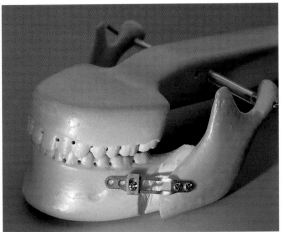

a   b

Fig. 1.23 a, b

This special orthognathic plate (SplitFix Plate or Adjustable Sagittal Split Plate) facilitates temporary and permanent fixation of the bone segments after a sagittal split osteotomy. It allows intraoperative correction of the joint-bearing fragment without removal of the plate. The plate is used especially for mandibular advancement procedures.

a Preliminary fixation before advancement of mandible.
b Situation after advancement. Definite fixation can now be performed, with two additional screws in the distal fragment.

Universal Fracture Plates 2.4

a

b

Fig. 1.24 a, b

Universal fracture plates for 2.4 screws. Their design is similar to reconstruction plates, but they are weaker. They should be used only in load-sharing situations. They must be protected by bone. They can also be used for the fixation of microvascular grafts. Plate thickness: 2.0 mm.
a Straight universal fracture plates.
b Prebent angulated universal fracture plate for the left side.
c Plate/screw profile of 2.4 screw with Universal Fracture Plate.

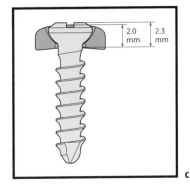

2.0 mm   2.3 mm

c

Reconstruction Plates 2.4

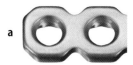

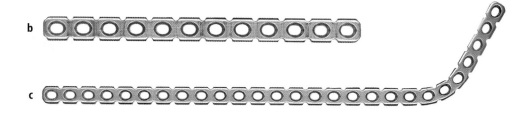

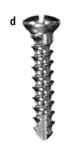 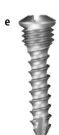

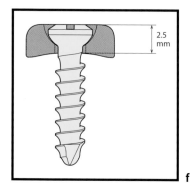

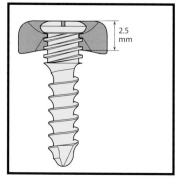

Fig. 1.25 a–g

Reconstruction plates 2.4 are much stronger than universal fracture plates. Plate thickness 2.5 mm. These are used for temporary load bearing situations.

Note: Plates cannot be used as permanent load-bearing implants.

If supplied with threaded holes, they can be used either in the regular manner with the regular 2.4 screw or as a locking system together with the special locking 2.4/3.0 screws.

a Oval-shaped plate holes with thread.
b Straight plate.
c Prebent angulated reconstruction plate for the right or left side (left side shown).
d 2.4 MF cortical screw for reconstruction plates.
e UniLOCK screw with additional thread for plate hole and threaded inset for plate hole protection during bending.
f Plate/screw profile of reconstruction plate without thread and regular 2.4 screw.
g Plate/screw profile of UniLOCK system. Reconstruction plate with threaded hole and special 2.4 locking srew.

Reconstruction Plates 2.7

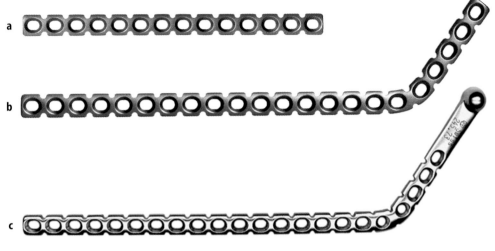

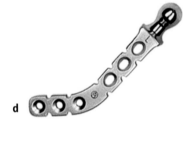

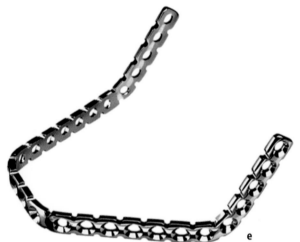

Fig. 1.26 a–e

Reconstruction plates for 2.7 screws are slightly stronger than 2.4 reconstruction plates. Plate thickness 3.1 mm. These are the only implants available in stainless steel as well as titanium.
a Straight reconstruction plate.
b Angulated reconstruction plate left side.
c Angulated reconstruction plate with condylar head left side. Available in three different sizes.
Note: Not yet (1997) approved by the United States Food and Drug Administration.
d Condylar implant left side, available in three different sizes.
e Reconstruction plate for replacement of almost complete mandible.

THORP Reconstruction Plates 4.0

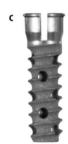

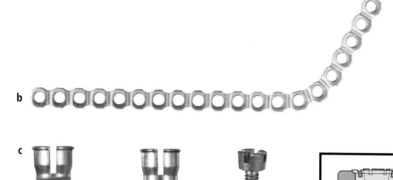

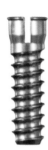

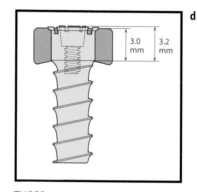

THORP

Fig. 1.27 a–d

Titanium hollow reconstruction plate (THORP). Plate thickness 3.0 mm. Screws with special heads can be locked in plate hole with special locking screws.

a Straight plate.
b Angulated plate left side.
c Hollow and solid 4.0 screws with additional locking screw.
d Plate/screw profile of THORP system. Plate with special 4.0 screw with locking screw in place.

Fig. 1.28 a–d

Recapitulation of plate/screw profiles:

a 2.4 screw with universal fracture plate

b Reconstruction plate without threaded holes and regular 2.4 screw.

c UniLOCK system. Reconstruction plate with threaded holes and special 2.4 locking screw.

d THORP system. Plate with special 4.0 screw with locking screw.

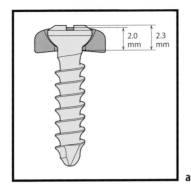

Fracture

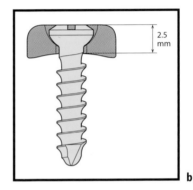

Recon

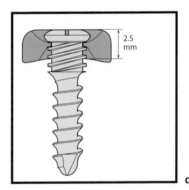

UniLOCK

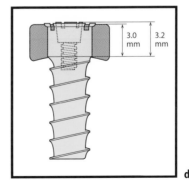

THORP

Single Vector Percutaneous Distraction Device

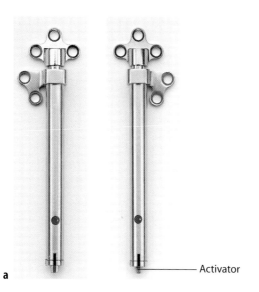

a

Activator

Fig. 1.29 a–d

a Single vector percutaneous distraction device for mandibular ramus distraction; available with a left or right foot to facilitate anterior or posterior position of screws on the mandible. Fixation to the mandible with 2.0 screws. Distractor with two feet which can be separated by activation of the head of the internal shaft at its end and lengthengs up to 30 mm.

b Activation screwdriver with internal hexagonal drive. One full turn counterclockwise equals 0.5 mm advancement. The marking on the screwdriver indicates rotational direction for lengthening.

c,d Schematic drawing of applied distractor device which functions transbuccally.

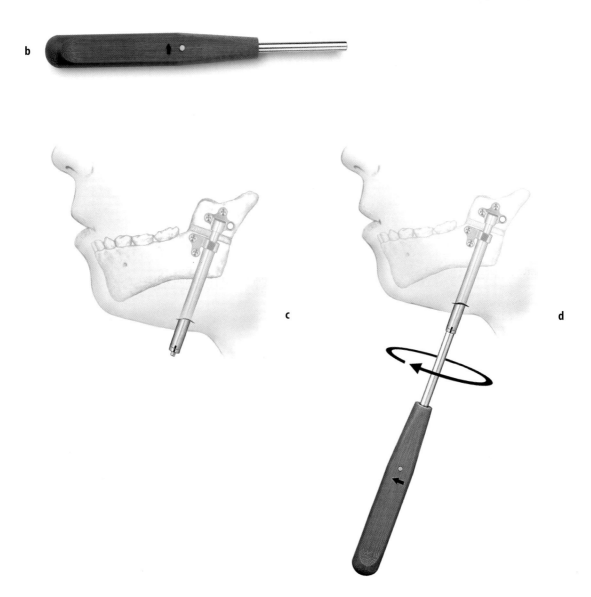

b

c

d

Plate Cutting Instruments

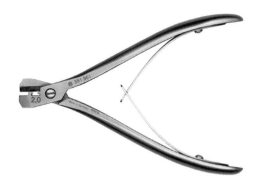

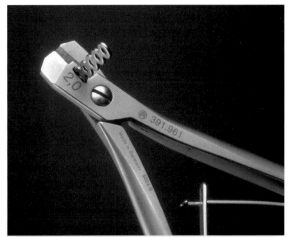

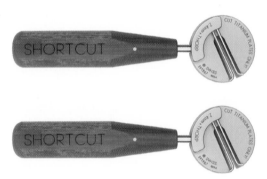

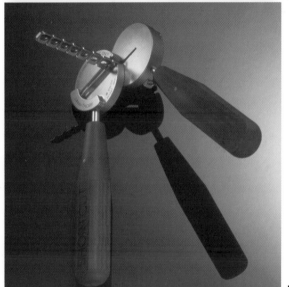

1.6.3 Instruments (Figs. 1.30–1.34)

Special instruments for correct and precise adaptation of the plates onto the surface of the bone are necessary. These include bending and cutting devices, which differ in size for the various systems.

Difficult contouring of plates should be carried out with the aid of separate malleable templates which can be bent manually to the shape of the bone and are available for all mandibular plates and the 2.0 and 1.5 craniofacial system.

Fig. 1.30 a, b

a Plate cutting forceps for all plates from 1.0 to 2.0.
b Plate cutter for 2.4 plates and THORP reconstruction plates (Shortcut™ 2.4/THORP). The device must be used in pairs.

Bending Instruments for 1.0–2.0 Plates

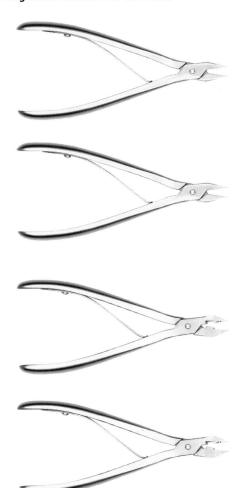

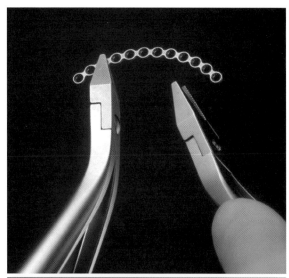

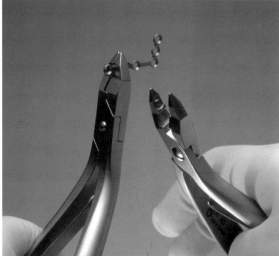

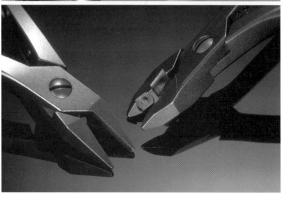

Fig. 1.31 a–c

a Pair of bending pliers, pointed, for 1.0 to 2.0 plates.
b Pair of bending pliers with special inset for the plate hole, thus preventing the deformation of the plate hole during bending.
c *Left*: close up of mouth of bending pliers shown in **a**.
Right: mouth of bending pliers shown in **b**.

Bending Instruments for 2.4, 2.7 and THORP-Plates

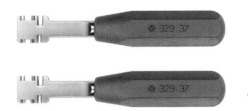

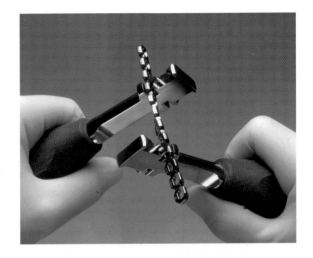

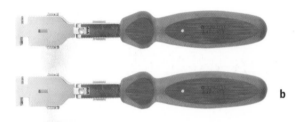

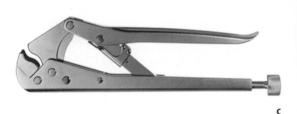

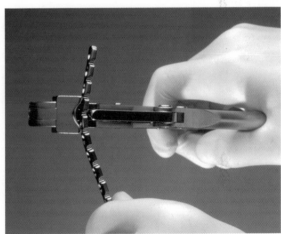

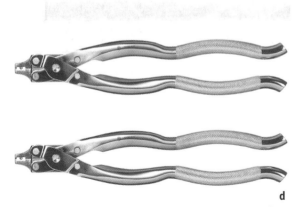

Fig. 1.32 a–d

a Bending irons for 2.4 plates.

b Bending irons for 2.4 plates with locking mechanism, available only in North America

c Bending pliers which can be adjusted to the thickness of the plate and to the grip of the surgeon by turning the knob at the end of the handle. Plates should be bent between the holes and in small steps to avoid sharp indentations. Especially for reconstruction plates bending templates are often first molded to the bone and then used as a model when contouring the plate.

d Pair of bending pliers with insets for the plate hole to prevent deformation of the plate hole.

Transbuccal Instruments

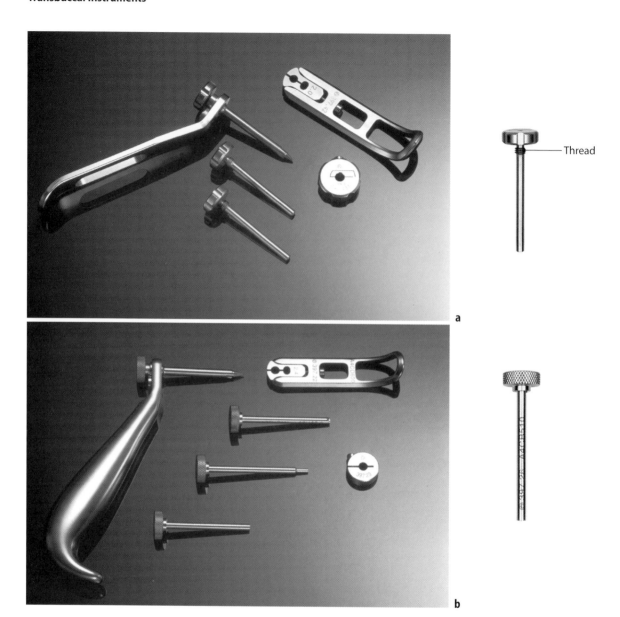

Thread

a

b

Fig. 1.33 a, b

Transbuccal instruments. For technique see Fig. 1.34 a–c.
a Set of instruments for transbuccal placement of 2.0 or smaller systems. As cheek retractor a ring or a blade is available. Sleeves are fixed to the handle via a thread.
b Set of instruments for transbuccal placement of 2.4 system. As cheek retractor a ring or a blade is available.

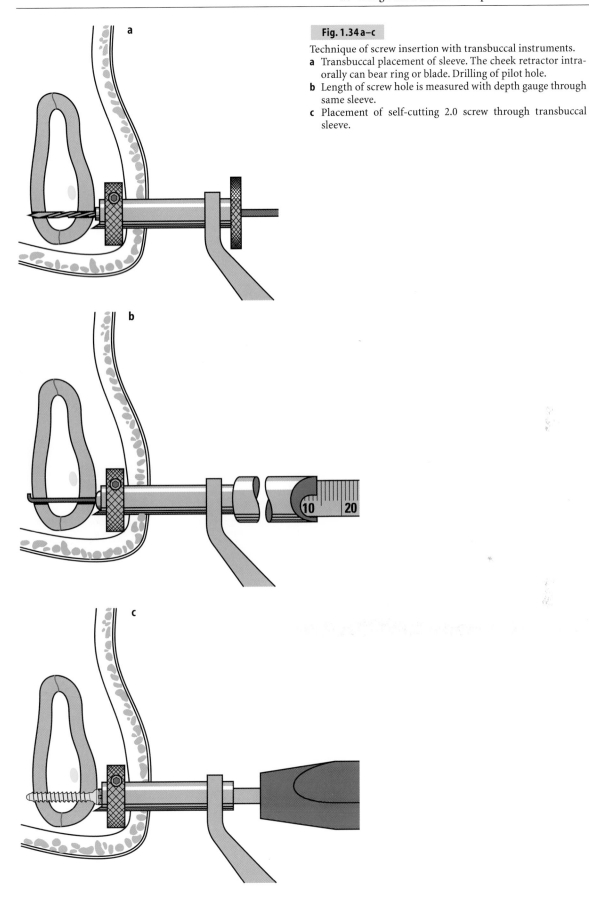

Fig. 1.34 a–c

Technique of screw insertion with transbuccal instruments.

a Transbuccal placement of sleeve. The cheek retractor intraorally can bear ring or blade. Drilling of pilot hole.

b Length of screw hole is measured with depth gauge through same sleeve.

c Placement of self-cutting 2.0 screw through transbuccal sleeve.

Power Tools

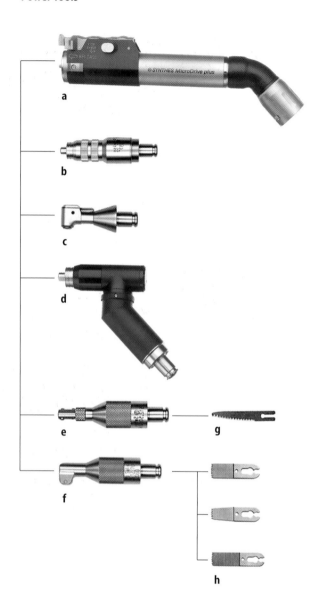

Fig. 1.35 a–h

a Micro Drive plus air drill for facial, hand, and foot applications. Forward and reverse. Speed: 0–15 000 1/min.
b Drill attachment, straight. Maximum speed 3 000 1/min.
c Drill attachment 90°. Maximum speed 7 500 1/min.
d Oscillating drill attachment 45°. Oscillating motion around 270°.
e Reciprocating saw. Piston stroke 3 mm. Maximum speed 6 000 oscillations 1/min.
f Oscillating saw. Sawblade deviation 15°. Maximum frequency 6 000 oscillations 1/min.
g Saw blade for reciprocating saw.
h Saw blades in different widths and lengths for oscillating saw.

1.6.4 Power Tools (Figs. 1.35, 1.36)

Power Tools

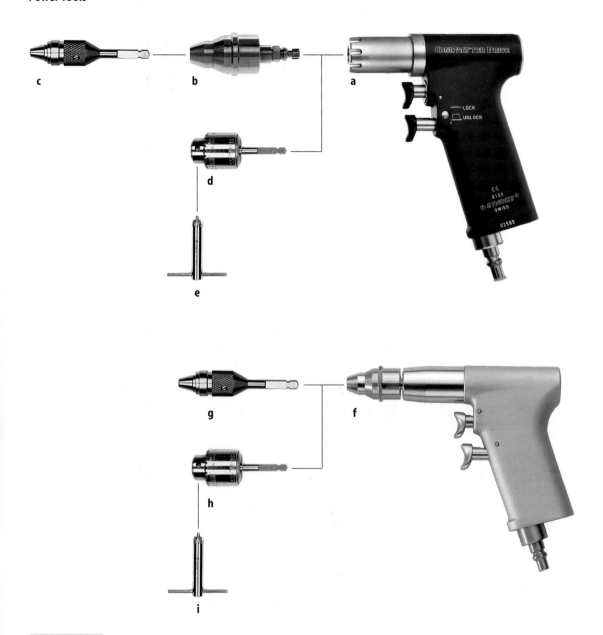

Fig. 1.36 a–i

a COMPACT™ AIR DRIVE II. Air-driven power tool, forward and reverse without work interruption. Power and speed can be regulated by a soft button placed at the air inlet. This allows a good control and precise working. Speed 500 1/min. Cannulation diameter 3.2 mm.

b–e Various attachments for Compact air drive.

b Chuck with quick coupling: can be coupled with COMPACT™ AIR DRIVE; accepts AO/ASIF instruments with quick coupling geometry.

c Drill attachment for instruments with dental coupling (mini-quick coupling)

d Jacobs chuck with key; accepts tools with round shaft 1.0–6.0 mm, with triangular shaft 1.0–6.5 mm, Schanz screws.

e Key for Jabobs chuck.

f Small air drive. Air-driven power tool. Forward and reverse without work interruption. Drill speed is controlled with the lower trigger operated by the middle finger. The upper trigger allows reversing the drill and is operated with the index finger. Quick coupling for insertion of AO/ASIF instruments with quick coupling geometry. Speed 800 l/min

g Drill attachment for instruments with dental coupling (mini-quick coupling)

h Jacobs chuck.

i Key for Jacobs chuck.

1.7 Set Configurations

1.7.1 Set Configuration Exept North America (Figs. 1.37, 1.38)

1.7.2 North American Set Configuration (Fig. 1.39)

Fig. 1.37 a–d

a Compact MF™. The craniofacial system includes implant modules in the dimensions 1.0, 1.3, 1.5, 2.0 mm and a 2.0 mm mandible system. The whole system can be stored in a large Vario Case™.

b Modules and instrument tray are shown open. The modules contain plates, screws, and the dimension-specific instruments, such as drill bits and screw driver

c Standard instrument tray contains only the most necessary instruments for the operation like the bending and cutting devices, screwdriver handles, plate holding forceps, and transbuccal instruments. All the implant modules in four different dimensions can be used with the same instrument tray.

d Additional instrument tray contains instruments such as drill sleeves, reduction forceps, depth gauge.

Set Configuration (except North America)

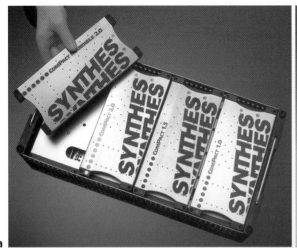

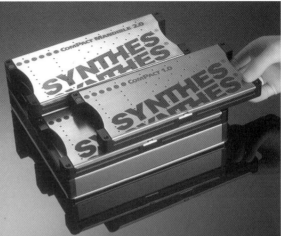

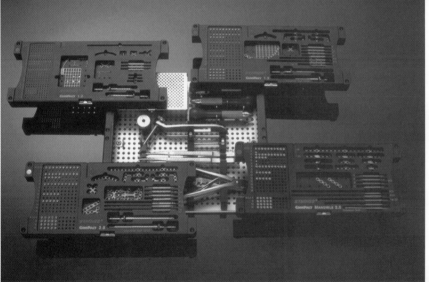

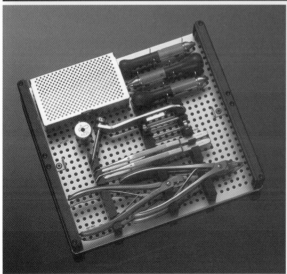

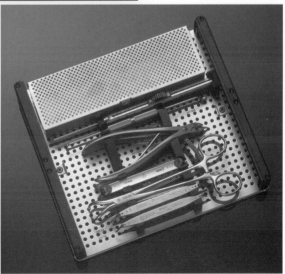

Set Configuration (except North America)

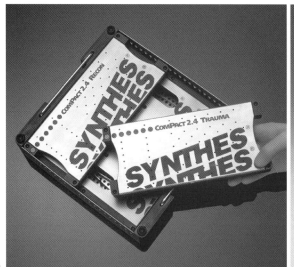
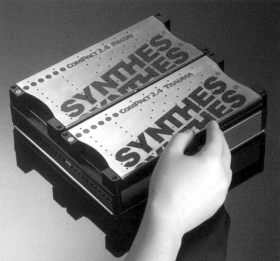

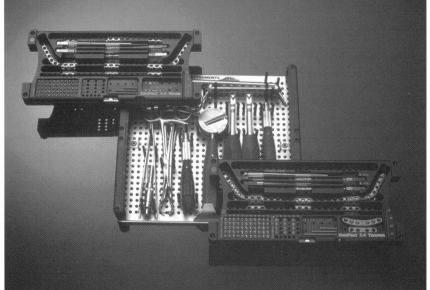

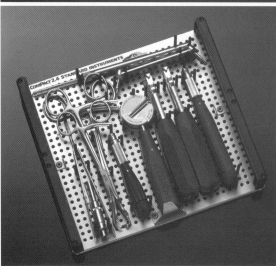

Fig. 1.38 a, b

a Compact 2.4™. A mandible system containing a reconstruction module and a trauma module. The system can be stored in a small Vario Case™.

b Modules and instrument tray shown open.

The reconstruction module (*above left*) contains rigid reconstruction plates 2.4, and the dimension-specific instruments (drill bits, screwdrivers)

The trauma module (*bottom right*) contains Universal Fracture plates 2.4, LC-DC plates 2.4, drill bits, and screwdriver.

The instrument tray contains the most necessary instruments such as cutting and bending device, screwdriver handles, drill sleeve, depth gauge, reduction forceps, and plate-holding forceps.

Set Configuration (North America)

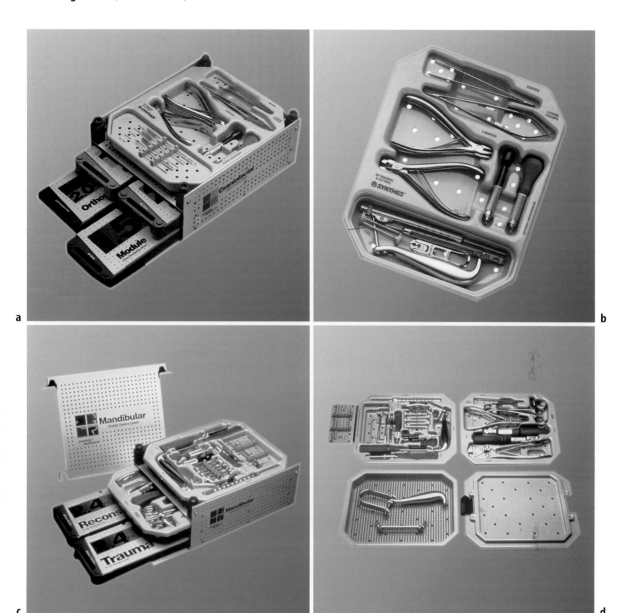

Fig. 1.39

a The Craniofacial Modular Fixation System available on the North American market contains one instrument and four implant modules with the dimensions 1.0, 1.3, 1.5, and 2.0. The set can be used for all fractures and orthognathic operations in the midface and cranium.

b The instrument tray for the craniofacial modular fixation system concentrates on the most necessary universal instruments for the application of the screws and plates in the different sizes.

c The Mandibular Modular Fixation System available on the North American market contains two instruments trays and two implant modules for all rigid internal fixation applications in the mandible: trauma, reconstruction, and orthognathics.

d The instrument trays for the mandibular modular fixation system contains all universal instruments such as bending and cutting instruments, transbuccal instruments needed for the trauma and the reconstruction module

External Fixation Devices

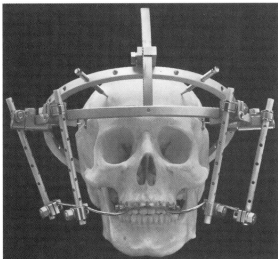

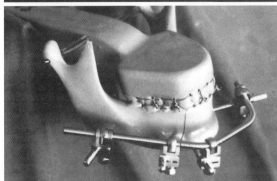

Fig. 1.40 a, b

a External HALO Frame Fixator as it was used in the 1980s. No more available.

b External Pin Fixation Device, developed 1985. At the moment not available because of lack of indications.

References and Suggested Reading

Anderson R (1936) Femoral bone lengthening. Am J Surg 31:479

Ashhurst DE (1986) The influence of mechanical conditions on the healing of experimental fractures in the rabbit. A microscopical study. Philos Trans R Soc Lond B Biol Sci 313:271–302

Assael LA (1990) Considerations in rigid internal fixation of midface trauma. Oral Maxillofac Surg Clin North Am (2) 1:103–119

Brunner U, Kessler S, Cordey J, Rahn B, Schweiberer L, Perren SM (1990) Defektbehandlung langer Röhrenknochen durch Distraktionsosteogenese (Ilizarov) und Marknagelung. Theoretische Grundlagen, tierexperimentelle Ergebnisse, klinische Relevanz. Unfallchir 93:244–250

Champy M, Lodde JP (1971) Synthesis mandibulare. Location de synthèse aux function de contraints mandibulaires. Stomat (Paris)

Claes L, Palme U, Palme E, Kirschbaum U (1982) Biomechanical and mathematical investigations concerning stress protection

Coleman J (1994) Osseous reconstruction of the mid-face and orbits. Clin Plast Surg 21:113

Cordey J, Schwyzer HK, Brun S, Matter P (1985) Bone loss following plate fixation of fractures? Helv Chir Acta 52:181–184

Cordey J, Perren SM, Steinemann S (1987) Parametric analysis of the stress protection in bone after plating. In: Bergmann G, Kölbel R, Rohlmann A (Eds) Biomechanics: basic and applied research. Nijhoff, Dordrecht, pp 387–392

Danckwardt-Lilliestrom G, Grevsten S, Olerud S (1972) Investigation of effect of various agents on periosteal bone formation. Ups J Med Sci 77:125–128

Dannis R (1979) Théorie et pratique de l'osteosynthèse. Masson, Paris

Day et al (1995) Calvarial Bone Grafting in Craniofacial Reconstruction. Facial Plast Clinics North Am (3) 3:241–257

Frodel J, Marentette L (1993) Lag screw fixation of the upper craniomaxillofacial skeleton. Arch Otolaryngol Head Neck Surg 119:297

Fuji N, Yamashiro M (1983) Classification of malar complex fractures using computed tomography. J Oral Maxillofac Surg 41:562–567

Gautier E, Cordey J, Lüthi U, Mathys R, Rahn BA, Perren SM (1983) Knochenumbau nach Verplattung: biologische oder mechanische Ursache? Helv Chir Acta 50:53–58

Gautier E, Cordey J, Mathys R, Rahn BA, Perren SM (1984) Porosity and remodelling of plated bone after internal fixation: result of stress shielding or vascular damage? Elsevier Science, Amsterdam

Goodship AE, Kenwright J (1985) The influence of induced micromovement upon the healing of experimental fractures. J Bone Joint Surg Br 67:650–655

Gotzen L, Haas N, Strohfeld G (1981) Zur Biomechanik der Plattenosteosynthese. Unfallheilk 84:439–443

Greenberg AM, Prein J (eds) (1997) Craniomaxillofacial reconstruction and corrective bone surgery. Springer, Berlin Heidelberg New York

Gruss JS, Mackinnon SE (1986) Complex maxillary fractures. Role of buttress reconstruction and immediate bone grafts. Plast Reconstr Surg 78:9–22

Gunst MA, Suter C, Rahn BA (1979) Die Knochendurchblutung nach Plattenosteosynthese. Helv Chir Acta 46:171–175

Haas N, Gotzen L, Riefenstahl L (1985) Biomechanische Untersuchungen zur Plattenfixation an die Hauptfragmente. Orthopedics 123:591

Haug (1993) Basics of stable internal fixation of maxillary fractures craniomaxillofacial fractures: principles of internal fixation using the AO/ASIF technique. pp 135–157

Hayes WC (1980) Basic biomechanics of compression plate fixation. In: Uhthoff HK, Stahl E (eds) Current concepts of internal fixation of fractures. Springer, Berlin Heidelberg New York, pp 49–62

Hutzschenreuter P, Perren SM, Steinemann S, Geret V, Klebl M (1969) Some effects of rigidity of internal fixation on the healing pattern of osteotomies. Injury 1:77–81

Ilizarov GA (1989) The tension-stress effect on the genesis and growth of tissues. Clin Orthop 238:249–281

Jackson IT (1989) Classification and treatment of orbitozygomatic and orbitoethmoidal fractures. The place of bone grafting and plate fixation. Clin Plast Surg 16:77–119

Kellman R (1995) Recent advancements in facial plating techniques. Facial Plast Clin North Am (3) 3:227.239

Klotch DW, Gilliland R (1987) Internal fixation vs. conventional therapy in midface fractures. J Trauma 27:1136–1145

Krompecher S, Kerner E (1979) Callus formation. Symposium on the biology of fracture healing. Academiai Kiado, Budapest

Kroon FMH, Mathisson M, Cordey JR, Rahn BA (1991) The use of miniplates in mandibular fractures: an in vitro study. J Craniomaxillofac Surg 19 (6):199–204

Kuhn A, McIff T, Cordey J, Baumgart FW, Rahn BA (1996) Bone deformation by thread-cutting and thread-forming cortex screws. Injury 26 [Suppl 1]:12–20

Küntscher G (1970) Das Kallus-Problem. Enke, Stuttgart

Lane WA (1913) The operative treatment of fractures. Medical Publishing, London

Lanyon LE, Rubin CT (1985) Functional adaptation in skeletal structures. Harvard University Press, Cambridge, pp 1–25

Manson PN (1986) Some thoughts on the classification and treatment of the Le Fort fractures. Ann Plast Surg 17:356–363

Manson PN, Hoopes JE, Su CT (1980) Structural pillars of the facial skeleton: an approach to the management of Le Fort fractures. Plast Reconstr Surg 66:54

Marx RE (1994) Clinical application of bone biology to mandibular and maxillary reconstruction. Clin Plast Surg 21:377

Matter P, Brennwald J, Perren SM (1974) Biologische Reaktion des Knochens auf Osteosyntheseplatten. Helv Chir Acta [Suppl] 12:1

Müller ME, Nazarian S, Koch P (1987) Classification AO des fractures. 1 Les os longs. Springer, Berlin Heidelberg New York

Müller ME, Nazarian S, Koch P, Schatzker J (1990) The comprehensive classification of fractures of long bones. Springer, Berlin Heidelberg New York

Müller ME, Allgöwer M, Schneider R, Willenegger H (1991) Manual of internal fixation. Springer, Berlin Heidelberg New York

Pauwels F (1980) Biomechanics of the locomotor apparatus. Springer, Berlin Heidelberg New York

Perren SM, Cordey J (1980) The concept of interfragmentary strain. In: Uhthoff HK, Stahl E (eds) Current concepts of internal fixation of fractures. Springer, Berlin Heidelberg New York, pp 63–70

Perren SM, Rahn BA, Lüthi U, Gunst MA, Pfister U (1981) Aseptische Knochennekrose: sequestrierender Umbau? Orthopäde 10:3–5

Phillips JH, Rahn BA (1989) Comparison of compression and torque measurements of self-tapping and pretapped screws. Plast Reconstr Surg 83:447

Rahn BA (1987) Direct and indirect bone healing after operative fracture treatment. Otolaryngol Clin North Am 20:425–440

Rhinelander FW (1978) Physiology of bone from the vascular viewpoint, vol 2. Society for Biomaterials, San Antonio, pp 24–26

Rudderman RH, Mullen RL (1992) Biomechanics of the facial skeleton. Clin Plast Surg 19 (1):11–29

Rüedi T (1975) Titan und Stahl in der Knochenchirurgie. Hefte Unfallheilk 3

Schatzker J, Tile M (1987) The rationale of operative fracture care. Springer, Berlin Heidelberg New York

Schenk R (1987) Cytodynamics and histodynamics of primary bone repair. In: Lane JM (ed) Fracture healing. Churchill Livingstone, New York

Schenk RK (1992) Biology of fracture repair. In: Browner BD, Jupiter JB, Levine AM, Trafton PG (eds) Skeletal trauma. Saunders, Philadelphia, pp 31–75

Schenk RK, Willenegger H (1963) Zum histologischen Bild der sogenannten Primärheilung der Knochenkompakta nach experimentellen Osteotomien am Hund. Experientia 19:593

Schmoker RR (1992) Management of infected fractures in nonunions of the mandible. In: Yaremchuk M, Gruss J, Manson P (ed) Rigid fixation of the craniomaxillofalcial skeleton. pp 233–244

Schwenzer N, Steinhilber W, Traumatologie des Gesichtsschädels, Banaschweski, München-Grafelfing

Spiessl B (1988) Osteosynthese des Unterkiefers. Springer, Berlin Heidelberg New York

Spiessl B (1989) Internal fixation of the mandible - manual of AO/ASIF principles. Springer. Berlin Heidelberg New York

Spiessl B, Schroll K (1972) Spezielle Frakturen- und Luxationslehre, vol I. Gesichtsschädel. Thieme, Stuttgart

Steinemann S (1998): In Greenberg AM, Prein J (eds) Craniomaxillofacial reconstructive and conective bone surgery. Metal for craniomaxillofacial internal fixation implants and its physiological implication. Springer NY

Steinemann S, Mäusli PA (1988) Titanium alloys for surgical implants - biocompatibilitty from physico-chemical principles. Sixth World Conference on Titanium, Cannes

Tonino AJ, Davidson CL, Klopper PJ, Linclau LA (1976) Protection from stress in bone and its effects. Experiments with stainless steel and plastic plates in dogs. J Bone Joint Surg Br 58:107–113

Uhthoff HK, Dubuc FL (1971) Bone structure changes in the dog under rigid internal fixation. Clin Orthop 81:165–170

Weber BG, Brunner C (1981) The treatment of nonunions without electrical stimulation. Clin Orthop 161:24–32

Weber BG, Cech O (1973) Pseudarthrosen. Pathophysiologie – Biomechanik – Therapie – Ergebnisse. Huber, Bern

Wolf J (1892) Das Gesetz der Transformation der Knochen. Hirschwald, Berlin

Wolff J (1986) The law of bone remodelling. Springer, Berlin Heidelberg New York

Woo SLY, Akeson WH, Coutts RD, Rutherford L, Jemmott GF, Amiel D (1976) A comparison of cortical bone atrophy secondary to fixation with plates with large differences in bending stiffness. J Bone Joint Surg Am 58:190–195

Yamada H, Evans FG (1970) Strength of biological materials. Williams and Wilkins, Baltimore

Yaremchuk MF, Gruss JS, Manson PN (1992) Rigid fixation of the craniomaxillofacial skeleton. Butterworth-Heinemann, London

Chapter 2

Anatomic Approaches

2

Chapter Author: Joachim Prein
Contributor: Nicolas J. Lüscher

Good exposure to the fracture site is the key to anatomic reposition and stable osteosynthesis. Nerve or vascular damage by surgical approaches to the bone must be strictly avoided. A careful neurological evaluation of sensory (supraorbital, infraorbital, or mental nerve) and motor nerves (facial or occulomotorius nerve) is therefore mandatory before operating on the patient. The most often damaged nerve is the marginal branch of the facial nerve during osteosynthesis of the horizontal branch of the mandible. The open fracture treatment with osteosynthesis must include the careful planning of the skin incisions for optimal cosmetic and functional results.

For good planning of the skin incision it is important to have a wide exposure of the complete face during the operation. The nasal intubation tube is fixed over the nose and the frontal midline in mandibular fractures. In simple midface fractures the intraoral tube goes downwards to the chest wall. In panfacial fractures different routes for intubation may be necessary, such as nasal, oral submental, and, exceptionally, tracheotomy, depending on the local and individual situation. We perfer to cover the gastric and the intubation tube with a translucent, sterile sheet (e.g., Op-Site).

After the operation the wounds are usually drained with Redon suction drains in a closed system using a small skin incision in the skinlines for better scarring of the drainage holes. The wound is always closed in layers, and the muscles are carefully adapted with resorbable suture material. For skin closure we use separate stitches, 3.0 or 4.0 for the coronary approach (or staples), 5.0 for the face and mandible, and 6.0 for the eyelids with monofil nonresorbable suture material.

Careful taping reduces the tension on the skin and edema. All patients are taught to massage their skin incisions starting 4 weeks after the operation, to apply pressure, and to avoid ultraviolet light as long as the scars are hyperemic and red.

Never forget that every patient considers the scars as the surgeon's signature.

Explanation of Abbreviations

BPI	Blepharoplasty incision
CI	Coronary incision
EBI	Eyebrow incision
FA	Facial artery
FB	Frontal branch of the facial nerve
FLI	Face lift incision
FN	Facial nerve
FSO	Foramen supraorbitale
GI	Glabellar incision
ION	Inferior orbital nerve
LBI	Lower blepharoplasty incision
LCL	Lateral canthal ligament
LD	Lacrimal duct
LEI	Low eyelid incision
LG	Lacrimal gland
MA	Malar arch
MB	Marginal branch of facial nerve
MCL	Medial canthal ligament
MCS	Monocortically placed screws
MN	Mental nerve
NLS	Nasal lacrimal sack
OF	Orbital fat
SCI	Subciliar incision
SI	Stab incision
SL	Skin lacerations
SM	Submental skin fold
SON	Supraorbital nerve
TCI	Transconjunctival incision
UBI	Upper blepharoplasty incision

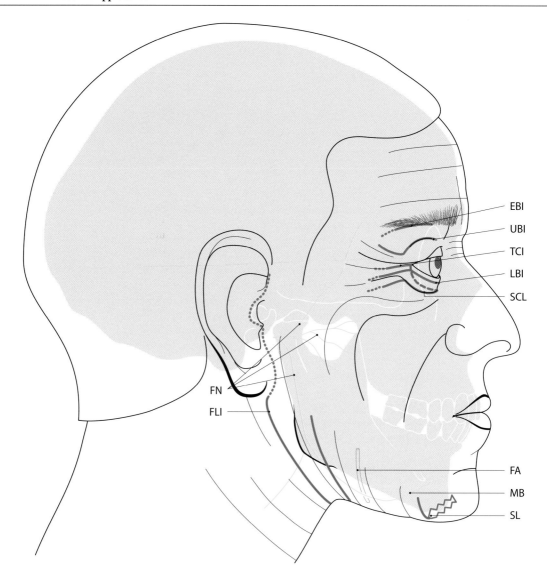

Fig. 2.1

Lateral approaches to the facial skeleton.
Mandible: The lobule of the ear, angle of the mandible, and mouth must always be visible during the operation to allow perfect orientation for correct skinline incisions.

The modified face lift incision for the approach to the mandibular joint turns around the lobule and can be extended downwards to the horizontal skin folds of the neck to allow exposure of the angle of the mandibula (*FLI*). The main stem of the facial nerve may be damaged (*FN*) during the osteosynthesis of condylar neck fractures and should be, whenever possible, exposed. Careful use of the Langenbeck hook is mandatory to avoid nerve damage.

Exposure of the horizontal branch of the mandible follows the skin lines, which may cross the margin of the mandible or not. The marginal branch (*MB*) may overlap the margin of the mandible by 1 cm. Therefore after incising the skin the platysma and fascia colli must be incised 1 cm below the skin incision to avoid proximity to the nerve. If the facial artery (*FA*) is dissected, the plane of the marginal branch is always above the vessel.

Skin lacerations (see Fig. 2.3, *SL*) may be used for the approach to fractures and can be extended into the direction of skin lines or combined with separate incisions.
Orbit and Zygoma: The subciliar incision (*SCI*) is the most common exposure for the malar bone, inferior orbital rim, and orbital floor. The orbicularis muscle is separated in its fibers 5 mm below to the skin incision.

Lower blepharoplasty incision (*LBI*) is less advisable because of the danger of postoperative ectropion, especially in elderly patients. Too much traction on the skin margins during drilling must be avoided.

The skin extension of a transconjunctival incision (*TCI*) disinserts the lateral canthal aponeurosis and gives a very direct approach to the bone.

The eyebrow incision (*EBI*) for the exposure of the lateral orbital rim is nicely hidden in the hair, but we prefer the upper blepharoplasty incision (*UBI*) for a direct and very atraumatic approach to the lateral and superior orbital rim.

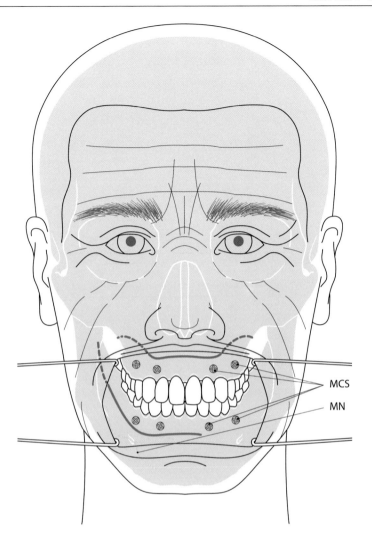

MCS

MN

Fig. 2.2

Intraoral approaches to the facial skeleton.
All mucosal incisions are placed 2 mm above or below the attached gingiva. To give good exposure, transmucosal approaches must be very long. In the mandible care must be taken to avoid damage to the mental nerve (*MN*), which perforates the bone between and below the tooth roots 4 and 5. Proximal to the mental foramen the nerve canal goes down 2–3 mm to raise up again posteriorly in the mandible. Therefore in the horizontal area the screws must be placed very low to avoid nerve damage.

Intermaxillary fixation can either be via dental splints, with the help of unicortically placed short screws (*MCS*), or with miniplates fixed with screws in the alveolar ridge of the maxilla and mandible.

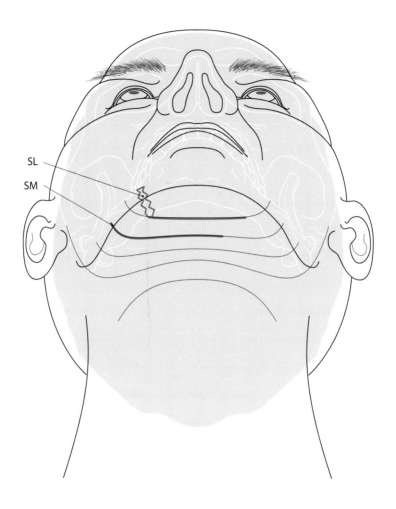

Fig. 2.3

Submental approach.
Use of the submental skin fold (*SM*). The skin is separated from
the muscle to give way to the bone with minimal bleeding. Skin
lacerations (*SL*) can be included in the skin line incisions or
used as a second and separate approach.

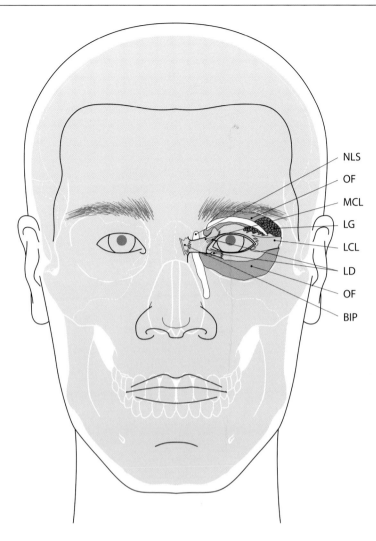

NLS
OF
MCL
LG
LCL
LD
OF
BIP

The canthal ligaments and the lacrimal system.
The medial canthal ligament (*MCL*) is a well-defined anatomic entity with a very strong attachment to the bone. The bony insertion point (*BIP*) of the medial ligament must be placed in correct position during osteosynthesis.

The lacrimal duct (*LD*) and the nasal lacrimal sack (*NLS*) are deep to the ligament and can most often be preserved. The lateral canthal ligament (*LCL*) is not a ligament but a broad aponeurotic structure. For exposure of the orbital cavity and floor the lacrimal gland (*LG*) and the orbital fat (*OF*) are mobilized via the subperiosteal plane.

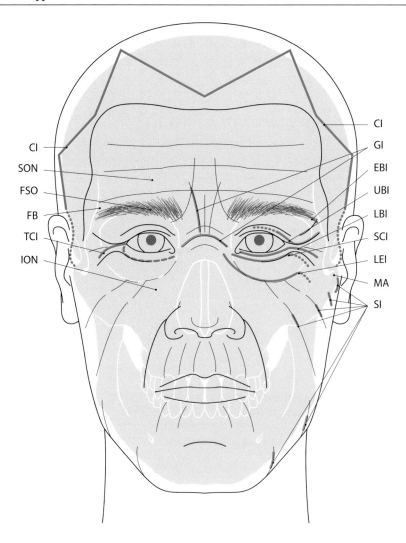

Fig. 2.5

Anterior approaches to the facial skeleton.

In all complex fractures of the midface the coronary incision (*CI*) is mandatory. The W incision of the skin margins respects the hairline and can easily be sutured back at the end of the operation. The plane of dissection is subgaleal and subperiosteal, about 2 cm above the orbital rim. The supraorbital nerve (*SON*) must be identified and occasionally burried out of a small foramen (*FSO*).

Lateral dissection is deep on the temporal fascia to avoid damage to the frontal branch (*FB*) of the facial nerve, exposing easily the malar arch (*MA*).

The glabelar incision (*GI*) either vertical or horizontal exposes the root of the nose and can be used to place a nasal bone graft with screw fixation.

Four incisions are possible to approach the *lower margin of the orbit*. We prefer either the subciliar incision (*SCI*) in the first eyelid fold 4–5 mm below the rim that may be extended laterally up to 2 cm [cave frontal branch of the facial nerve (*FB*)!] or the transconjuctival incision (*TCI*) that may be extended cutting the lateral canthus.

Lower blepharoplasty incision (*LBI*) may lead to postoperative ectropion. The low eyelid incision (*LEI*) gives a good and direct view to the orbital rim, but the scar may be visible and produce an eyelid edema.

Most of the malar fractures include the intraorbital foramen, therefore the infraorbital nerve (*ION*) must always be shown for decompression. Avoid nerve compression by an osteosynthesis plate.

The frontal branch (*FB*) of the facial nerve lays in the deep subcutaneous layer and goes up to the frontal muscle about 1.5 cm posterior to the lateral canthus.

To approach the upper orbital rim we perform a lateral upper blepharoplasty incision (*UBI*), which leads directly to the zygomaticofrontal suture. The eyebrow incision (*EBI*) is an alternative. Lacerations can be included in the skinline approach to the orbit.

Stab incisions (*SI*) are cut in the skinlines for closed reduction with the hook in malar fractures or for wound drains.

CHAPTER 3

Mandibular Fractures

Chapter Author: Wilfried Schilli
Contributors: Peter Stoll
               Wolfgang Bähr
               Joachim Prein

3.1 Introduction

The aim of adequate internal fixation of facial fractures including mandibular restoration of form and function with plates and screws is to provide for undisturbed healing under the condition of function and without any period of intermaxillary fixation (IMF). It is therefore necessary to carry out an adequate fixation for each individual fracture type. The question of how to perform adequate fixation depends on the different fracture types, the general health and compliance of the patient, and the timing of the operation. While one fracture can adequately be fixed with one miniplate only, another fracture may have to be stabilized with a reconstruction plate in order to be adequately fixed. In addition to these factors, the choice of fixation depends on the experience and judgement of the surgeon. When in doubt, it is always safer to select a stronger plate and screw or go for a double plate fixation instead of a single plate fixation. Failures are almost always due to a misjudgement of the surgeon and not to the hardware. It is of utmost importance to recognize and understand failures in order to provide for a safe and quick repair.

An absolute prerequisite is the ability of the surgeon to identify and secure the correct occlusion prior to stable fixation of facial fractures with plates and screws. During surgery intermaxillary fixation is a must.

3.2 Treatment Planning

Not only the type of fracture but also the patient's personality, age, sex, and general condition is of great importance for treatment planning.

Personality of Patient. Highly educated and intelligent patients show better compliance with therapeutic measures and advice while those with a low social standard may be negligent in their postoperative behaviour. These patients require more supervision. It is our experience that persons with a low social standard often do not present for implant removal. Therefore it is neces-sary to use inert osteosynthesis material, for example, titanium, which makes implant removal unnecessary.

Age and Sex of Patient. Postoperative healing is generally better when the patient is young. This is also the case with bone healing. On the other hand, elderly patients frequently exhibit diminished osseous density due to osteoporosis. The biting strength of young men is generally greater than that of women. The consequence is that a more stable fixation device should be preferred in young men.

General Remarks. Medically compromised patients with metabolic diseases such as diabetes, allergies, and hemorrhage and patients addicted to drugs must be treated with particular caution. Metabolic diseases may affect otherwise uneventful postoperative wound healing. Allergic reactions to titanium are not known.

In addition, patients with cardiac or pulmonary diseases may exhibit problems with general anesthesia. These patients should be treated under particular anesthesiological care either in general or local anesthesia.

Psychiatric and neurological diseases (e.g., epilepsia) do not allow IMF and require open reduction of the fracture.

3.3 Cost Effectiveness

Number of Plates and Screws. The number of plates and screws used for fracture treatment should be limited to achieve adequate stability. Overtreatment (oversize!) should be avoided.

Return to Work. The overall aim of fracture treatment is safe restoration of form and function. By utilizing open reduction and adequate internal fixation IMF for several weeks can be avoided. In economic terms this may be cheaper in numerous cases because the patient is allowed to return to work earlier.

3.4 Adequate Stability

The definition of this parameter is difficult. While one fracture may be adequately fixed with only one miniplate, the other may have to be fixed with a strong reconstruction plate. The choice depends on the experience and judgement of the surgeon, the condition of the patient, and the specific fracture type.

Reasons for failure are almost always due to the surgeon, rather than to the hardware used. It is very important to reanalyze failures in order to recognize and understand the reason for the complication. The aim is to carry out a safe and quick repair.

Compression is only an additional tool for stabilization, not the prerequisite. Compression supports – at least in the initial phase of fracture healing – sharing of functional load between hardware and bone. Nevertheless exact and meticulous reduction of the fragments is compulsory.

In all cases mentioned it is not antibiotic treatment but stability of the fragments which is the prerequisite for uneventful bone healing. It must be stressed that antibiotic cover is only a supporting factor.

Whenever possible the third molar should not be removed prior to open reduction and fixation of the fracture, as it facilitates to some extent exact repositioning of the fracture surfaces. Osteotomies to remove a third molar should be avoided if possible in order not to loose bony support of the fragments.

3.5 Mistakes in Application and Technique

Insufficient Reduction of the Fracture With Incongruency of the Fracture Surfaces and Interposition of Soft Tissue. Good visibility of the fractured area during open reduction is important. For example, in subcondylar fractures it is inappropriate to use an intraoral approach under all circumstances with poor visibility and loss of the ability to control reduction. If there is any doubt, it is better to prefer an extraoral approach.

Poor Positioning of Screw (→ Nerve Damage, Root Damage). To avoid nerve and root damage the plate must be placed adequately, for example, not at the level of the mandibular nerve channel or the tooth roots. If this is not possible, the direction of the screw holes must be in such a way that the screw bypasses these structures, or it must be placed in a monocortical manner.

Choice of Inadequate Hardware (Too Weak, Too Small), Especially When in Combination With Subcondylar Fractures. Young men generally require stronger hardware. The functional forces in elderly patients with edentulous and atrophic mandibles should not be underestimated,

however. Here a load-bearing osteosynthesis with a stronger fixation device must be performed (see Sect. 3.15). Defect or comminuted fractures require bridging osteosynthesis via reconstruction plates. In this context it must be stressed that even the strongest plate may fracture with time (due to fatigue) when the bony continuity is not restored.

Compression in Comminuted Areas. Comminution means a lack of bony support. Compression in comminuted areas is impossible and leads to dislocation of the fragments. It is therefore necessary at first to simplify the fracture via reduction of the small bone pieces and fixation with small plates and screws and to bridge the whole area thereafter with a reconstruction plate. The screws of the reconstruction plate should not engage the small bone pieces in the comminuted area ("bridging osteosynthesis").

Insufficient Fixation of the Plate (Too Few Screws). If compression of the fragments is not achievable, it is better to use more screws for fixation of the plate. In cases of a defective or comminuted fracture at least three screws on each sides of the defect or the comminution are mandatory. Thin and weak bone generally requires the use of more screws than thick and hard bone.

Screw in the Fracture Gap. Good visibility helps to avoid the positioning of a screw in a fracture gap. Nevertheless in oblique fractures the postoperative X-ray may reveal poor position of a screw, i.e., in the fracture gap, which was not realized during the operative procedure. Therefore it is necessary to supervise also the lingual aspect of the fracture before drilling the screw holes.

Stripping of the Screw Holes. Drill bit, tap (if necessary), and screw should be used in the same direction. Repeated insertion and removal of screws is to be avoided. In weak and demineralized bone, tapping may not be advisable.

Plate Bending Error (→ Gapping, Torsion, Increased Intercondylar Distance). Bending errors can be produced especially by using stronger plates. It is therefore important to supervise not only the buccal aspect of the fracture after fixation of the plate but also the lingual. A gap on the lingual side can be avoided by overbending the plate. Lingual gaps especially in the chin area may result in a cross-bite situation and increased intercondylar distance.

Torsion of the plate may produce occlusal interference, for example, tilting of the smaller fragment or an open bite. Therefore final intraoperative supervision of occlusion is compulsory.

3.6 Failures

Nonunion/Pseudarthrosis

Infection/Osteomyelitis. The above situations require surgical revision. Nonunion and pseudarthrosis must be stabilized by using a reconstruction plate. If there is bone loss, the fibrous tissues within the gap may be removed and replaced by corticocancellous bone grafts.

Infection and osteomyelitis must be treated as soon as possible. It is not advisable to manage local infection with fistulation by using antibiotics. Antibiotics play only a supporting role. The reason of infection/osteomyelitis in the majority of the cases is instability of the fracture and loose hardware. Therefore the only effective measure to manage the situation is reoperation, cleaning of the infected area and application of a reconstruction plate. It is important to use at least three screws on each side of the fracture. The screws must not be placed in the infected area.

Broadening of the Face (Increased Intercondylar Distance), Especially in Combination With Condylar and Subcondylar Fractures. Broadening of the face is esthetically and functionally unacceptable. Therefore this complication also requires reosteosynthesis by using a strong plate. Overbending is compulsory.

Malocclusion. Malocclusion may be seen postoperatively as the result of an insufficient intermaxillary fixation during surgery. While slight occlusal interferences after open reduction and internal fixation of mandibular fractures may eventually be corrected by grinding the occlusal surfaces of the teeth, serious malocclusion requires reosteosynthesis in the correct position of the fragments.

Hardware Fracture (Plate/Screw). Hardware fractures require removal and in the case of instability reosteosynthesis.

3.7 Indications for Osteosynthesis

Fractures Requiring Open Reduction and Adequate Fixation

- Severely dislocated fractures
- Open fractures
- Complicated/comminuted fractures
- Infected fractures
- Mandibular fractures in combination with condylar or subcondylar fractures
- Panfacial fractures
- Fractures in patients with edentulous jaws
- Fractures in uncooperative patients
- Fractures in medically compromised patients
- Patients in which IMF is not advocated
- On patient's request

3.8 Indications for Perioperative Antibiotic Cover

- Medically compromised patients
- Severely comminuted fractures
- Heavily contaminated fractures
- Severely lacerated soft tissues
- Difficult fractures with predictably long operation time
- Delayed fracture treatment (more than 24 h)

The intravenous administration starts prior to surgery and lasts not longer than 24 h. This antibiotic prophylaxis is not sufficient as therapy for a preoperatively infected fracture. It cannot replace insufficient mechanical stability. Mechanical stability remains the best protection against infection.

3.9 General Remarks

- The first step in reduction is restoration of occlusion. The reduction must be secured with IMF either by splints or other fixation devices.
- Selection of access depends mainly on the localization and type of fracture and the possibility of fracture reduction and supervision.
- In dentate patients supervision of occlusion is mandatory. In edentulous patients it is very advisable to use the prosthesis as a guideline for the correct intermaxillary relation.
- General anesthesia, mostly via nasal or submental intubation, is therefore necessary.
- Tension band plates are fixed whenever possible with bicortical screws. In situations in which tooth roots or the mandibular nerve can be lacerated, these screws are placed in a monocortical manner. Compression and reconstruction plates used at the inferior margin of the mandible are fixed with bicortical screws.

3.10 Localization and Types of Fracture

The localization and type of fracture define the treatment strategy and the surgical access and are described in the following sections. The various options for fixation according to the severity of the fractures are described for each localization.

3.11 Fractures of the Symphysis and the Parasymphyseal Area

Definition. Fractures of the symphysis and parasymphyseal area are those located in the anterior part of the mandible between the canine teeth. They include the area of the chin and the insertion of the anterior muscles of the floor of the mouth. Since these fractures are often not dislocated, they can cause diagnostic problems. Clinically a sublingual hematoma may be the only symptom. Furthermore, especially in connection with these fractures condylar or subcondylar fractures must be excluded.

Radiographically the fracture can be hidden by the overprojection of the vertical spine. Clinically in dentate patients this type of fracture is considered an open fracture since the fracture line runs through the alveolus.

Special Conditions Influencing Adequate Internal Fixation. The intraoral approach allows sufficient supervision of the reduction. All types of osteosynthesis can be applied via this approach. The creation of a gap on the lingual aspect of the fracture must be avoided. The danger of widening of the mandibular arch and thus broadening of the face is especially present in symphyseal fractures in combination with subcondylar fractures (see Fig. 4.1.7 a). In the chin area jaw function produces tortional as well as compressive and tensile forces. The largest tensile loads are located at the area of the alveolar crest and at the inferior border (Rudderman 1992).

Procedure. Generally the intraoral approach is used via an incision of the mucosa in the vestibulum. The extraoral approach may be used in cases with skin laceration.

Simple fractures may be carried out under local anesthesia.

3.11.1 Transverse Fracture Line Without Dislocation
(Fig. 3.1)

At least three types of fracture fixation are possible:

- A dental splint including at least three teeth on either side of the fracture in combination with a four-hole miniplate (2.0) or a four-hole LC-DC plate, placed just underneath the apices of the tooth roots (Fig. 3.2).
- Two four-hole miniplates (2.0), fixed with monocortically applied screws for the superior plate and bicortical screws for the inferior plate. The superior plate neutralizes the tensile forces (Fig. 3.3).

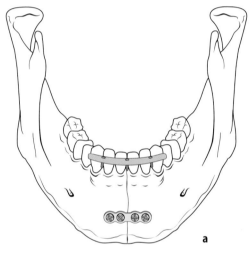

a

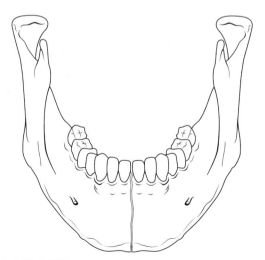

Fig. 3.1

Transverse fracture of the symphyseal area without dislocation.

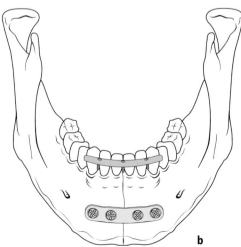

b

Fig. 3.2 a, b

a Open reduction and internal fixation with a four-hole miniplate (2.0) in combination with a dental splint.
b Open reduction and internal fixation with a four-hole 2.4 LC-DC plate in combination with a dental splint.

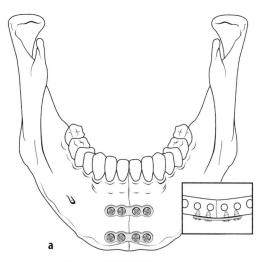

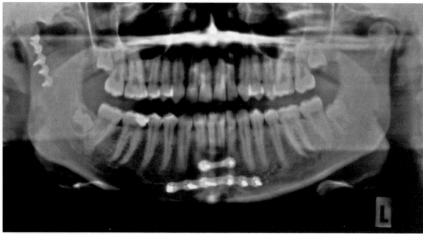

- Two or three long lag screws that cross the fracture line in a horizontal direction. These screws must generally be longer than 20 mm. For an optimal placement of the screw head the countersink must be used (Fig. 3.4). Both screws are placed in the bone below the tooth roots.
- Stronger plates such as reconstruction plates (Uni-LOCK or THORP) may be necessary when these fractures occur in combination with subcondylar fractures or with panfacial fractures.

Fig. 3.3 a, b

a Open reduction and internal fixation by using two four-hole miniplates (2.0). The superior plate must be fixed with monocortically placed screws (as indicated in *inset*).

b A 19-year-old woman. Postoperative radiograph showing two miniplates (2.0) in a symphyseal fracture. In this situation the surgeon chose to apply a short two-hole plate superiorly and therefore a longer six-hole miniplate inferiorly. The right subcondylar fracture was stabilized with a five-hole miniplate (2.0), whereas the condylar fracture on the left could not be internally fixed. Therefore IMF for 10 days with elastics was used.

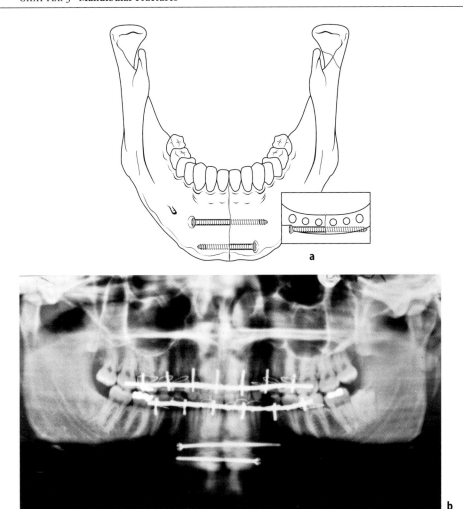

Fig. 3.4 a, b

a Open reduction and internal fixation by using at least two horizontal 2.4 lag screws. The superior screw must be placed within the external cortex in in order not to damage the tooth roots (see *inset*).

b Postoperative radiograph showing two horizontal lag screws. The splint was installed for intraoperative fixation of the occlusion and postoperative functional treatment of the subcondylar fracture on the left side.

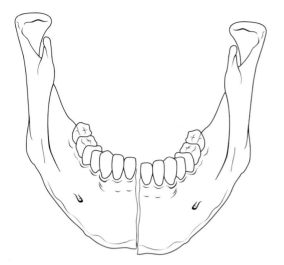

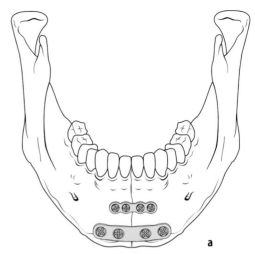

a

Fig. 3.5

Transverse fracture of the symphyseal area with dislocation.

3.11.2 Transverse Fracture Line With Dislocation
(Fig. 3.5)

This type of fracture requires wider surgical access to supervise reduction. Fixation of the reduced fracture with either a dental splint or a 2.0 plate in the area of the alveolar crest (tensile area), together with temporary IMF. Fixation of the fracture at the inferior border with either a 2.4 LC-DC plate (Fig. 3.6) or a Universal Fracture plate is necessary. When the LC-DC plate is preferred, the compression device is used via the excentric drill guide (see Fig. 1.17 b, c). Slight overbending is necessary. In physically strong and/or uncooperative patients the 2.4 DC plate may be too weak to close the lingual gap. In such cases the slightly stronger 2.4 Universal Fracture plate is advisable (Fig. 3.7). A reconstruction plate with at least six holes may be more appropriate in the presence of a concomitant uni- or bilateral subcondylar fracture.

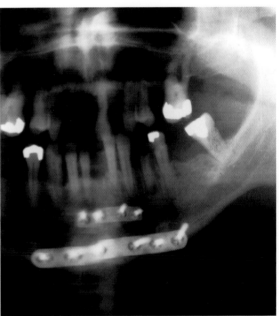

b

Fig. 3.6 a, b

a Open reduction and internal fixation with a four-hole mini-plate (2.0) and a four-hole 2.4 LC-DC plate. The superior plate is fixed with monocortically placed screws.
b Postoperative radiograph showing a four-hole miniplate (2.0) and a six-hole LC-DC plate.

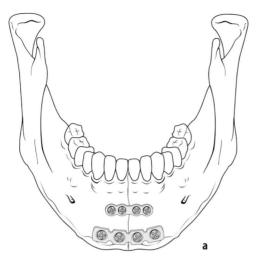

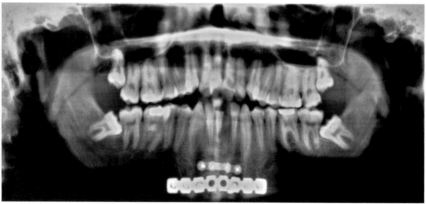

Fig. 3.7 a, b

a Open reduction and internal fixation by using a four-hole miniplate (2.0) and a four-hole 2.4 Universal Fracture plate.

b Fracture of the symphyseal area stabilized with a miniplate (2.0) and an eight-hole 2.4 Universal Fracture plate. The two inner holes have been left empty because of some bone comminution in this area. The stronger plate was especially necessary because of this comminution and the loss of the left lower incisor.

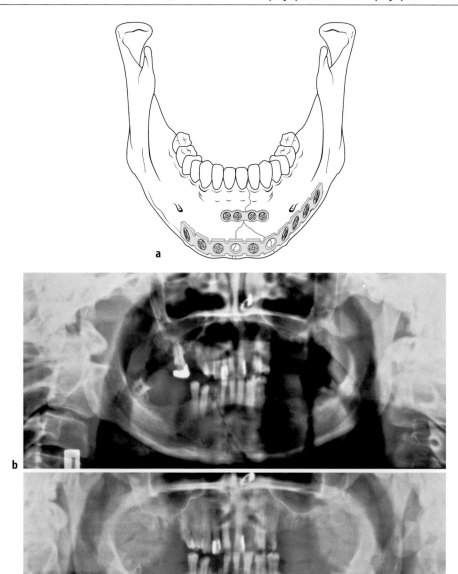

3.11.3 Fracture Line With Basal Triangle

In this situation a 2.4 Universal Fracture plate at the base is used. The main fracture ends should at least be fixed with three screws. The triangular piece of the base can further be fixed with 2.4 screws to the plate or with 2.0 or 2.4 screws acting as lag screws in a vertical direction. In the tensile area a miniplate (2.0) is used (Fig. 3.8).

Fig. 3.8 a–c

a Fracture of the symphyseal area with basal triangle. Open reduction and internal fixation by using a four-hole miniplate (2.0) and a ten-hole 2.4 Universal Fracture plate.

b Radiographic appearance of a symphyseal fracture with basal triangle in a partially edentulous mandible.

c Fixation with a six-hole miniplate (2.0) for adaptation and a 2.4 Universal Fracture plate at the base for stabilization. The screw holes in the area of comminution are left empty. Note: three screws on each side.

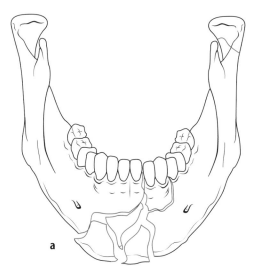

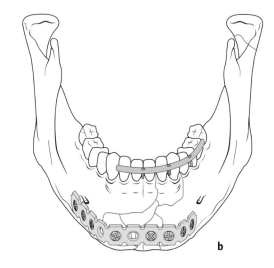

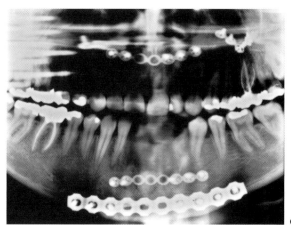

Fig. 3.9 a–c

a Comminuted fracture of the symphyseal area.
b Open reduction and internal fixation with a dental splint and a ten-hole 2.4 reconstruction plate.
c Comminuted symphyseal fracture after open reduction and internal fixation with an eight-hole adaptation plate in combination with a ten-hole 2.4 reconstruction plate. Plate holes above the comminuted fracture area are left empty. Load-bearing osteosynthesis!

3.11.4 Comminuted Fracture (Fig. 3.9 a)

The fragments are reduced by using a dental splint and IMF. Bridging of the fracture area is with a 2.4 reconstruction plate. Distortion of the main fracture ends must be avoided by using the plate holes in a neutral manner. This is of great importance, especially in patients with teeth. Care must be taken not to use screws too close to a fracture line. The thicker bony pieces may be fixed with screws to the plate (Fig. 3.9 b, c). Stripping of the lingual periosteum is not advised in order to avoid disturbance of the blood supply of the small bone pieces.

Special attention must be given to the condylar area since most of these comminuted chin fractures are observed in combination with condylar or subcondylar fractures. Especially when bilateral or in combination with panfacial fractures, these fractures should be internally stabilized, if anatomically possible.

3.12 Fractures of the Horizontal Ramus

Definition. Fractures of the horizontal ramus are those located between the canines and the last molar. Particular attention must be given to the mental nerve. Both AP projection and orthopantomogram are mandatory since the type of fracture directs the surgical approach. In dentate patients this type of fracture is always an open fracture since the fracture line runs through the alveolus.

Special Conditions Influencing Adequate Internal Fixation. The intraoral approach allows sufficient supervision in the anterior part of the horizontal ramus. In the posterior part a gap of both the inferior and the lingual aspects of the fracture cannot always be supervised via the intraoral approach. An extraoral approach may then be more appropriate. This is also a question of the experience of the surgeon and is therefore his decision.

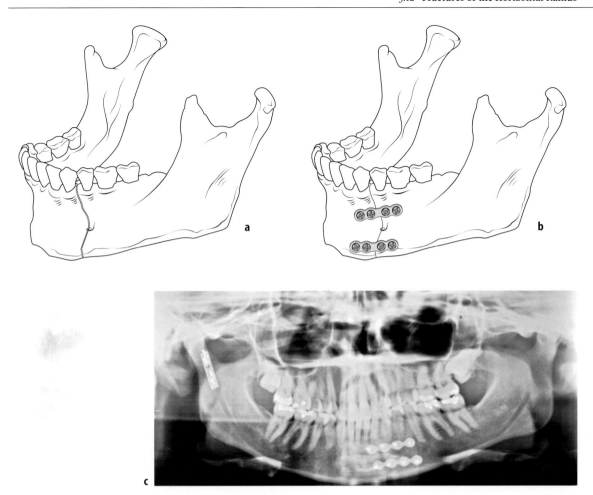

Fig. 3.10 a–c

a Fracture of the horizontal ramus without dislocation.
b Stabilization with two four-hole miniplates (2.0).
c Repair of a horizontal ramus fracture with two four-hole miniplates (2.0). The subcondylar fracture on the opposite side has been stabilized with a four-hole mini DC plate (2.0).

Procedure. An intraoral approach is generally chosen. In the molar area additional stab incisions may be necessary for the transbuccal placement of the screws. In heavily comminuted fractures an extraoral approach is seldom avoidable. Of course, cases with overlying skin lacerations are approached through the wound ("occasional approach").

Special attention must be given to the mental nerve when using the intraoral approach and to the marginal branch of the facial nerve when using the extraoral approach. For this reason a transbuccal approach is often chosen (see Fig. 1.34).

Generally all these fractures are operated on under general anesthesia.

3.12.1 Transverse Fracture Line Without Dislocation
(Fig. 3.10 a)

Two four-hole miniplates (2.0), monocortically applied screws for the tension-band plate, and bicortical screws for the plate at the inferior mandibular border are used (Fig. 3.10 b, c). In strong male patients and in uncooperative patients it may be necessary to use a 2.4 plate with bicortical screws at the inferior border. As tension band a dental splint may also be used (see Fig. 3.2).

3.12.2 Transverse Fracture Line With Dislocation
(Fig. 3.11 a)

This type of fracture requires wider surgical access to supervise reduction. Reduction is secured with a 2.0 miniplate in the alveolar crest (tensile area) or a tension band-splint. Fixation of the fracture in the inferior border with a 2.4 LC-DC plate (Fig. 3.11 b, c). Overbending in this area is less important than in the anterior part of

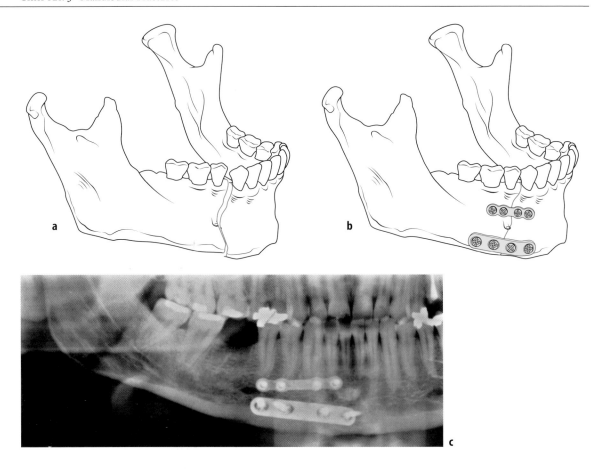

the mandible. In stronger male patients the 2.4 LC-DC plate may be too weak to withstand the functional forces and to close the lingual gap. In such cases a stronger 2.4 Universal Fracture plate is advisable (Fig. 3.12).

Fig. 3.11 a–c

a Fracture of horizontal ramus with dislocation.
b Repair of a fracture of the horizontal ramus with a four-hole miniplate (2.0) as tension band and a four-hole 2.4 LC-DC plate.
c Repair of a lateral fracture with a four-hole miniplate (2.0) as tension band and a four-hole LC-DC plate.

Fig. 3.12 a–e

a Preoperatively the same situation as in Fig. 3.11 a on the right ▶ side, but in combination with an angular fracture on the left side. Fixation with a miniplate (2.0) as tension band in combination with a 2.4 Universal Fracture plate.
b, c Radiographic appearance pre- and postoperatively. Two dislocated fractures in a young dentate man. Fixation with a miniplate (2.0) with monocortically placed screws and a 2.4 Universal Fracture plate with bicortically placed screws. Angular fracture see in Fig. 3.19 b.
d, e (see page 70)

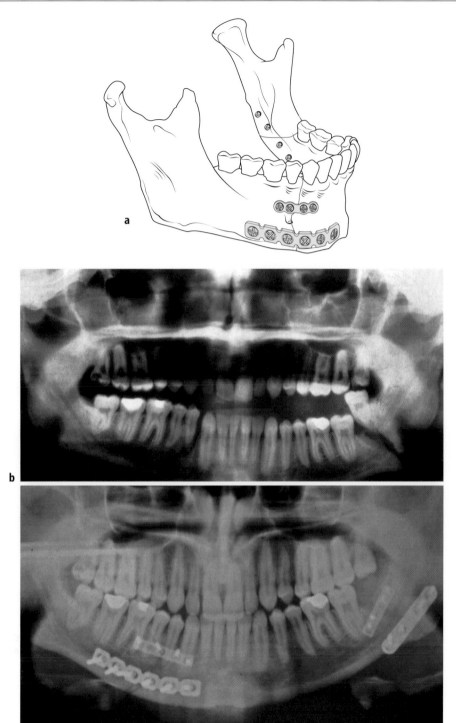

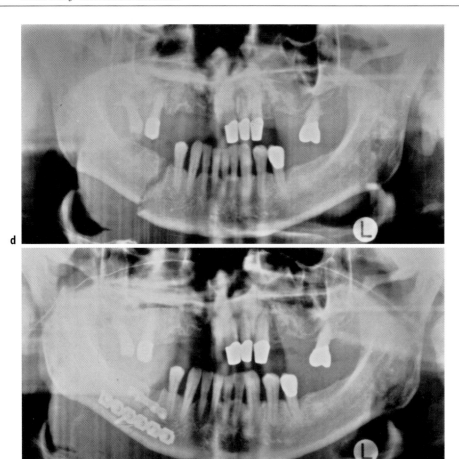

d

e

Fig. 3.12 d, e

d,e Pre- and postoperative X-rays of horizontal ramus fracture in edentulous area in a strong man. Fixation with a miniplate (2.0) in combination with a 2.4 Universal Fracture plate. Most of the screws are bicortically placed.

Fig. 3.13 a–e

a Oblique fracture of the horizontal ramus. Repair with three ▶ lag screws.

b,c Pre- and postoperative X-ray of a severely dislocated oblique fracture of the horizontal ramus. After open reduction adequate fixation with three 2.4 lag screws was achieved.

d Clinical example of an oblique fracture of the horizontal ramus in the premolar area. Typically, the fracture is hardly visible on the OPT.

e Ideal stabilization in this case with four 2.7 lag screws.

3.12.3 Oblique Fracture Line With/Without Dislocation

Fractures with an oblique fracture line have a wide surface and can therefore be fixed either only with lag screws or a lag screw in combination with plates. If stabilization with screws only is performed, three screws should be placed (Fig. 3.13). The area underneath the screwhead should be flattened, and therefore the countersink is used. If only two lag screws can be placed, a combination of these lag screws with a 2.4 LC-DC plate or a Universal Fracture plate is necessary, together with a splint for tension-banding (Fig. 3.14).

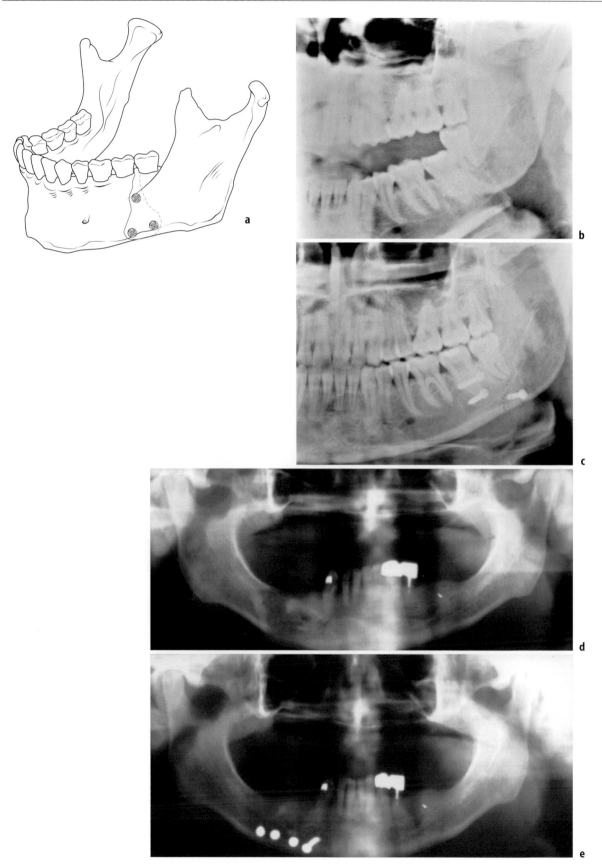

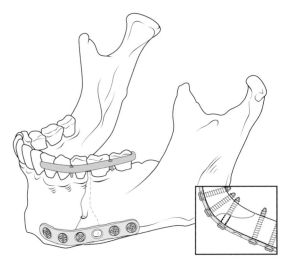

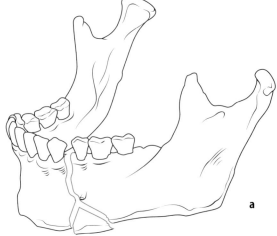

a

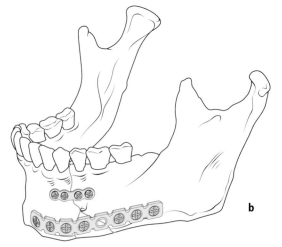

b

Fig. 3.14

Repair of an oblique fracture with one lag screw in combination with a 2.4 LC-DC plate at the lower border and a dental splint as tension band. Note: placement of lag screw in *inset*. The lag screw must be placed first and thereafter the remaining screws are placed in a neutral position.

Fig. 3.15 a–d

a Fracture of the horizontal ramus with basal triangle.
b Open reduction and adequate fixation with a four-hole miniplate (2.0) as tension band and an eight-hole Universal Fracture plate.
c Stabilization of a dislocated fracture with basal triangle with a miniplate (2.0) as tension band in combination with a 7 hole 2.4 Universal Fracture plate. Empty hole above the fracture line in between triangle and corpus.

3.12.4 Fracture Line With Basal Triangle (Fig. 3.15 a)

Osteosynthesis is performed with a 2.4 LC-DC plate or a 2.4 Universal Fracture plate at the base of the mandible. In appropriate situations the triangle can be fixed either to the plate with a 2.0 or 2.4 lag screw or to adjacent bone with a separate lag screw. In the tensile area a 2.0 miniplate with monocortically placed screws or a tension band splint is used (Fig. 3.15 b, c).

3.12.5 Comminuted Fractures (Fig. 3.16 a)

The fragments are reduced and approximated by using 1.5 or 2.0 miniplates or lag screws. The fracture area then is bridged with a 2.4 or 2.7 reconstruction plate. Of course, the screws must be placed in a neutral position since compression in the presence of a comminuted fracture is inappropriate and may lead to distortion and consequently to malocclusion (Fig. 3.16 b, c).

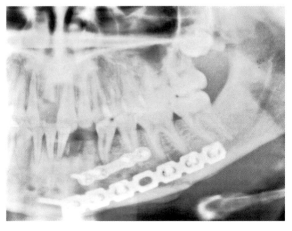

c

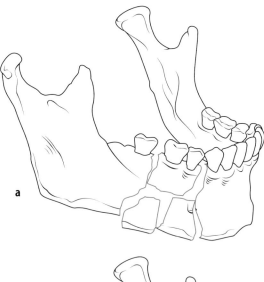

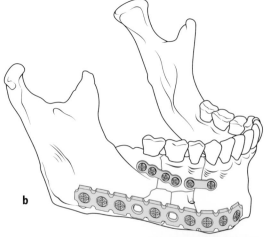

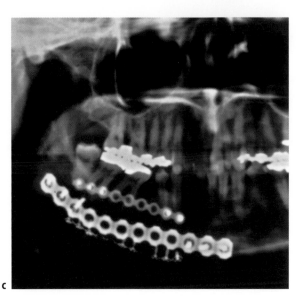

Fig. 3.16 a–c

a Comminuted fracture of the horizontal ramus.

b Open reduction and rigid fixation with two miniplates (2.0) for fracture adaptation and a 2.4 reconstruction plate. Note: three screws on each side of the nonfractured area are mandatory.

c Stabilization of a comminuted fracture of the horizontal ramus with two long mini adaptation plates for primary fixation of the various fragments. Bridging of the comminuted area with a 12-hole reconstruction plate. Note: three screws on either side.

3.13 Fractures of the Mandibular Angle

Definition. Fractures of the mandibular angle are those located posterior to the second molar and comprising the triangle between horizontal and ascending ramus. Frequently the fracture line runs through the area of an impacted third molar. Since the orthopantomogram alone often does not show the degree of dislocation, additional AP projections are mandatory.

The type of the fracture, the degree of dislocation, and the experience of the surgeon determine the surgical approach. If a third molar is partly impacted or in contact with the second molar, the fracture must be regarded as an open fracture.

Special Conditions Influencing Adequate Internal Fixation. Control of the inferior fracture aspect is limited when using the intraoral approach. The need for intraoperative intermaxillary fixation may be an additional obstacle in reduction of the fragments.

Procedure. The intraoral approach can be used in cases with no or only slight dislocation. While some of the screws for the plate fixation in the tension-band area can be placed via this approach, it is often necessary to use an additional stab incision for correct transbuccal placement of the screws at the base of the mandible.

Fractures with a high degree of dislocation or comminuted fractures need an extraoral approach for correct reduction and supervision of the placement of the plate. The correct application of longer and stronger plates is extremely difficult via an intraoral approach.

When using the extraoral approach, special attention must be given to the mandibular branch of the facial nerve (see Fig. 2.1).

In some instances local anesthesia may be sufficient for the treatment of a simple and nondislocated fracture when using a one-plate fixation in the area of the linea obliqua. All other cases, however, are usually carried out under general anesthesia.

It is not compulsary to remove a third molar which is located in the fracture line (especially not with an osteotomy) since this procedure might hinder the correct reduction and lessen stability of the fixation. This may

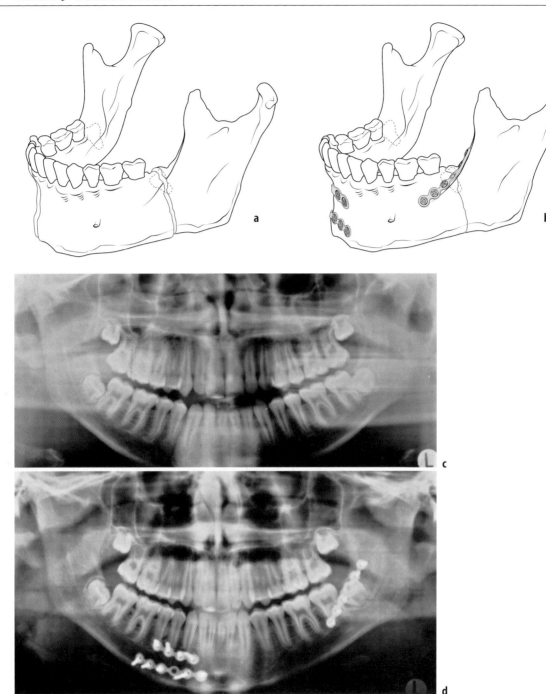

mean weakening of the tension zone. In cases in which removal of the wisdom tooth is advisable it should be performed after fixation of the fracture with plates.

a Transverse angle fracture without dislocation with fully retained wisdom tooth.
b Fracture repair with a single six-hole miniplate (2.0).
c,d Pre- and postoperative X-ray of fracture situation in a young woman, as shown in **a,b**. The fully retained wisdom tooth was not removed.

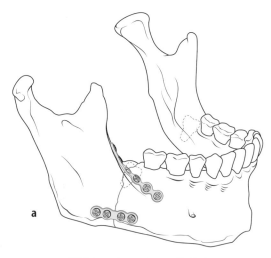

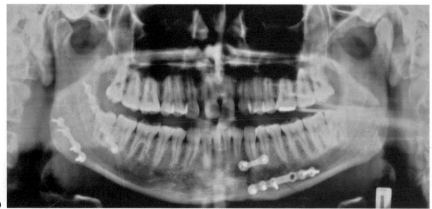

Fig. 3.18 a, b

3.13.1 Transverse Fracture Line Without Dislocation
(Fig. 3.17 a)

One-plate fixation is possible using a 2.0 miniplate (four or six holes; two or three screws on each side) with monocortically applied screws, when necessary (area of tooth roots) at the area of the linea obliqua, but this kind of fixation cannot neutralize all the forces that may occur during function (Fig. 3.17 b–d).

Especially in men this fracture is better managed using two 2.0 miniplates, one in the area of the linea obliqua and the second at the inferior border (Fig. 3.18). Again, the plate should be fixed with bicortically placed screws whenever possible. In stronger men it might be necessary to use a 2.4 LC-DC plate with bicortical screw fixation at the inferior border in combination with the 2.0 miniplate in the tension-band area (Fig. 3.19).

Fixation of the fracture is also possible using a single lag screw in anteroposterior oblique direction (Fig. 3.20) if the bone is strong and not osteoporotic. This technique, however, requires considerable experience on the part of the surgeon since there is danger of damaging the inferior alveolar nerve during drilling and tapping.

a Transverse angle fracture. Repair with a six-hole miniplate (2.0) at the superior border and a four-hole miniplate (2.0) at the inferior border.

b Postoperative X-ray. Fixation of the nondislocated angular fracture with two miniplates (2.0). A six-hole plate for the tension band at the superior border and a four-hole plate at the inferior border. Note: the wisdom tooth was not removed.

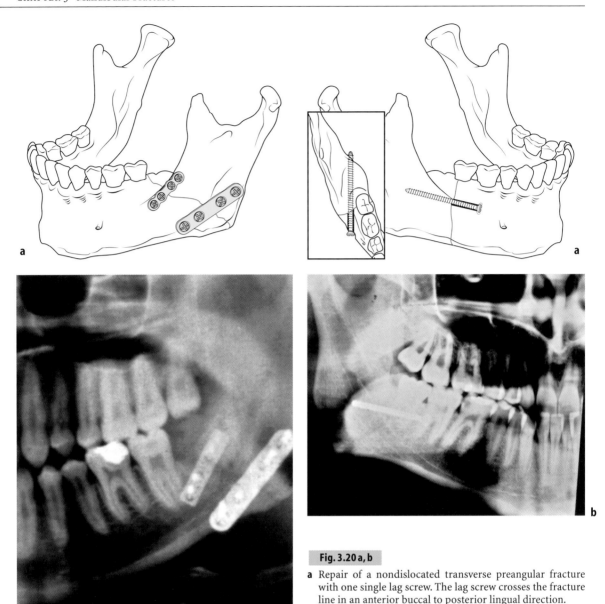

Fig. 3.20 a, b

Fig. 3.20 a, b

a Repair of a nondislocated transverse preangular fracture with one single lag screw. The lag screw crosses the fracture line in an anterior buccal to posterior lingual direction.
b Clinical situation as shown in **a**.

Fig. 3.19 a, b

a Transverse angle fracture. Repair with a four-hole miniplate (2.0) as tension band and a four-hole 2.4 LC-DC plate at the inferior border.
b Postoperative X-ray showing the fixation of a transverse angle fracture, as indicated in **a**. Strong male patient!

3.13.2 Transverse Fracture Line With Dislocation
(Fig. 3.21 a)

This type of fracture shows damage of the periosteal and the pterygoid/masseter "bandage." Interposition of muscle fibers makes the reduction more difficult. In these cases a one-plate fixation using a 2.0 miniplate might not be sufficient. An additional 2.0 (see Fig. 3.18a,b) or 2.4 LC-DC plate (see Fig. 3.19a,b) is placed at the inferior border of the mandibular angle. Stronger patients require a 2.4 Universal Fracture plate (Fig. 3.21 b–d).

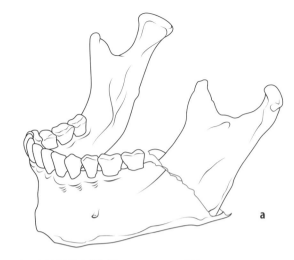

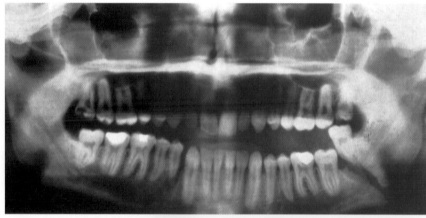

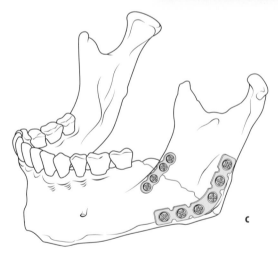

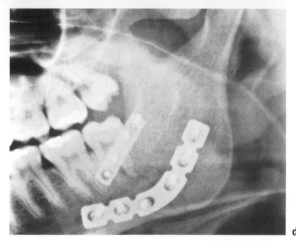

Fig. 3.21 a–d

a Angle fracture with dislocation. The muscle sling of masseter and pterygoideus pulls the proximal fragment cranially.

b Dislocated angular fracture on the left side. Anterior-superior dislocation of the proximal fragment because of the traction of the muscle sling is well visible.

c Open reduction and adequate fixation of dislocated angle fracture with a four-hole miniplate (2.0) as tension band and a six-hole 2.4 Universal Fracture plate.

d Postoperative X-ray. Repair of a dislocated angle fracture by means of a four-hole miniplate (2.0) as tension band and a six-hole 2.4 Universal Fracture plate. Note: the wisdom tooth has been left in place.

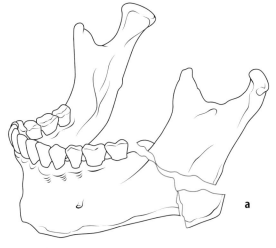
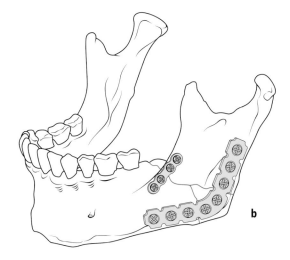

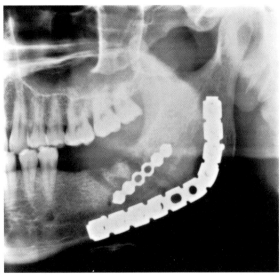

Fig. 3.22 a–c

a   Angle fracture with basal triangle.
b   Open reduction and adequate fixation with a four-hole mini-
    plate (2.0) at the superior border and an eight-hole angu-
    lated 2.4 Universal Fracture plate.
c   Postoperative X-ray of an angle fracture with basal triangle.
    Repair with a six-hole miniplate (2.0) and in this case a ten-
    hole 2.7 reconstruction plate.

3.13.3 Angular Fractures With Basal Triangle
(Fig. 3.22 a)

An angulated 2.4 Universal Fracture plate or a 2.4 Reconstruction Plate with six to eight holes is used at the base
of the mandible. The triangle can either be fixed to the
plate or with lag screws (2.0 or 2.4) to the main fragments. In the tensile area a 2.0 miniplate is generally
used (Fig. 3.22 b, c). As always, care must be taken not to
place the screws too close to the fracture line. If in doubt,
it is always safer to use a longer plate and leave the hole
close to the fracture line empty.

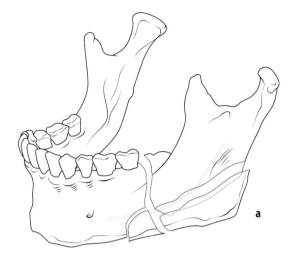

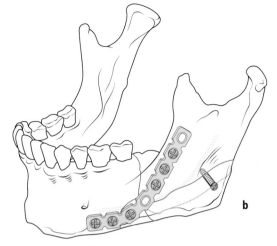

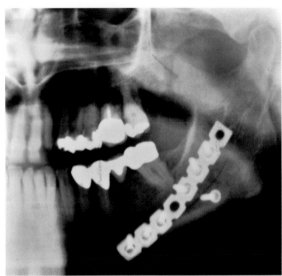

3.13.4 Comminuted Angular Fractures (Fig. 3.23 a)

Comminuted fractures of the angular area are often observed in combination with other mandibular fractures and maxillary fractures. After temporary intermaxillary fixation all mandibular fractures must be exposed before the reduction and fixation of the fragments is done. This can be performed either with lag screws (Fig. 3.23 b) or with 1.5 or 2.0 miniplates (see Fig. 3.25). Simpler fractures should be fixed first. In comminuted areas, such as in Fig. 3.24 (right angle) and Fig. 3.25, at first adaptation is performed with miniplates, and thereafter the fractured area is completely bridged with the stronger 2.4 reconstruction plate. Secondary distortions of the fracture area are prohibited by using the plate holes in a noncompressive manner (Figs. 3.23–3.25). The fixation of coexisting subcondylar fractures in these instances is very important.

Fig. 3.23 a–c

a Comminuted fracture in the left mandibular angle. The fracture is both transverse and longitudinal.

b,c Internal fixation of a comminuted fracture, in the left mandibular angle with a lag screw for the longitudinal fracture and an eight-hole reconstruction plate (2.7), bridging the comminuted area. Since it was a wide open fracture and the mandibular nerve well visible, fixation could easily be performed with the anterior screws placed below the nerve and the posterior screws placed above the nerve.

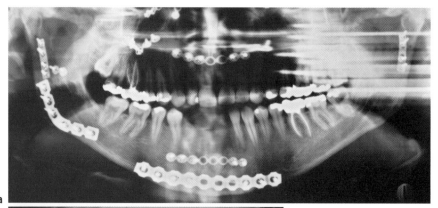

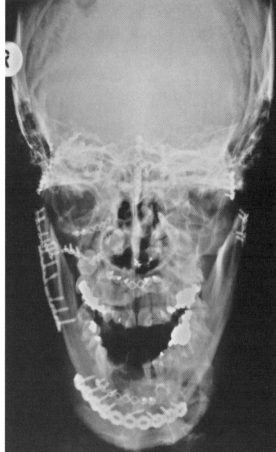

Fig. 3.24 a, b

Postoperative X-ray after stabilization of a panfacial fracture. The comminuted fracture of the right mandibular angle was stabilized with miniplates (2.0) together with a prebent angulated Universal Fracture plate. Note: stabilization of both subcondylar fractures with DC miniplates. Combination of miniplate fixation together with reconstruction plate for the chin fracture.

3.13.5 Comminuted Fractures of the Ascending Mandibular Ramus

This type of fracture may require a combined submandibular and preauricular approach. The fracture is simplified by using 2.0 miniplates and subsequent bridging and the whole fracture stabilized by a 2.4 Universal Fracture plate or 2.4 reconstruction plate (Fig. 3.25).

Fig. 3.25 a–g

a Comminuted fracture of the ascending mandibular ramus.
b Open reduction and adaptation of the fragments with different miniplates (2.0).
c Subsequent bridging of the comminuted area with a 2.4 Universal Fracture plate.
d–g (see page 82).

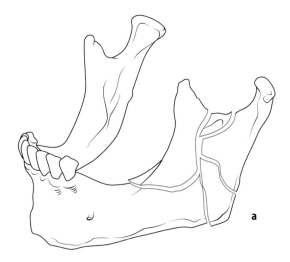

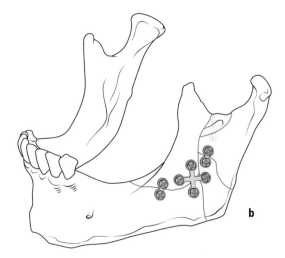

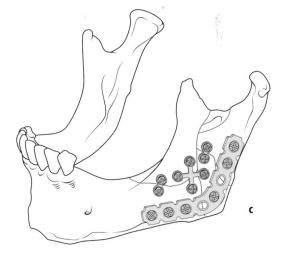

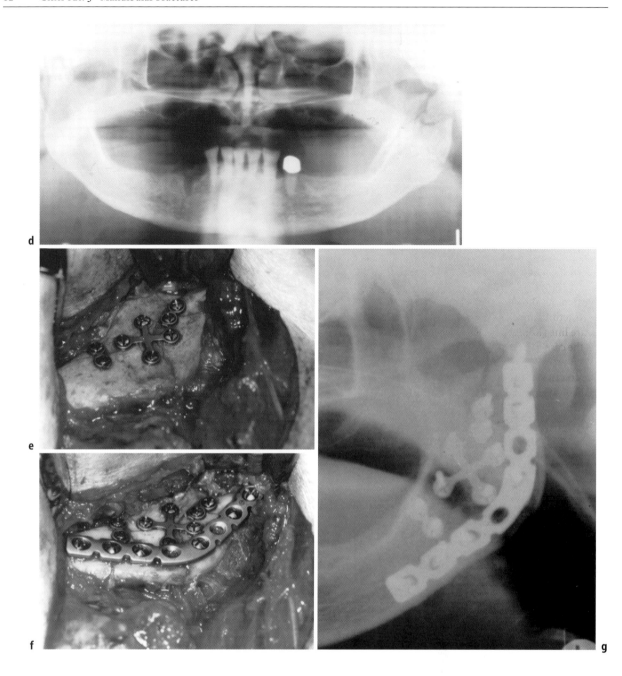

Fig. 3.25 d–g

d Preoperative X-ray showing the comminuted fracture of the ascending mandibular ramus, as shown in **a**.

e Open reduction and simplification of the fracture with several mini adaptation plates (2.0).

f Bridging of the comminuted area with a 2.4 Universal Fracture plate.

g Postoperative X-ray exhibiting the different fragments in their regular position.

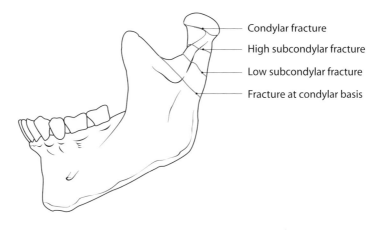

Condylar fracture
High subcondylar fracture
Low subcondylar fracture
Fracture at condylar basis

Fig. 3.26

Fracture classification according to Köhler.

3.14 Condylar and Subcondylar Fractures

Definition. As shown in Fig. 3.26, condylar and subcondylar fractures are classified according to the level of the fracture line (Köhler 1951).

In the case of condylar fractures the fracture line runs inside the capsule of the temporomandibular joint. These fractures cannot be fixed with plates or screws.

Subcondylar fractures are situated below the capsule. They are classified into high and low condylar fractures as well as fractures of the basis of the condylar process.

Fractures on the basis of the condylar process are at the level of the bottom of the sigmoid knotch (incisura semilunaris).

Various patterns of dislocation and luxation of the proximal fragment are possible.

For treatment planning both AP projections and an orthopantomogram are mandatory. Generally these fractures are closed fractures.

Special Conditions Influencing Internal Fixation. As a rule condylar fractures are treated conservatively, one of the reasons being the danger of necrosis of the proximal fragment (condylar head). This is due to interruption of the vascular supply by denudation during an open-reduction procedure.

The decision about the kind of treatment for subcondylar or fractures at the base of the condylar neck depends on several factors. These are:

- Status of dentition
- Degree of dislocation
- Condition of the patient
- Concomitant fractures of the mandible, such as corpus fractures and bilateral subcondylar fractures
- Bimaxillary fractures or panfacial fractures. (For more precise information about indications for internal fixation of subcondylar fractures, see "References and Suggested Reading").

In general, especially nondislocated fractures are treated conservatively, as this shows excellent long-term results.

In the case of a high-grade dislocation or luxation of the small fragment, conservative treatment with at least 2 weeks of intermaxillary fixation or direct or indirect extension is possible. However, a reduction of fragments is almost never achieved. Therefore in some special instances open reduction and internal fixation are desirable.

Either an intra- or an extraoral approach to the subcondylar area is possible. Using an intraoral approach, however, makes the reduction of the fragments and especially the application of plates and screws extremely difficult. In addition, it does not allow sufficient supervision of the reduction. The extraoral approach is performed via a submandibular (Risdon) or preauricular incision; sometimes the combination of both approaches is necessary (see Fig. 2.1). When using the preauricular access alone, the necessary extension of the fracture exposure for a better reduction and fixation may not be possible. Care must be taken not to lacerate the frontal branch of the facial nerve when using the preauricular approach, and the marginal branch of the facial nerve when using the submandibular approach. All procedures are performed under general anesthesia.

3.14.1 Transverse Fracture Line With Dislocation

After exposing the fracture from either approach, pulling the mandibular angle in a caudal direction may facilitate reduction of the dislocated or luxated small fragments. If necessary, reduction is secured using one or two reduction forceps. Fixation of the fracture at the posterior border of the ascending mandibular ramus and the condylar process with a four-hole mini-DC plate and bicortical screws. In general, one plate is sufficient.

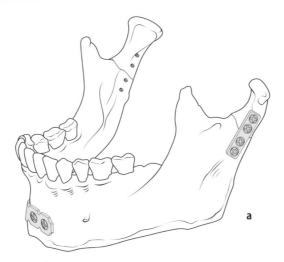

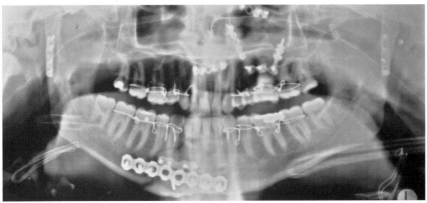

Care must be taken not to use a plate that is too thin, as this may lead to plate fracture (Hammer 1997). Regular miniplates that are ordinarily used for midface fractures are too thin. It is also important that there is room for two bicortical screws on each side of the fracture (Fig. 3.27).

In fully dentured patients with fractures of the base of the condylar process, which may also be considered as the ascending ramus, Universal Fracture plates for stabilization may be advisable (Fig. 3.28).

Fig. 3.27 a, b

a Internal Fixation of bilateral low subcondylar fractures with DC miniplates (2.0).
b Postoperative X-ray after adequate fixation of bilateral low subcondylar fractures with DC miniplates (2.0) in a panfacial fracture situation.

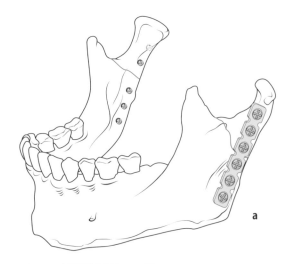

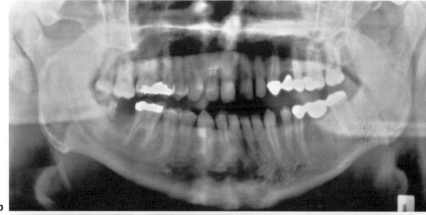

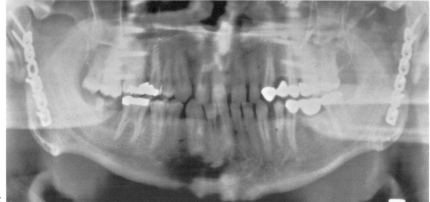

Fig. 3.28 a–c

a Adequate fixation of bilateral fractures of the base of the condylar process (ascending ramus) in a fully dentured strong man with six-hole 2.4 Universal Fracture plates.

b, c Pre- and postoperative X-rays of bilateral fractures of the base of the condylar process. Fixation with 2.4 Universal

Fracture plates. Note the malocclusion visible on the preoperative X-ray. These strong plates for that situation were indicated because fracture repair had to be performed 3 weeks after the accident. Under these circumstances the considerable scar contracture must be taken into account.

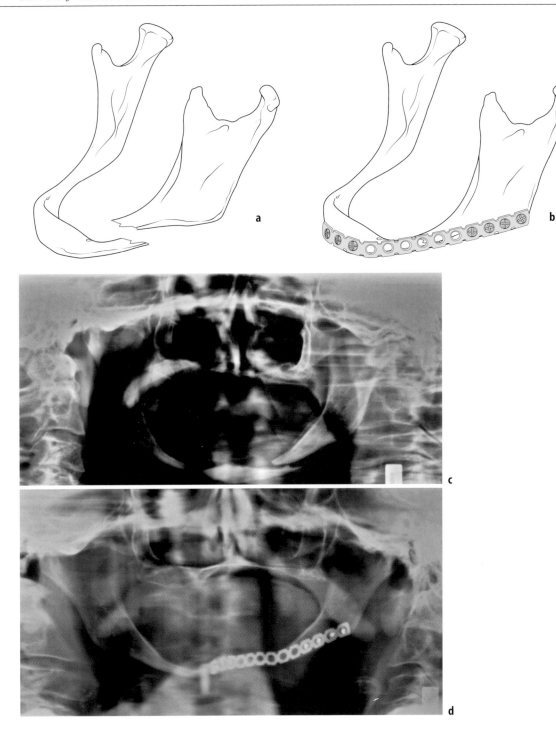

Fig. 3.29 a–d

a Dislocated fracture of the horizontal ramus of an extremely atrophic mandible.

b Adequate fixation of the fracture with a 2.4 Universal Fracture plate. Note: screw placement in vicinity of the fracture is not possible. Therefore the screw must be placed in angle and chin area.

c,d Pre- and postoperative X-ray of a dislocated fracture of the horizontal ramus in an extremely atrophic mandible. Fixation with a long 2.4 Universal Fracture plate. Note: the height of the mandible in the very atrophic area is lower than the width of the plate.

3.15 Fractures of the Atrophic Mandible (Fig. 3.29a)

Definition. An atrophic mandible shows resorption of the alveolar process. Atrophic edentulous mandibles can be extremely thin. The muscular forces acting upon the bone are incomparable to forces acting upon dentate mandibles. In fractures of the atrophic and edentulous mandible functional load must be transmitted by using a stable fixation device. In contrast to dentate mandibles, tension – neutral – and compression zones are situated closely together due to the reduced height of the bone. Therefore only one plate can be applied, which should counteract the masticatory forces and take over the functional load.

In addition to its reduced dimension the quality of the edentulous and atrophic mandibular bone must also be taken into consideration. Osseous density is frequently diminished due to osteoporosis. The bone is weak and fragile; screws can fail due to stripping of the bone threads. In very weak bone it is advisable to use the screws without pretapping.

Since atrophy occurs mainly in the area of the alveolar process and here especially in the lateral horizontal branch, fracture management differs from that described earlier in this chapter. In some instances screws can be placed only in the angular and chin areas. Therefore long plates must often be used.

Procedure. If available, the prosthesis should also be used in edentulous patients for correct establishment of the intermaxillary relation. The prosthesis can be fixed temporarily with wires or screws to the jaw.

Since the plates must carry a full functional load, it is recommended to use 2.4 Universal Fracture plates or Reconstruction plates. Anterior fractures without comminution can be approached by an intraoral access, whereas posterior fractures of the horizontal ramus and comminuted fractures are subject to an extraoral approach. The plate must be long enough so that the screws do not need to be placed to very low or thin areas of the mandible (Fig. 3.29). The rule is: The weaker the bone, the stronger the plate must be.

Even if these elderly patients do not wear dentures, one should not underestimate the functional load. Fatigue fractures of miniplates are often observed and are therefore not considered for fracture stabilization in these instances.

3.16 Infected Fractures (Fig. 3.30a)

Definition. Open fractures can generally be regarded as contaminated. Since fractures in the dentate area have communication with the oral cavity, they are also regarded as open fractures.

Infections with clinical relevance show swelling, pain, hyperthermia, reddening and secretion of pus. In the case of acute infection radiographic signs can be missing. Chronic cases exhibit the typical signs of osteomyelitis.

Special Conditions Influencing Adequate Internal Fixation. Instability produces and maintains the infectuous process. In the case of inappropriate osteosynthesis and screw loosening the hardware acts as a foreign body and must be removed. An osteosynthesis can be inappropriate because of the wrong plate selection (too short, too weak) or loosening of screws.

Osteosynthesis of an acutely infected fracture or pseudarthrosis must be a safe procedure. Under these conditions absolute immobility is mandatory. Therefore the 2.4 reconstruction system is recommended (Fig. 3.30). It is important not to place any screws into infected bone. This area must be spared from insertion of screws. The reconstruction plate acts as a bridging device. Large areas of infected or necrotic bone require curettage and immediate cancellous bone grafting.

Antibiotic therapy alone does not eliminate the infection as long as the fracture is unstable.

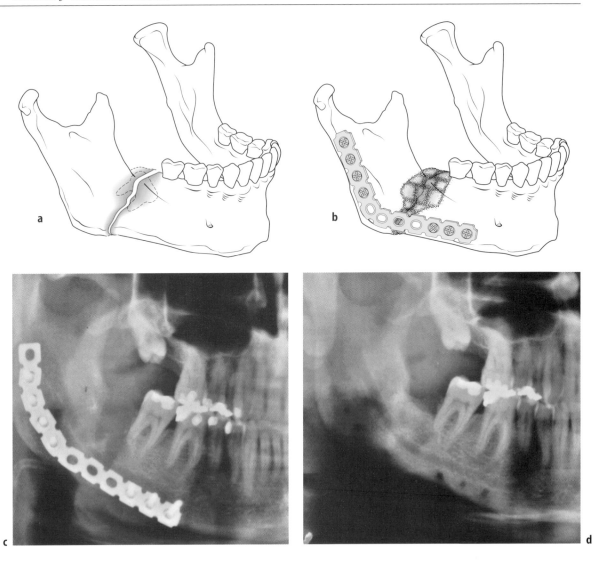

Fig. 3.30 a–d

a Acutely infected fracture of the mandibular angle, 6 weeks after removal of an infected wisdom tooth.

b Bridging of the infected area with a 2.4 reconstruction plate. Note: screws must not be placed into infected bone. At least three screws must be used outside the fractured area.

c Adequate fixation of acutely infected fracture of the mandibular angle, as shown in **b**. Simultaneously a bone graft was placed into the empty infected socket.

d On special request of the patient, the plate was removed 4 - months after fixation. Note: complete reossification.

3.17 Defect Fractures (Fig. 3.31 a)

Definition

Defect fractures exhibit loss of bone in the fractured area. A "jigsaw puzzle" reduction and simplification by 2.0 plates is not possible. The only orientation for the correct distance of the remaining bone stumps is given by IMF in the case of a nonfractured and dentate maxilla.

Even with soft-tissue defects and when a plate cannot be covered with soft tissue primarily, the bone fragments must be stabilized by bridging osteosynthesis with a reconstruction (UniLOCK or THORP) plate (Fig. 3.31 b–d and Fig. 3.32). It is advisable to perform the fixation with at least three, or if possible four, screws on each side. Primary bone grafting is performed only when the defect area can be closed well with soft tissues.

Fig. 3.31 a–d

a Defect fracture of the mandible in the area of chin and left horizontal ramus. The chin segment with the incisor teeth is extremely dislocated. The premolars are lost.

b X-ray of above situation.

c Postoperative X-ray showing bridging osteosynthesis for the defect area with a 21-hole reconstruction plate. The segment of the alveolar ridge in the chin area was stabilized with one lag screw. Because of unfavorable soft-tissue conditions primary bone grafting was not performed.

d X-ray after bone grafting of left mandibular corpus, as well as several tooth extractions, bridge work, and plate removal. Nowadays, if not especially requested, these plates are not removed.

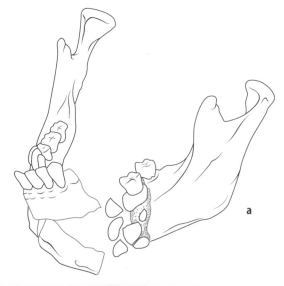

a

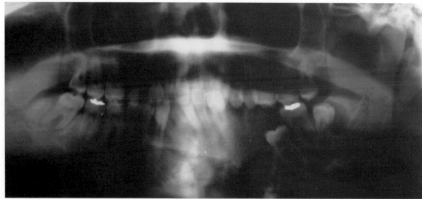

b

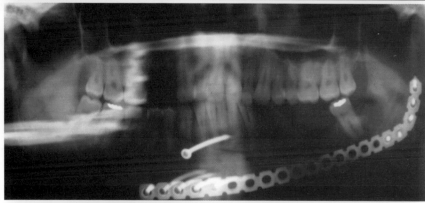

c

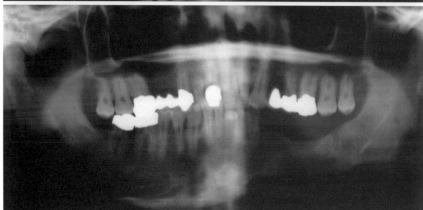

d

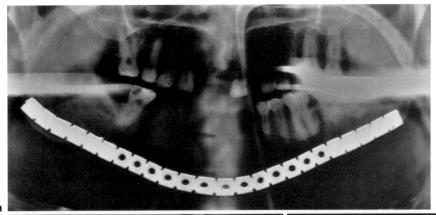

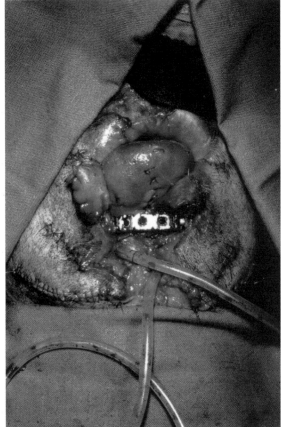

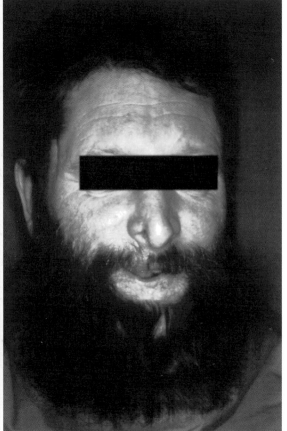

Fig. 3.32 a–c

a Bridging osteosynthesis with 24-hole reconstruction plate from angle to angle after a wide open defect fracture of the mandible, due to a gunshot laceration.

b The bridging plate was used for stabilization of both horizontal ramus and chin area. Although due to the soft-tissue loss the plate could not be covered primarily, there was no problem with infection.

c Bone and soft-tissue reconstruction was performed later.

Fig. 3.33 a–e

a Diagram showing bilateral mandibular fractures in a 7-year-old child.

b Diagram showing stabilization of bilateral mandibular fracture in a 7-year-old child with 2.4 plates and screws.

c OPT showing fixation of bilateral mandibular fractures with 2.7 system. Today the 2.4 system, as shown in **b**, would be appropriate. There is barely room to place these plates and screws at that young age.

d OPT showing the same patient as in **c** 5 years later. The plates were removed 1 year after osteosynthesis. The X-ray shows no tooth damage due to plate and screw placement, but due to the fracture.

e Postoperative X-ray in a 8-year-old child. Internal fixation of a paramedian fracture with a DC miniplate (2.0) because of comminution.

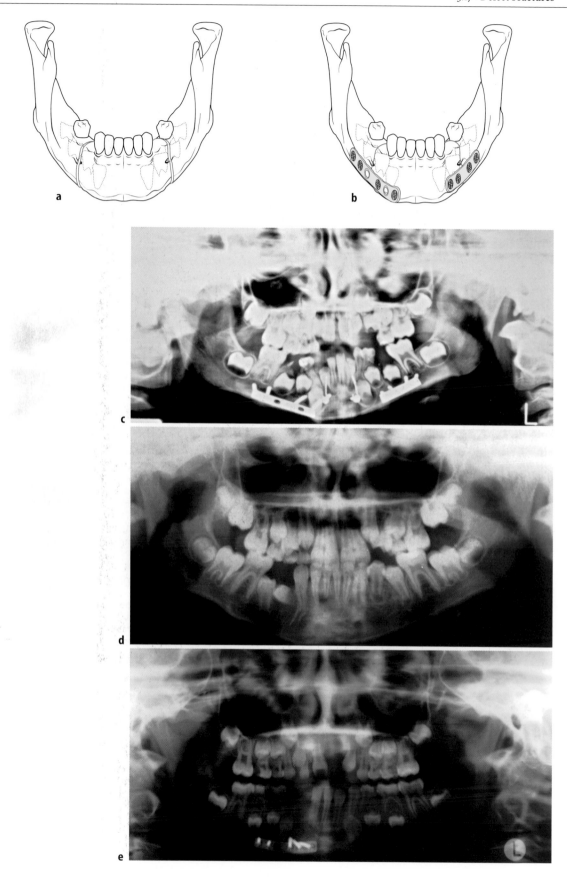

3.18 Mandibular Fractures in Children

Definition. Fractures in mandibles of children occur in either deciduous dentition, early mixed dentition, or late mixed dentition. All types of fractures can occur.

Special Conditions Influencing Internal Fixation. In early childhood the anatomic conditions for internal fixation are generally unfavorable due to small dimensions, bone weakness, localization of the tooth buds, and inferior alveolar nerve. Therefore as a rule mandibular fractures in deciduous dentition and early mixed dentition are with few exceptions (2.0 miniplates) treated conservatively. Only in late mixed dentition is the space for application of plates and screws sufficient. Here 2.0 or 2.4 plates can be used (Fig. 3.33).

Indications for internal fixation in decidous dentition and early mixed dentition are severely dislocated and comminuted fractures with or without soft-tissue laceration. Another indication for internal fixation is in mentally retarded children in whom intermaxillary fixation is not feasible. Screws are applied monocortically if tooth buds or the mental nerve are endangered, and there is enough bony substance for the placement of a screw. Generally, however, titanium screws and plates must not necessarily be taken out; removal of osteosynthesis material in children seems advisable. Research results have shown, however, that titanium implants most probably do not interfere with the growth of the membranous skeletal bones. Due to the appositional growth, plates may finally be completely incorporated.

References and Suggested Reading

Alpert B, Anderson T (1992) Experience with rigid fixation of mandibular fractures and immediate function. J Oral Maxillofac Surg 50:555–561

Ardary WC (1989) Prospective clinical evaluations of the use of compression plates and screws in the management of mandibular fractures. J Oral Maxillofac Surg 47:1150–1153

Assael LA (1994) Treatment of mandibular angle fractures: plate and screw fixation. J Oral Maxillofac Surg 52:757–761

Bähr W (1992) Comparison of torque measurements between cortical screws and emergency replacement screws in the cadaver mandible. J Oral Maxillofac Surg 50:46–49

Bähr W, Stoll P (1991) Pre-tapped and self-tapping screws in children's mandibles. – A scanning electronic microscopy examination of the implant beds. Br J Oral Maxillofac Surg 29:330–332

Beckers HL (1979) Treatment of initially infected mandibular fractures with bone plates. J Oral Surg 37:310–313

Cawood JI (1985) Small plate osteosynthesis of mandibular fractures. Br J Oral Maxillofac Surg 23:77

Champy M, Pape HD, Gerlach KL (1986) The Strasbourg miniplate osteosynthesis. In: Krüger E, Schilli W (eds) Oral and maxillofacial traumatology, vol 2. Quintessence, Chicago, pp 19–41

Chuong R, Donoff RB, Guralnick WC (1983) A retrospective analysis of 327 mandibular fractures. J Oral Maxillofac Surg 41:305–309

Dodson TB, Perrott DH, Kaban LB et al (1990) Fixation of mandibular fractures: a comparative analysis of rigid internal fixation and standard fixation techniques. J Oral Maxillofac Surg 48:362–366

Ellis E (1993) Treatment of mandibular angle fractures using the AO reconstruction plate. J Oral Maxillofac Surg 51:250

Ellis E, Ghali G (1991) Lag screw fixation of anterior mandibular angle fractures. J Oral Maxillofac Surg 49:13–21

Ellis E, Ghali G (1991) Lag screw fixation of mandibular angle fractures. J Oral Maxillofac Surg 49:234–243

Ellis E, Karas N (1992) Treatment of mandibular angle fractures using two mini-dynamic compression plates. J Oral Maxillofac Surg 50:958–963

Ellis E, Sinn DP (1993) Treatment of mandibular angle fractures using 2.4 dynamic compression plates. J Oral Maxillofac Surg 51:969–973

Ellis E, Tharanon W (1992) Facial width problems associated with rigid fixation of mandibular fractures: case reports. J Oral Maxillofac Surg 51:969–978

Ellis E, Walker L (1994) Treatment of mandibular angle fractures using two non-compression miniplates. J Oral Maxillofac Surg 52:1032–1036

Hammer B, Schier P, Prein J (1997) Osteosynthesis of condylar neck fractures: a review of 30 patients. Br J Oral Maxillofac Surg 35:288–291

Hardt N, Gottsauner A (1993) The treatment of mandibular fractures in children. J Craniomaxillofac Surg 21:214–219

Hoffmann W, Barton R, Price M et al (1990) Rigid internal fixation. J Trauma 30:1032

Iizuka T (1992) Rigid internal fixation of mandibular fractures with special reference to complications of different techniques. Thesis, University of Helsinki

Iizuka TL, Lindqvist C (1991) Sensory disturbances associated with rigid fixation of mandibular fractures. J Oral Maxillofac Surg 49:1264–1268

Iizuka T, Lindqvist C (1992) Rigid internal fixation of mandibular fractures: an analysis of 270 fractures treated using the AO/ASIF method. Int J Oral Maxillofac Surg 21:65–69

Iizuka T, Lindqvist C, Hallikainen D et al (1991) Infection after rigid internal fixation of mandibular fractures: a clinical and radiological study. J Oral Maxillofac Surg 49:585–593

James RB, Fredrickson C, Kent JN (1981) Prospective study of mandibular fractures. J Oral Surg 39:275–281

Jones JK, Van Sickels JE (1988) Rigid fixation: A review of concepts and treatment of fractures. Oral Surg Oral Med Oral Pathol 65:13

Joos U, Schilli W (1985) Complications after osteosynthesis of the mandible. In: Hjorting-Hansen E (ed) Oral and maxillofacial surgery: Proceedings from the 8th International Conference on Oral and Maxillofacial Surgery. Quintessence, Chicago

Kearns G, Perrott DH, Kaben LB (1993) Rigid fixation of mandibular fractures. Does operator experience reduce complications? J Oral Maxillofac Surg 52:226

Klotch DW, Bigger JR (1979) Plate fixation for open mandibular fractures. Laryngoscope 95:1374

Klotch DW, Prein J (1987) Mandibular reconstruction using AO plates. Am J Surg 154:384–388

Koury M, Ellis E (1992) Rigid internal fixation for the treatment of infected mandibular fractures. J Oral Maxillofac Surg 50:434–443

Levy F, Smith R, Odland R et al (1991) Monocortical mini plate fixation of mandibular angle fractures. Arch Otolaryngol Head Neck Surg 117:149–154

Lindqvist C, Kontio R, Pihakari A et al (1986) Rigid internal fixation of mandibular fractures – an analysis of 45 patients treated according to the ASIF method. Int J Oral Maxillofac Surg 15:657–664

Lung JR, Graham WP, Miller SH (1976) Pericortical compression clamps for mandibular fixation. Plast Reconstr Surg 57:487

Messer EJ, Hayes DE, Boyne PJ (1967) Use of intraosseous metal appliances in fixation of mandibular fractures. J Oral Surg 25:493–502

Nakamura S, Takenoshita Y, Oka M (1994) Complications of miniplate osteosynthesis for mandibular fractures. J Oral Maxillofac Surg 52:233–239

Niederdellmann H (1982) Rigid internal fixation by means of lag screws. In: Krüger E, Schilli W (eds) Oral and maxillofacial traumatology, vol 1. Quintessence, Chicago, pp 371–386

Niederdellmann H, Shetty V (1987) Solitary lag screw osteosynthesis in the treatment of fractures of the angle of the mandible: a retrospective study. Plast Reconstr Surg 80:68–74

Niederdellmann H, Akuamoa-Boateng E, Uhlig G (1981) Lag screw osteosynthesis: a new procedure for treating fractures of the mandibular angle. J Oral Surg 39:938–940

Passeri LA, Ellis E, Sinn DP (1983) Complications of non-rigid fixation of mandibular angle fractures. J Oral Maxillofac Surg 51:382

Prein J, Beyer M (1990) Management of infection and nonunion in mandibular fractures. Oral Maxillofac Surg Clin North Am 2(1):187–194

Prein J, Hammer B (1990) Stable fixation of mandibular fractures in accordance with the AO principles. In: Fonseca RJ, Walker RV (eds) Oral and maxillofacial trauma. Saunders, Philadelphia, pp 1172–1232

Prein J, Kellman RM (1987) Rigid internal fixation of mandibular fractures – basics of AO technique. Otolaryngol Clin North Am 20:441–456

Raveh J, Vuillemin T, Lädrach K et al (1987) Plate osteosynthsis of 367 mandibular fractures. J Craniomaxillofac Surg 15:244–253

Rix L, Stevenson AR, Punni-Moorthy A (1991) An analysis of 80 cases of mandibular fractures treated with mini plate osteosynthesis. Int J Oral Maxillofac Surg 20:337–341

Rudderman RH, Mullen RL (1992) Biomechanics of the facial skeleton. Clin Plast Surg 19(1):11–29

Schilli W (1982) Compression plate osteosynthesis through the ASIF system. In: Krüger W Schilli W (eds) Oral and maxillofacial traumatology, vol 1, Quintessence, Chicago, pp 308–365

Schilli W, Härle F (1976) Die funktionsstabile Osteosynthese – ein Problem des operativen Zugangs. Fortschr Kiefer Gesichtschir 21:300–303

Smith WP (1991) Delayed miniplate osteosynthsis for mandibular fractures. Br J Oral Maxillofac Surg 29:73–76

Spiessl B (ed) (1976) New concepts in maxillofacial bone surgery. Springer, Berlin Heidelberg New York

Spiessl B (1989) Internal fixation of the mandible. A manual of AO/ASIF principles. Springer, Berlin Heidelberg New York

Stoll P, Ewers R (1980) Kiefergelenkssituation nach Collumfrakturen, kombiniert mit Frakturen am Unterkieferkörper. Fortschr Mund-Kiefer-Gesichtschir 25:93–95

Stoll P, Wächter R (1996) Functional and morphological results after conservative and operative treatment of condylar neck fractures. J Craniomaxillofac Surg 24, Suppl 1, 110

Stoll P, Niederdellmann H, Sauter R (1983) Zahnbeteiligung bei Unterkieferfrakturen. Dtsch Zahnärztl Z 38:349

Stoll P, Wächter R, Schlotthauer U, Türp J (1996) Spätergebnisse bei 15 Jahre und länger zurückliegenden Kiefergelenkfortsatzfrakturen – Eine klinisch-röntgenologische Studie. Fortschr Mund-Kiefer-Gesichtschir 41:127–130

Takenoshita Y, Oka M, Tashiro H (1989) Surgical treatment of fractures of the mandibular condylar neck. J Craniomaxillofac Surg 17:119–124

Tu H, Thenhulzen D (1985) Compression osteosynthesis of mandibular fractures: a retrospective study. J Oral Maxillofac Surg 48:585–589

Türp JC, Stoll P, Schlotthauer U et al. (1996) Computerized axiographic evaluation of condylar movements in cases with fractures of the condylar process: a follow-up over 19 years. J Craniomaxillofac Surg 24:46–52

Wächter R, Stoll P (1996) Long-term results after application of the THORP-system in tumor surgery and traumatology: 12-year experience report. J Craniomaxillofac Surg 24, Suppl 1, 123

Wächter R, Stoll P, Bähr W, Schilli W (1996) Versorgung der komplexen infizierten Unterkieferfraktur mit dem THORP-System – eine prospektive Studie. Fortschr Mund-Kiefer-Gesichtschir 41

CHAPTER 4

Craniofacial Fractures

Chapter Author: Paul N. Manson
Contributers: C. R. Forrest
B. Hammer
P. N. Manson
B. Markowitz
J. H. Phillips
J. Prein
P. Sullivan

4.1 Organization of Treatment in Panfacial Fractures

Contributor: Paul N. Manson

4.1.1 Introduction

In the case of multiple facial fractures an order of treatment should be developed. In the past "inside out," "top to bottom," or "bottom to top" philosophies have prevailed, each with its own vigorous proponents [1]. Recently an "outside to inside" management scheme for the midface has been proposed emphasizing the zygomatic arch [2]. The exact order of treatment is not as important as the development of a plan which permits accuracy of anatomic positioning of the various facial segments. Exposure, identification, and fixation of the facial buttresses (Fig. 4.1.1a), guarantees best correct alignment and stabilization of facial fractures. Because of the face's complexity and multiple parts it is important that an order of facial fracture treatment be developed to address Le Fort (midface) and accompanying fractures. Such midface "extended" fractures (combining two or more areas) are referred to as "panfacial" fractures.

The approach described provides a uniform format for recreating facial dimensions, and proceeds from intact cranial vault and cranial base landmarks through the entire anterior portion of the face. The treatment of all Le Fort and any associated fractures may be integrated into this plan, which provides for both simple and panfacial injuries of all degrees of complexity. The treatment plan minimizes extraneous prepping and brings order to operative intervention by efficient, sequential manipulation.

4.1.2 Surgical Sequencing of Le Fort Fracture Treatment

The face is divided into upper and lower halves at the Le Fort I level (Fig. 4.1.1b). Each facial half is divided into two facial units. In the lower face are the occlusal and mandibular units. The occlusal unit consists of the teeth, palate, dentition, and alveolar processes of the maxilla and the mandible. The mandibular unit consists of horizontal and vertical sections. The vertical section includes the condyle, ramus, and angle. The horizontal section is the body and symphysis and parasymphysis areas.

In the upper face are the frontal and upper midfacial units. The frontal unit consists of the most superior frontal and temporal bones, the supraorbital rims, the orbital roofs, and the frontal sinus. The upper midfacial unit is composed of the zygomas laterally, the nasoethmoid area centrally, and the internal portion of the orbits bilaterally (Fig. 4.1.1c). The upper and lower midface meet at the Le Fort I level. Each unit is therefore divided into sections based on central, lateral and horizontal and vertical divisions.

Midface fracture treatment is predicated on an accurate physical examination and on evaluation with a thorough computed tomography (CT) scan. Although it may seem obvious, patients must have other significant injuries evaluated prior to undertaking facial surgery. The airway is protected by intubation or tracheostomy. The endotracheal tube should either be placed through the nose, through a gap in the dentition, behind the molar teeth, submentally, or a tracheostomy (possibly endoscopically) may be employed.

4.1.3 Occlusion

Attention is directed first to the dentition. Arch bars are applied to the teeth of the maxilla and the mandible. If fractured, the hard palate must be reduced and stabilized with stable fixation before intermaxillary fixation (Fig. 4.1.2; see also Figs. 4.2.6, 4.2.10). One or two mini-plates (2.0) are applied in the roof of the mouth and at the piriform aperture. Two-dimensional palate stabilization of the maxillary dental arch is therefore completed. This step sets a template for the correct width of the whole lower face by providing an anatomically reduced maxillary arch as a template for mandibular reconstruction. Similarly, alveolar fractures of the mandible may be reduced with small 2.0 or 1.5 plates, or perhaps the 1.3 or microsystem (Fig. 4.1.3). This step stabi-

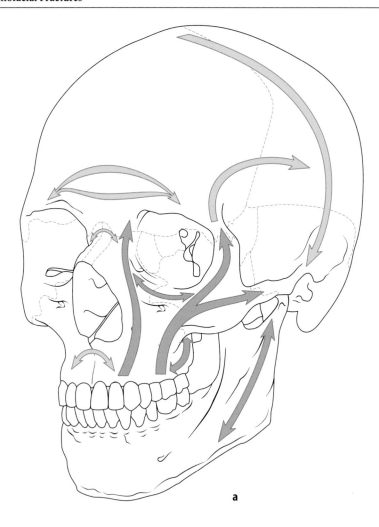

a

Fig. 4.1.1 a–c

a Horizontal and vertical buttresses of the facial skeleton (arrows)

b View of face with division line for upper and lower facial halves at the Le Frt I level.

c View of face: identification of the four facial units: frontal, upper midface, occlusal, and mandibular units.

Occlusal unit: components are the teeth, the palate, the alveolar processes of the maxilla and the mandible.

Units of the mandible: vertical, horizontal; vertical consists of condyle, ramus and angle; horizontal consists of body, symphysis, and parasymphysis.

The upper face consists of the frontal sinus area medially and two lateral frontal-temporal-supraorbital segments.

The upper midface unit consists of the zygomas laterally, and the nasoethmoid areas centrally, and the internal portion of the orbits bilaterally.

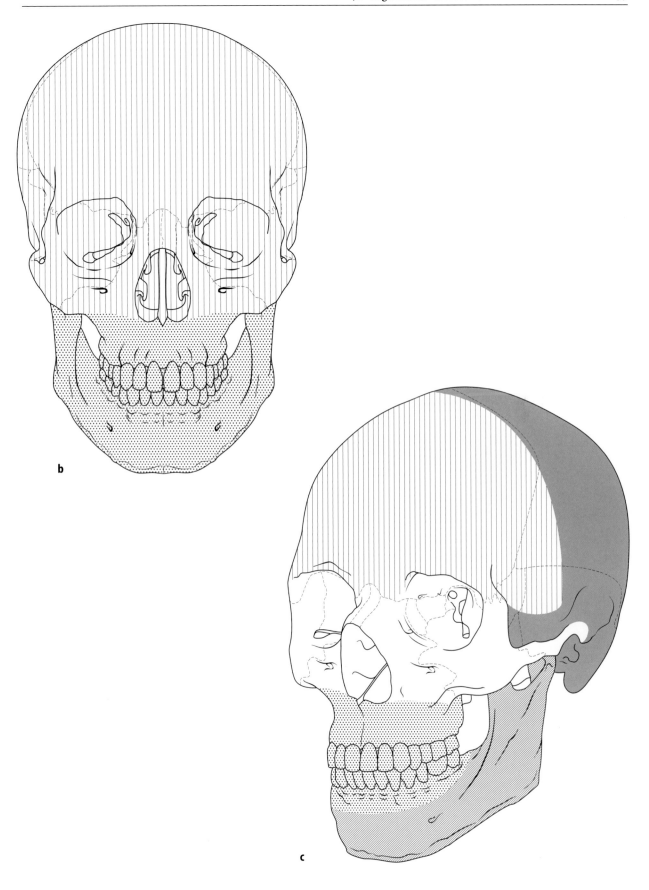

b

c

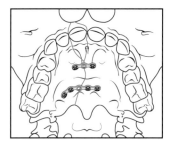

Fig. 4.1.2

Sagittal fractures of the maxilla should be stabilized by an approach through the roof of the mouth. The maxillary alveolus is stabilized at the pyriform aperture. One or two plates of the 2.0 system are used.

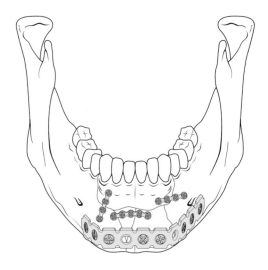

Fig. 4.1.3

Alveolar fractures of the mandible should be reduced with small monocortically placed screws of the midface system.

lizes dentition. Alginate impressions of the dentition are obtained and aid in the preparation of models or splints that key any remaining fractures for an accurate reduction. The patient is then placed in intermaxillary fixation. The occlusal relationship obtained is then compared to the ideal as determined from an analysis of dental models. In patients who are edentulous or partially edentulous it is necessary to use the original dentures for intermaxillary fixation (see Fig. 4.1.8). Special attention should be paid to the presence of subcondylar fractures. If present, they may lead to errors in the transverse or vertical dimension.

Preinjury photographs can be helpful in establishing the facial dimensions to be achieved. They also document preexisting facial asymmetry.

4.1.4 Upper Face: The Cranial Unit

Frontal bone fracture fragments, as removed, are marked in sequence after exposure is provided by a coronal incision (see Fig. 2.5). After neurosurgical exploration any remaining mucosa of the fracture involved frontal and ethmoid sinuses is removed. The frontal sinus is obliterated or cranialized depending on the presence or absence of a relatively intact posterior wall (see Sect. 4.1.6). Obliterative sinus and cranial base bone grafting must be complete to eliminate the sinus cavity and isolate the nose from the intracranial cavity. The frontal bar is reconstructed and the anterior sinus wall reassembled. The lower section of the supraorbital rim and lower anterior frontal sinus form the "frontal bar" (Fig. 4.1.4a), and this provides the inferior stable landmark in frontal bone reconstruction. Temporal bone alignment must be correct in narrowness (facial width) and length through the anterior cranial fossa to ensure proper projection of the frontal bar (Fig. 4.1.4b).

Using the frontal bar and intact superior cranial vault as guides, the remainder of the frontal bone segments are assembled and checked for symmetry. The frontal vault segments may need expansion for proper contour, assessed for symmetry with both sides. Bone fragments, initially linked with wires or small plates and screws, are then stabilized to adjacent intact bone. The initial frontal bone assembly may be performed on a back table while neurosurgery is in progress.

Orbital roof reconstruction is then completed by either replacement or bone grafts as required, and roof reconstruction stabilized to the frontal bar (Fig. 4.1.4c) and placed in a largely extraorbital position. Care must be taken to stabilize the orbital roof fragments in anatomic position and not to "overgraft" the superiorly arching orbital roof too far inferior by utilizing flat or intraorbitally placed bone which produces a downward and forward deformity of globe position (see Sect. 4.5).

4.1.5 Upper Midfacial Unit

Initially all fragments of the orbital rims including the superior, lateral, inferior, and medial segments are linked with interfragment wires. In the upper midfacial unit the nasoethmoidal area is reduced first as it is important to secure a narrow intercanthal distance by tightening the transnasal wire (Fig. 4.1.5). This step is the most important procedure in nasoethmoidal fracture reduction, as the wire links one medial orbital rim to the other. The nasoethmoidal area, reduced with interfragment and transnasal wires, is then linked superiorly to the frontal bar reconstruction and inferiorly to the maxillary alveolus with stable fixation, a technique called "junctional" rigid fixation (see Fig. 4.1.5).

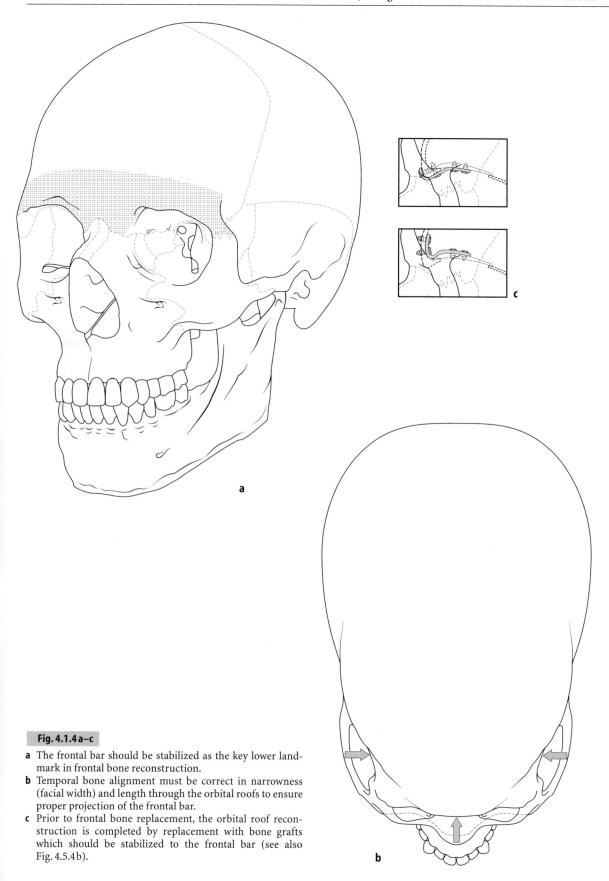

Fig. 4.1.4 a–c

a The frontal bar should be stabilized as the key lower land-mark in frontal bone reconstruction.

b Temporal bone alignment must be correct in narrowness (facial width) and length through the orbital roofs to ensure proper projection of the frontal bar.

c Prior to frontal bone replacement, the orbital roof recon-struction is completed by replacement with bone grafts which should be stabilized to the frontal bar (see also Fig. 4.5.4 b).

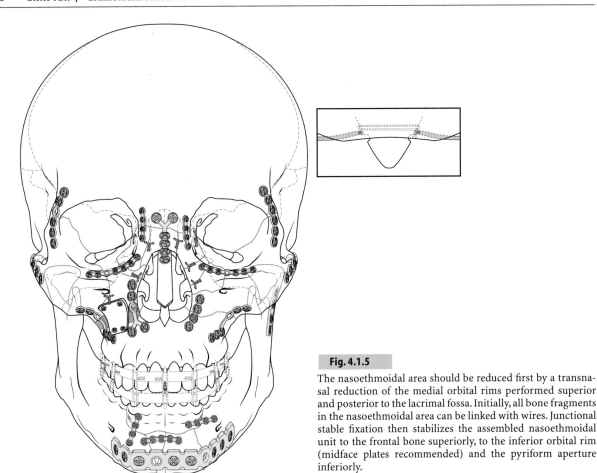

The nasoethmoidal area should be reduced first by a transnasal reduction of the medial orbital rims performed superior and posterior to the lacrimal fossa. Initially, all bone fragments in the nasoethmoidal area can be linked with wires. Junctional stable fixation then stabilizes the assembled nasoethmoidal unit to the frontal bone superiorly, to the inferior orbital rim (midface plates recommended) and the pyriform aperture inferiorly.

This step stabilizes projection of the nasoethmoidal complex; Le Fort I level and orbital rim fixation stabilize the lower projection. Plates extending along the medial orbital rim anterior to the canthal ligament produce an unnatural thickness and should be avoided.

Stable fixation of the zygoma begins by exposing all articulations of the zygoma with adjacent bones (see Fig. 4.4.1). These are the zygomaticofrontal suture, the inferior orbital rim, the zygomaticomaxillary buttress, the zygomatic arch and the lateral and inferior internal orbit. Placing wires in the zygomaticofrontal suture and the inferior orbital rim provides initial positioning of the zygoma (Fig. 4.1.6). The zygomaticomaxillary buttress is visualized to confirm approximate position. Next the arch is reduced beginning with the intact segment posteriorly, holding the anterior arch segments in a flat reduction which emphasizes the anterior projection of the zygoma. If the most posterior fracture in the zygomatic arch is oriented sagittally, a lag or tandem screw technique should be used, or perhaps the superior aspect of the glenoid fossa plated (see Fig. 4.4.6, insets 4 and 5). A 2.0 midface plate is placed over the remaining arch segments. Before arch reduction is begun, the

Fig. 4.1.6 a, b

a Initial alignment of the zygoma is achieved by positioning ▶ its five peripheral articulations. Positioning wires are placed at the zygomaticofrontal suture, the inferior-orbital rim, and eventually the zygomatic arch.
b The arch is then reduced, holding the malar eminence forward, compressing the arch inward, which stabilizes midfacial width and emphasizes anterior projection of the malar eminence.

zygoma at the inferior orbital rim and in the lateral orbit, must be checked for alignment, especially in the naso-orbital-ethmoidal segment (see Sects. 4.3, 4.5).

The zygoma is then stabilized with a midface or 1.3 plate at the inferior orbital rim in panfacial fractures as the use of a microplate in this region is not sufficient for cases in which nasoethmoid support is lost (see Fig. 4.1.5). When multiple segments of the inferior orbital rim are present, the segments are initially linked with interfragment wires or with smaller microplates with one loose screw in each segment. They should then be held superiorly and anteriorly as stable fixation is completed. The zygomaticofrontal suture is then reduced

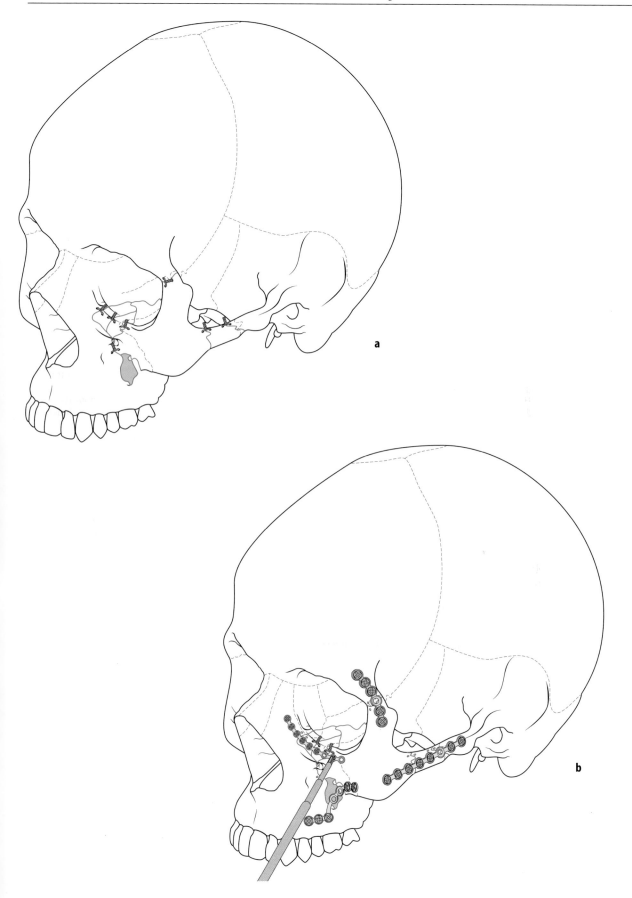

with a midface plate after the inferior orbital rim is related anteriorly. Proper zygomatic reduction can be confirmed only by simultaneously visualizing multiple areas of alignment with adjacent bones. After stabilization of the orbital rim is complete, the inferior orbit must be reconstructed with split cranial, rib, or iliac crest grafts. Stable posterior bone "ledges" are identified medially, laterally, and inferiorly. Bone grafts should then be strutted between the reconstructed rim and the stable posterior ledges, completing the reduction of the internal orbit and, in so doing, the upper midface. If desired, the bone grafts may be stabilized behind the orbital rim with miniplates or screws.

4.1.6 Lower Face

At first intermaxillary fixation in the patient's regular occlusion is performed (see Chap. 3). Fractures in the horizontal portion of the mandible are exposed through intraoral or extraoral incisions (see Figs. 2.1–2.3) and, if necessary for primary and temporary approximation, linked with interfragment wires. Comminuted fractures can also be simplified with miniplates. Internal fixation is performed allowing at least three screws for each fragment. The occlusion is checked before and after both the wire and plate reduction. After the initial wire reduction, adjustments in bone position are made, and stable plate fixation is completed in the horizontal mandibular segment. Simple angle fractures may be reduced through intraoral incisions. Complicated angle fractures are more easily reduced with extraoral approaches. The width of the mandible is supervised by using the anatomically reduced maxillary arch and dental inclination as guides to prevent rotation and excessive width at the angles. The lingual cortex of the mandible is not routinely visualized in fracture reduction; the fracture tends to gap if complete approximation of the entire thickness of the mandible fracture surfaces is not achieved. There is a tendency (in parasymphysis fractures in combination with bilateral subcondylar fractures) for the bicondylar width to be too wide and to have an excessive width and flaring at the mandibular angles. The lateral mandibular dentition tends to rotate lingually and to "flare" at the angle increasing the lower facial width (Fig. 4.1.7).

Open reduction of the vertical (ramus and condylar) segment of the mandible is required if significant malalignment or overlapping of ramus or subcondylar fractures exists. Condylar head dislocation produces a loss of ramus height which may change facial dimensions, complicating the treatment of multiply fractured patients. Condylar dislocation in the presence of a loose Le Fort fracture is an indication for open reduction to stabilize the height of the ramus and the forward projection of the mandible. Depending on the location of the

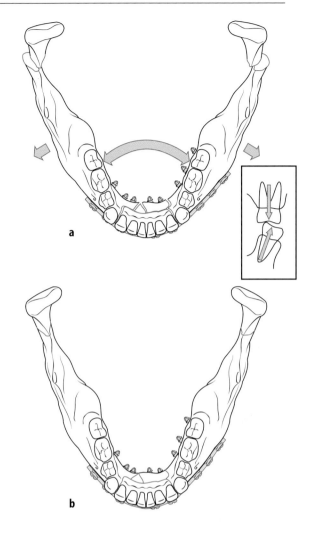

Fig. 4.1.7 a, b

As the proper width of the mandible is achieved, fractures in the anterior symphysis/parasymphysis area tend to "gap" on their buccal surface.

a If insufficient correction of mandibular width is obtained, the fracture may appear to be in reduction on the buccal surface anteriorly, but actually there is an excessive width at the angles allowing the lateral mandibular segments to rotate lingually, tipping the dentition, creating an open bite by bringing the lingual and palatal cusps out of alignment.

b Situation as in **a** but with correct fixation of the chin fracture by means of a correctly bent reconstruction plate.

fracture of the ramus, exposure is performed via either a preauricular or a Risdon incision. In questionable cases the facial nerve is best identified and protected. The temporomandibular joint is examined at the time of open reduction through a preauricular incision, and meniscus injury is assessed and corrected. The use of a temporoparietal flap is indicated if the meniscus is destroyed. Reconstruction of the ramus precedes the horizontal mandible and stabilizes it in proper position in relation to the cranial base (projection). Open reduction assists in supervising facial width at mandibular angles.

4.1.7 Linking the Upper and Lower Face

The lower and the upper facial units are then united at the Le Fort I level by plating the four anterior maxillary buttresses (see Fig. 4.1.5). Midface height and facial length are set by using an intact or an anatomically reconstructed buttress as a guide. One or more buttresses can almost always be reconstructed anatomically by piecing together existing fragments. In the absence of a reconstructed buttress, lip-tooth position provides the best clue to facial height. Old photographs may suggest the correct lip-tooth relationship.

The Le Fort I level fixation of the nasomaxillary buttress is the third area in which nasoethmoidal projection is stabilized. The other two areas are the frontal bar and inferior orbital rim.

Buttress bone gaps exceeding 5 mm are grafted for both functional and esthetic reasons. It is currently our recommendation to bone graft defects in the anterior sinus wall (see Fig. 4.1.5) as this prevents prolapse of soft tissue into the sinuses. Nasal bone grafting to improve the height in the nose or to smooth the dorsal nasal contour completes the facial reconstruction (see Figs. 4.1.5, 4.2.5 b, d). Nasal bone grafting is performed most accurately after the nasomaxillary buttress reconstruction and anterior nasal spine stabilization of the septum have been completed. If the medial canthal ligaments have been detached, they should be reattached following bone grafting of the medial orbit and nose to a separate set of transnasal wires placed before the nasoethmoidal reduction is completed. These are passed transnasally posterior and superior to the lacrimal fossa and pulled tight just prior to closure of incisions (see Sect. 4.3; Figs. 4.1.5, 4.3.3 b, 4.3.4 b).

4.1.8 Edentulous Fractures

In edentulous maxillary fracture treatment there is a tendency to avoid intermaxillary fixation and merely align the four anterior maxillary buttresses. This technique may overlook posterior displacement of the maxilla despite what appears to be satisfactory alignment of the anterior maxillary buttresses as the maxilla is not related in anteroposterior dimensions to a properly positioned mandible. If available, the original dentures of the patient provide correct intermaxillary fixation (Fig. 4.1.8). If broken, these dentures may be repaired first. Plate and screw fixation in an edentulous maxilla may require the use of alveolar bone as a stable lower fix-

ation point, and the plates may then need to be removed before a denture can be tolerated. Proper maxillary projection is confirmed only by relating the maxillary and mandibular alveolar ridges with temporary splints and dentures. Maxillary buttress reconstruction is therefore a guide for maxillary height, but not projection.

4.1.9 Soft Tissue

Current facial fracture reduction schemes emphasize complete degloving of all bones by detaching soft tissue and incising fascial layers. It is important when closing incisions to close or reposition attachments to the reassembled craniofacial skeleton. Generally this is the best performed by first closing the periosteum. The areas for periosteal closure are the zygomaticofrontal suture, inferior orbital rim, medial and lateral canthus areas, periosteum over the frontal process of the zygoma, muscular layers of the gingival buccal sulcus and mandibular incisions, and incision in the temporal fascia for zygomatic arch exposure. Marking the edges of the periosteal incisions with sutures allows precise identification at the end of the case for periosteal closure. These areas are illustrated in Fig. 4.1.9.

This approach emphasizes multiple areas of alignment for each fractured bone with the possibility of initial wire and final stable fixation. The important dimension is facial width. Control of facial width involves dissection to established cranial base landmarks; supervision of facial width in fact reciprocally emphasizes facial projection. Control of facial width is the most important first step in injury restoration and is possible only with extended approaches.

4.1.10 Soft-Tissue Injury

The fundamental challenge in facial fracture treatment is restoring the preinjury facial appearance and not simply linking together edges of bone at fractures. Deformity following facial fractures results from both soft-tissue changes and from bone malalignment. Deformity of both bone and soft-tissue significantly increases in the presence of highly comminuted fractures, especially when they involve the upper midfacial and orbital areas. The contribution of blunt soft-tissue injury and soft-tissue contracture to residual facial deformity has not been emphasized in the literature on facial fracture. Contused soft tissue heals with a network of internal scaring whose configuration is dictated by the position of the underlying bone fragments. When soft tissue heals over malreduced fractures, shrinkage and contracture of the soft-tissue envelope occur. Scarring and internal rigidity occur in the pattern of the unreduced bone segments. The internal scaring thickens soft tissue, opposing res-

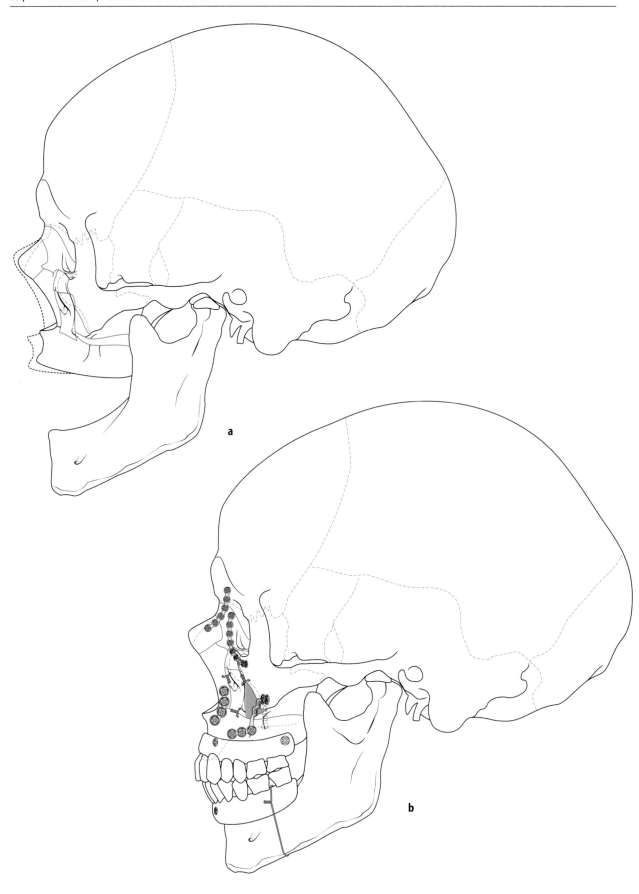

a

b

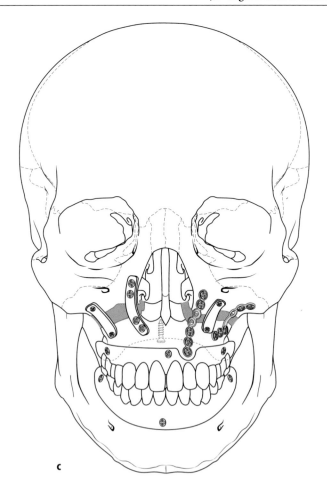

c

Fig. 4.1.8 a–c

In edentulous maxillary fracture treatment there is a tendency to avoid intermaxillary fixation and merely to align the four anterior maxillary buttresses. This technique tends to result in posterior displacement of the maxilla despite apparent alignment of the anterior maxillary buttresses as the maxillary dental arch is not brought into proper anterior/posterior relationship by positioning it to a properly positioned mandible.

a Midface fracture of an edentulous patient with dislocated midface in posterior-caudal direction.

b Same fracture as in **a** after correct reduction with correct mandibulomaxillary fixation with the patient's prosthesis and fixation with miniplates (2.0 and 1.3).

c Fixation of a Le Fort I fracture with miniplate and bone grafts, using the patient's dentures for correct alignment.

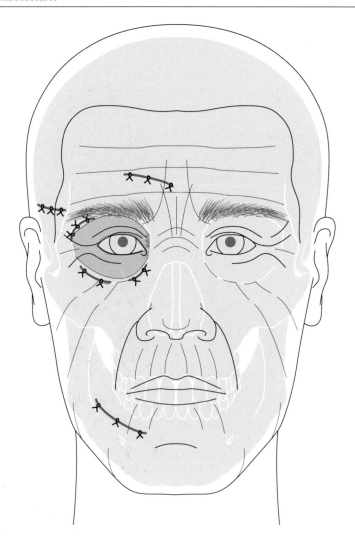

toration of the preinjury appearance, even if the underlying bone is finally replaced into its proper anatomic
position. Examples of soft-tissue rigidity accompanying
malreduced fractures include the conditions of enophthalmos, medial canthal ligament malposition, short
palpebral fissure, rounded canthus, and inferiorly displaced malar soft-tissue pad. Secondary management of
any one of these conditions is more challenging and less
effective than is primary reconstruction. A unique
opportunity thus exists in immediate fracture management to maintain expansion and position of the soft-tissue envelope and determine the geometry of soft-tissue
fibrosis by providing an anatomically aligned facial
skeleton as support. Excellent restoration of appearance
results from primary soft-tissue positioning.

Fig. 4.1.9

Positioning and refixation of soft tissues to the skeleton should
occur for each incision. The areas of closure are diagrammed
and include the temporal fascia, the frontal musculature, the
zygomaticofrontal suture, (the periosteum over the frontal process of the zygoma), the inferior orbital rim and the muscular
layers of the intraoral incisions. Refixation of the medial and
lateral canthal ligaments completes the reconstruction.

4.1.11 The "Double Insult" to Soft Tissue

Delayed reconstruction of facial fractures at 7–14 days post injury results in a second soft-tissue injury by dissection and incisions in healing areas of contusion and hemorrhage. Two injuries are created: the initial injury and the surgical manipulation. Delayed treatment creates a "double insult" to the already contused and damaged soft tissue. This is especially harmful, causing subcutaneous fibrosis. The skin, following delayed facial fracture repairs, is more thickened, rigid, lusterless, reddened, hyperpigmented, and fibrotic than skin from early injury repairs where the initial contusions, fractures, incisions, and dissection are all part of a single soft-tissue injury and recovery.

Accurate skeletal reconstruction requires anatomic assembly and stabilization of the basic configuration of the bone buttresses. Missing or unstable bone fragments should be replaced with bone grafts and the existing skeletal framework expanded with bone grafts, where required. The thorough reconnection of all buttress fragments must proceed from intact bone to intact bone and must be complete and accurate in three dimensions throughout the entire area of injury. Conceptualizing each unit of the facial skeleton in three dimensions and emphasizing supervision of width, restoration of projection and correction of the facial height in each unit allows assembly of the whole skeleton based on a conceptually precise framework for bone reconstruction. Performing the bone reconstruction early in complicated facial injuries allows the most natural restoration of the preinjury appearance to be determined by the combined relationship of bone and soft tissue.

References and Suggested Reading

Gruss J, Bubak PJ, Egbert M (1992) Craniofacial fractures: an alogorithm to optimize results. Clin Plast Surg 19:195–206

Gruss JS, MacKinnon SE (1986) Complex maxillary fractures: role of buttress reconstruction and immediate bone grafts. Plast Reconstr Surg 78:9–22

Gruss JS, MacKinnon SE, Kassel EE et al (1985) The role of primary bone grafting in complex cranio-maxillofacial trauma. Plast Reconstr Surg 75:17–24

Gruss JS, Pollock RS, Phillips JH, Antonyshyn O (1989) Combined injuries of the cranium and face. Br J Plast Surg 42:385–398

Gruss JS, Van Wyck L, Phillips JH et al (1990) The importance of the zygomatic arch in complex midfacial fracture repair and correction of post-traumatic orbito-zygomatic deformities. Plast Reconstr Surg 85(6):878–890

Kelly K, Manson PN, van der Kolk C, Markowitz B (1990) Sequencing Le Fort fracture treatment. J Craniofac Surg 1:168–178

Manson PN (1986) Some thoughts on the classification and treatment of Le Fort fractures. Ann Plast Surg 17:356–363

Manson PN, Glassman D, Van der Kolk C, Petty P (1990) Rigid stabilization of sagittal fractures of the maxilla and palate. Plast Reconstr Surg 85:711–716

Manson PN, Markowitz B, Mirvis S et al (1990) Toward CT-based facial fracture treatment. Plast Reconstr Surg 84:202–214

Markowitz BL, Manson PN (1989) Pan-facial fractures: organization of treatment Clin Plast Surg 16:105–114

Merville L (1974) Multiple dislocations of the facial skeleton. J Maxillofac Surg 2:187–203

Rorich R, Shewmake K (1992) Evolving concepts of craniomaxillofacial trauma management. Clin Plast Surg 19:1–10

4.2 Le Fort I–III Fractures

Contributors: **Lower Midface (Le Fort I)**
Christopher R. Forrest
John H. Phillips
Upper Midface (Le Fort II + III)
Joachim Prein

4.2.1 Lower Midface (Le Fort I)

4.2.1.1 Anatomy

The midface consists of the paired maxillae, palatine bones, and medial and lateral pterygoid processes of the sphenoid bone. It acts as a link between the cranial base and the occlusal plane and provides protection in an anterior-posterior plane for the face, protection for the skull base, and a site for muscle and ligament attachments.

Anatomic support for the midface is provided through a series of buttresses or struts that are used to distribute masticatory forces from the teeth to the skull base (Sicher and DeBrul 1970; Manson et al. 1980; Gruss and Mackinnon 1986). Buttresses exist in the horizontal and coronal planes (Gentry et al. 1983; see Fig. 4.1.1a), but the vertical struts of the midface are clinically most important with respect to the management of midface fractures. Although these vertical buttresses are quite strong in the sense of vertically directed stresses, they are unable to withstand equivalent forces directed in a transverse plane.

The three principle vertical buttresses of the maxilla consist of (Fig. 4.2.1):

- The nasomaxillary (medial) buttress which extends from the cuspid and anterior portion of the maxillary alveolus along the pyriform aperture, the medial side of the orbit through the anterior lacrimal crest, and the nasal process of the maxilla to the superior orbital rim and nasoethmoid region.
- The zygomaticomaxillary (lateral) buttress extends from the maxillary alveolus above the anterior molar

to the zygomatic process of the frontal bone and laterally to the zygomatic arch
- The pterygomaxillary (posterior) buttress which attaches the maxilla posteriorly to the pterygoid plates of the sphenoid bone.

The posterior support of the maxilla is derived from the pterygoid plates, while the anterior support comes from the medial and lateral anterior buttresses. Anatomic alignment and fixation of the medial and lateral buttresses is important in achieving anatomic reduction of the maxilla in relation to the cranial base and to restore proper vertical height and horizontal projection (Fig. 4.2.1).

4.2.1.2 Classification

Maxillary fractures have traditionally been classified according to lines of fracture based on anatomic lines of weakness as described by René Le Fort in 1901, as follows:

- Le Fort I fracture (Fig. 4.2.2): low horizontal fracture with disrupture of the tooth-bearing section of the maxilla
- Le Fort II fracture (Fig. 4.2.3a): triangular or pyramidal central midface fracture
- Le Fort III fracture (Fig. 4.2.4): high horizontal fracture alongside the junction between the cranial and facial skeleton.

Although this provides a uniform method to describe the general level of the major fracture line and allows references regarding the probable points of stability required in surgical treatment, these classic patterns are rarely encountered in clinical practice. In addition, this classification scheme does not incorporate vertical or segmental alveolar fractures or the issues of comminution or bone loss. Manson (1986) has elaborated on the Le Fort classification to take these issues into account:

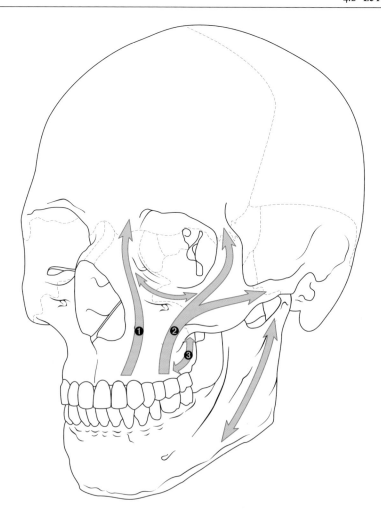

- Horizontal
  - Dentoalveolar fractures
  - Le Fort I (transverse, Guérin) fractures
  - Le Fort II (pyramidal) fractures
  - Le Fort III (craniofacial dysjunction) fractures
- Vertical (sagittal)
  - Medial palatal split
  - Lateral palatal (maxillary tuberosity) split

Fig. 4.2.1

Diagram of maxillary buttresses showing anterior maxillary buttress (medial; ❶), lateral buttress (zygomaticomaxillary; ❷), pterygomaxillary buttress (posterior; ❸). These represent regions of thicker bone designed to provide support for the maxilla in the vertical dimension.

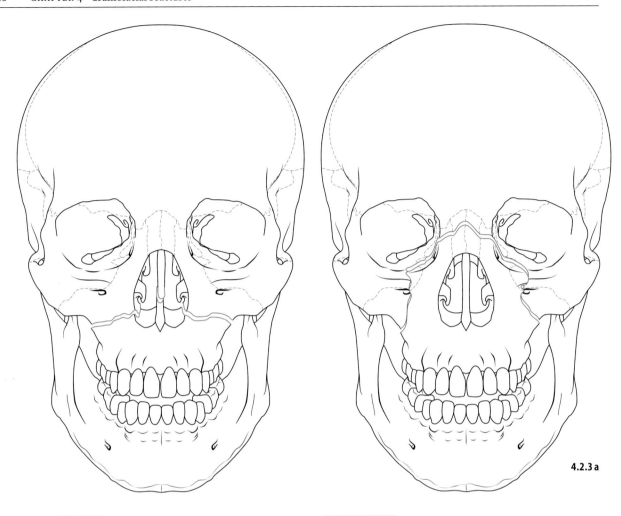

4.2.3 a

Fig. 4.2.2

Le Fort I fracture.

Fig. 4.2.3 a, b

Le Fort II fracture.
a Typical postero-caudal dislocation with open bite.
b Correct internal fixation with 2.0 L-plates for the lateral-vertical buttresses. 1.3 adaption plate infraorbitally and for the nasoethmoidal region. *Inset* showing fixation with one 2.0 Y-plate instead of two 1.3 mini plates.

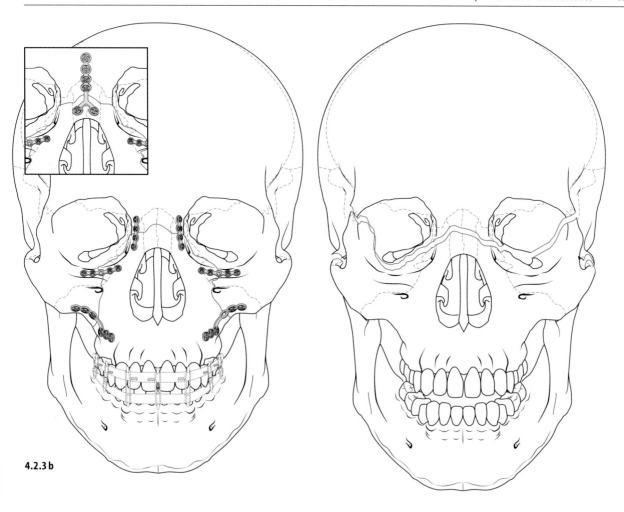

4.2.3 b

Fig. 4.2.4

Le Fort III fracture with postero-caudal dislocation and anterior open bite.

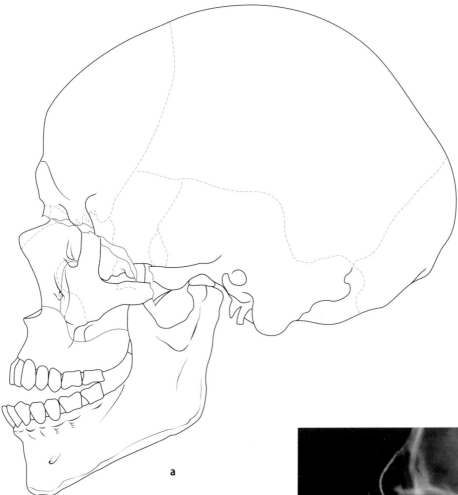

a

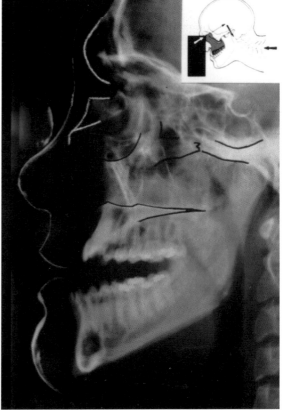

c

4.2.1.3 Diagnosis

The diagnosis of midface fractures is usually made clinically, although this may be more difficult if the maxilla
fracture is incomplete or impacted. Clinical signs of
bilateral ecchymosis, edema involving the midface, and
orbits should alert the clinician to examine the patient
for malocclusion, maxillary mobility, and missing teeth.
Digital examination of the hard palate may reveal evidence of a sagittal or maxillary tuberosity fracture. Res-
olution of facial swelling may reveal elongation ("equine
facies") or flattening ("dish face," see Fig. 4.2.5 a, c) of the
midface due to maxillary displacement. Dorsal and caudal pull by the medial pterygoid muscles may produce
an anterior open bite and tendency to class III malocclusion (Fig. 4.2.5 a, c). Sagittal palatal fractures may result
in lateral rotation and superior tilting of the maxillary
segments, producing increased transverse width of the
maxillary arch with cross-bite (Fig. 4.2.6).

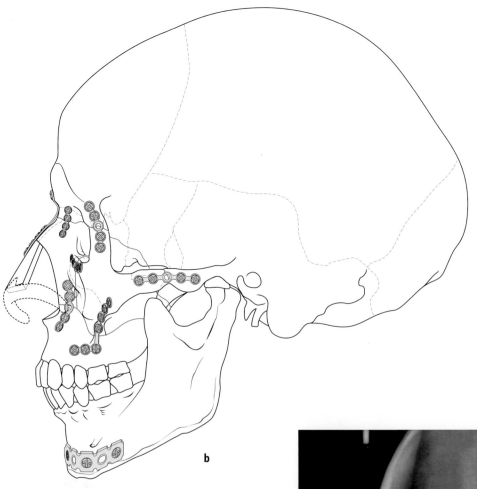

b

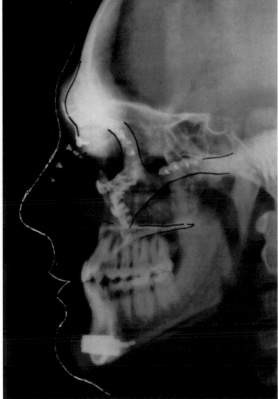

d

Fig. 4.2.5 a–d

a Diagram showing dorsal and caudal pull by the medial pterygoid muscles to produce an anterior open bite and tendency to class III malocclusion.
b Diagram after fixation of fracture situation as shown in
Fig. 4.2.5 a, including the reconstruction of the nasal dorsum
with a bone graft.
c Lateral cephalogram showing dorsal-caudal dislocation of
midface in Le Fort III fracture situation. Note: key area at
zygomatic arch fracture.
d Lateral cephalogram after reposition and correct stabilization of Le Fort III and I fractures. Note: stabilization with
miniadaption plate at zygomatic arch area and immediate
reconstruction of nasal ridge with a bone graft and stabilization with lag screws.

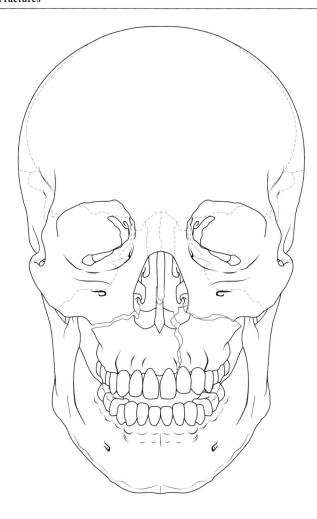

Diagram showing Le Fort I fracture and paramedian sagittal palatal fracture on the left side with lateral rotation and superior tilting of maxillary segments.

Clinical diagnosis of a maxillary fracture may be confirmed using plain facial radiographs, and especially the water's view. The latter projection gives the best information about midfacial structures. However, 5-mm axial CT images provide the best means of visualizing the fracture patterns, degree of comminution, and bone loss. In severe fracture situations three-dimensional CT images may provide additional information regarding displacement of the midface in relation to the mandible and orbits but should be used to satisfy clinical impressions. With chipped or missing teeth a chest film should be obtained to rule out aspiration.

4.2.1.4 Le Fort I Fractures

In 1866 Guérin described a pattern of maxillary fracture which has subsequently become more commonly referred to as the Le Fort I fracture (see Fig. 4.2.2). The line of the fracture extends transversely above the tooth roots through the maxillary sinus and nasal septum, posteriorly across the pyramidal process of the palatine bone and pterygoid process of the sphenoid bone.

The primary aims of treatment of Le Fort I maxillary fractures are the restoration of correct midfacial vertical height and anterior projection and restoration of occlusion.

Treatment

1. Systematic radiographical evaluation of the extent and pattern of injury, sometimes including CT.
2. Restoration of original occlusion using mandibulomaxillary fixation.
3. Direct exposure of all involved fractures.
4. Reduction and anatomic realignment of the maxillary buttresses to reestablish normal maxillomandib-

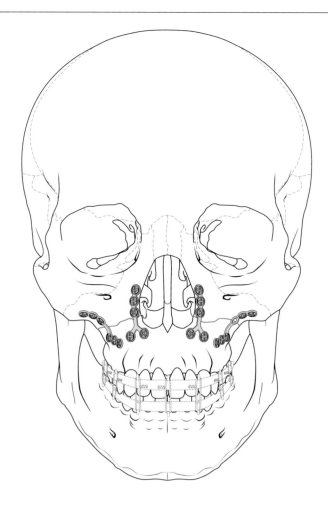

Fig. 4.2.7

Diagram showing ideal internal fixation of Le Fort I fracture with Y and L miniplates at anterior and medial buttresses. Note: Temporary IMF in correct occlusion during surgery.

ular and maxillo-zygomatico-orbital relationships to restore normal maxillary height, anterior projection, transverse width, and occlusion.

5. Internal fixation (osteosynthesis) using miniplate and screw fixation (Fig. 4.2.7).
6. Use of primary bone grafts to reconstruct and stabilize comminuted (absent) maxillary buttresses to prevent midface collapse or elongation (Figs. 4.1.5, 4.2.13).

The initial treatment of midface fractures incorporates the general principles of trauma management and includes establishment and maintenance of airway, supervision of hemorrhage, investigation, and management of associated injuries (cervical spine, neurological injury, etc.). Bleeding from the greater palatine or internal maxillary arteries may be life threatening and may require early maxillary reduction and intermaxillary fixation, including anterior and posterior nasal packing.

Surgical treatment of Le Fort I fractures should be performed as soon as possible. General oral hygiene is administered throughout the treatment period. Delay of surgical treatment for more than 7 days may result in difficulty in reducing the maxilla from its retruded position due to bony fragment impaction and soft-tissue contraction.

Airway Management. Airway management during surgery may be ideally secured using a reinforced nasotracheal tube sewn to the membranous nasal septum. This allows adequate exposure and facilitates application of intermaxillary fixation. However, severe swelling, nasal mucosal disruption, associated basal skull fracture, etc. may prevent placement of a nasotracheal tube. In cases of an isolated maxillary fracture the endotracheal tube may be secured to a molar with 26-gauge wire and positioned behind the third molar, thereby affording restoration of premorbid mandibulomaxillary occlusal relationships. In cases of combined maxillary and mandibular fractures judicious use of a tracheostomy may be necessary. The endoscopic placement of the tracheostomy is especially atraumatic and less visible postoperatively. In addition to this, submental placement of the endotracheal tube may be another very helpful way of anaesthezising these patients without interfearing with the occlusion.

Exposure. Maxillary fractures in the Le Fort I plane may be exposed through an upper gingivobuccal sulcus incision (see Fig. 2.2). Rarely, exposure may be obtained directly through soft-tissue lacerations. Both maxillae may be widely exposed subperiosteally to identify all four anterior buttresses. In segmental alveolar fractures preservation of vascular supply to tooth-bearing alveolar fragments may be achieved through a segmental upper buccal incision. Care must be taken in dissection to avoid the infraorbital nerve, which is located approximately 1 cm below the inferior orbital rim below the medial limbus. When comminution of the buttresses occurs, care is taken to identify and anatomically replace the fragments to achieve proper midface height. If these fragments are too small to be replaced with adequate fixation, they should be discarded and primary bone grafts employed to reconstruct the buttresses. Attempts to preserve vascular supply to small fragments hinders exposure to the buttresses and may preclude anatomic reduction. Small fragments should be retrieved from the maxillary antrum as they may act as sequestra and result in maxillary sinusitis. Torn maxillary sinus mucosa is removed, but a formal drainage of the sinus is seldom necessary.

Reduction. Prior to reduction of the maxilla arch bars should be affixed to the maxillary and mandibular dentition to facilitate restoration of the original occlusal relationship.

If surgical treatment is delayed, or the maxilla is severely impacted, reduction from the retrodisplaced position may be difficult without osteotomy. Disimpaction forceps or a 24-gauge wire loop placed through a drill hole near the thick bone of the anterior nasal spine followed by manual traction may be necessary. It is important to overstretch the anterior position of the midface relative to the mandible, such that passive repositioning of the midface results in anatomic reduction. Difficulties arise with posterior relapse postoperatively if force is required to hold the maxilla in position while applying the internal fixation plates. The external dynamic forces of scar tissue contraction and muscle pull may overcome the static forces of miniplate fixation and consequently result in relapse.

Failure to appreciate the importance of mandibulomaxillary fixation in the treatment of all midface fractures may result in postoperative malocclusion, commonly in the form of anterior open bite. This occurs in cases of noncomminuted fractures when the surgeon

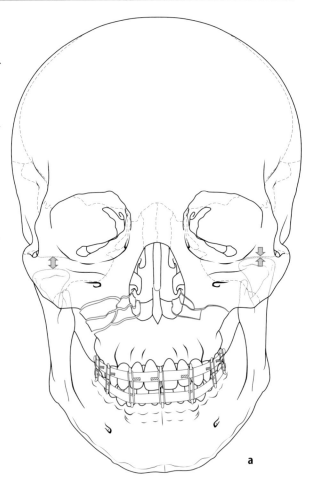

a

Fig. 4.2.8 a–c

a Diagram showing comminution in Le Fort I area on the right side and caudally dislocated joint. The occlusion is correct. Facial height on the right side on the comminuted area is too long.

b Fixation of Le Fort I fracture with premature contact on comminuted side and open bite on opposite noncomminuted side. Mandibular condyle now in correct position.

c Diagram showing fixation of the midface fracture in an edentulous patient with the help of patient's dentures to set the correct vertical hight. Fixation of Le Fort I area with plates and bone grafts because of fracture gap of more than 5 mm. The prostheses are fixed to the alveolar process and the palate with 2.4 screws. Anterior view.

believes that anatomic reduction of the medial and lateral buttresses will result in proper placement of the midface in three dimensions. If mandibulomaxillary fixation is not used, the posterior (pterygoid) buttress may be intruded, or more commonly extruded while appearing to be anatomically reduced at the anterior buttresses. This posterior extrusion results in premature

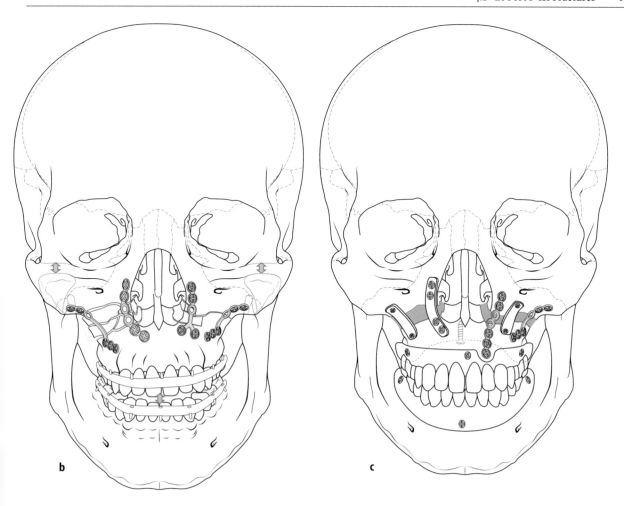

b

c

contact of the posterior molars, producing an anterior open bite, as shown on preoperative diagram (Figs. 4.2.2, 4.2.5 a). Mandibulomaxillary fixation is mandatory in the treatment of all Le Fort fractures so that the mandibular ramus can be used to set the height of the posterior (pterygoid) buttress prior to internal fixation. If treatment must be delayed, intermaxillary fixation alone prevents many of the deformities of the untreated fractured maxilla.

Care must be taken to ensure that no subcondylar fractures are present prior to fixation, and that the mandibular condyles are seated properly in the glenoid fossa. A unilateral open bite deformity may occur in cases in which the buttresses are comminuted on one side only. Inadvertent subluxation or dislocation of the temporomandibular joint inferiorly on the comminuted side may result in fixation of the lateral buttress with an increased vertical height. The opposite buttresses are reduced and fixed anatomically. When mandibulomaxillary fixation is released, and the condyle repositions, premature contact of the comminuted side occurs, resulting in open bite on the opposite noncomminuted side (Fig. 4.2.8 a, b). A similar situation may develop if a Le Fort I fracture occurs in conjunction with a zygomatic fracture. Care must be taken not to internally fix the zygoma in an inferiorly displaced position, or else a relative increase in vertical height exists in the maxilla on that side.

In the edentulous maxilla it may be necessary to use the patient's dentures or a Gunning splint to set the correct vertical height of the face (Fig. 4.2.8 c). If neither is available, anatomic buttress alignment may be followed by denture adjustment to account for minor occlusal discrepancies.

In conjunction with occlusion, anatomic alignment of the medial and lateral buttresses provides the key to the restoration of midface vertical height and horizontal projection. Comminution of all four anterior buttresses is fortunately rare. It is typical that there is at least one buttress in large enough fragments to allow for anatomic assessment of vertical height. This buttress may be plated first (Fig. 4.2.9) and the bone fragments rigidly fixed onto the plate using a lag screw technique. The other buttress heights are then set accordingly, and pri-

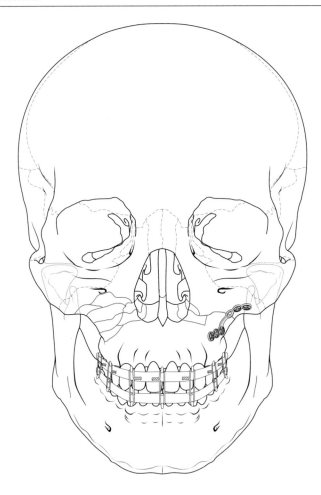

Fig. 4.2.9

Le Fort I fracture with comminution of both medical and one posterior buttress on the right. No comminution at left posterior buttress, which therefore is stabilized first. The height of the remaining buttresses is set according to this reconstruction. Lip-tooth position provides the best clue to facial height where no buttress can be reassembled from existing fragments. Note correct temporary IMF.

mary bone grafting may be performed (see Fig. 4.2.13). If all anterior buttresses are so severely comminuted that correct midface height cannot be determined at any of the buttresses, the surgeon may use the mandible to assess the appropriate anterior projection, and subjective judgement to set the relative midface height. Unfortunately, liptooth relation at rest may not be a reliable indicator depending on the amount of facial edema.

Occlusion. Restoration of occlusion is paramount to the appropriate treatment of midface fractures. Failure to reestablish the original occlusal patterns through the application of mandibulomaxillary fixation prior to internal fixation and reliance on anatomic positioning of the buttresses alone may result in postoperative malocclusion, as indicated above.

With an intact maxillary arch it is important to determine the patient's correct occlusion using information obtained by history, pretrauma photographs, dental records, and wear-facet patterns on the teeth. The use of acrylic wafer dental splints created from dental impressions taken under anesthesia may assist in determining normal occlusion and maintaining it during surgery.

Difficulty can arise when teeth are missing or the patient is edentulous. In these circumstances the surgeon's subjective judgement may be necessary to determine the "best fit." Sagittal fractures of the palate or segmental dentoalveolar fractures add further degrees of instability, making assessment and restoration of premorbid occlusion difficult. Careful palpation of the palate reveals unstable tooth-bearing segments to alert the surgeon of these difficulties.

Fixation. The use of miniplate fixation in treating maxillary fractures has eliminated the need for prolonged mandibulomaxillary fixation, allowing for improved oral hygiene, better nutrition, better airway, less weight

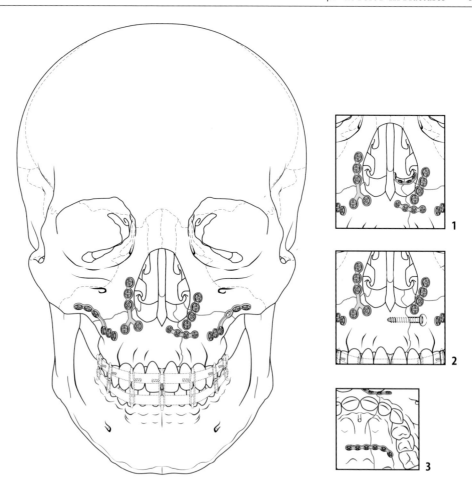

Fig. 4.2.10

Diagram showing fixation of Le Fort I fracture and paramedian sagittal palatal fracture. *Insets*, the various types of fixation for the sagittal palatal fractures.
Inset 1: Miniplate fixation anteriorly above incisor teeth and nasal floor inside left nose.
Inset 2: Lag screw fixation anteriorly.
Inset 3: Plate fixation anteriorly and palatal roof intraorally.

loss, and lower infection rates and may act to shorten the duration of hospitaliation. In addition, internal fixation keeps reduced fragments in position; there is less resorption of bone grafts and earlier return to function (Gruss and Phillips 1992; Schilli et al. 1981). Previous methods of buttress fixation using interosseous wires were intrinsically unstable and led to telescoping of segments and inability to withstand stresses, with bony relapse.

Compressive clamping of a miniplate to bone by the tensile force induced in the screw is the basis of fixation by bone plates. Compression was first advocated by Danis (1949) for stabilization of bone fractures. This has been shown to be benificial in treating long bone and mandibular fractures in which the use of compression plates promotes primary bone healing. However, in the midface compression is rarely employed due either to bony comminution or the thinness of the bone which would result in overlap of fragment ends with subsequent shortening. The exception to this is the use of compression with lag screw stabilization of a palatal split with screw placement anteriorly through the anterior nasal spine region (Fig. 4.2.10, inset 2).

Without compression the stability in the fracture site depends upon the inherent rigidity of the miniplate and friction between the fragment ends. If a small gap exists between the fragment ends, and the dynamic external forces from mastication are greater than the rigidity of the implant, movement in the gap can occur with detrimental effects on bone healing. The presence of movement may lead to a high-strain condition, which is not conducive to bone formation. As a result a fibrous nonunion and fragment end resorption may occur. However, in practice, nonunion of maxillary fractures is relatively rare.

Stripping of the bone thread is one of the commonest problems encountered during the insertion of a screw at

Screw

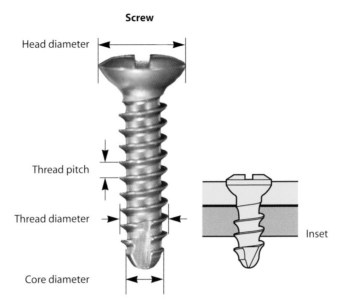

Head diameter

Thread pitch

Thread diameter

Core diameter

Inset

Fig. 4.2.11

Basic screw design showing the thread and core diameter as well as the pitch (distance between two threads).
Inset shows the relation in between pitch and thickness in bone. At least 2 threads should engage in cortical bone in order to provide sufficient holding capacity.

surgery. This is a problem especially when fixing plates to thin cortical bone in the midface area. Therefore it is important to position the buttress plates as far laterally and as close to the pyriform fossa as possible as these areas represent the thickest regions of bone in the midface and provide for good screw purchase and fixation (see Fig. 4.2.7).

The ability of the screw to provide holding power depends upon screw design, the changes in bone as the result of screw insertion, the reaction of the bone to the implant material, the resorption and remodeling of bone during fracture healing, and the reaction of bone to loading as the result of muscle forces. For proper screw anchorage one condition that must be met is that the bone cortex thickness be at least as thick as the distance separating two threads of the screw (pitch angle, Fig. 4.2.11 and inset; Diehl et al. 1974). Therefore in very thin bone, such as found in the maxilla, screws with smaller pitch angles may have some theoretical advantage as this results in more screw threads having contact with the bone. In addition, it has been demonstrated that screws with smaller pitch angles have slightly higher compressive values in 2-, 3-, and 4-mm bone thickness (Phillips and Rahn 1989; Kuhn et al. 1995).

The holding power of the fluted portion has been demonstrated to be 17%–30% less than that of the fully threaded nonfluted portion (Bechtol et al. 1959). This is seldom a problem in midface as the screw tip and cutting flutes can protrude safely into the maxillary antrum and maintain its holding power.

More torque is required to insert a self-tapping screw due to the cutting of the bone threads. This places increased stress on the screw which can lead to screw failures and microfracturing of the surrounding bone which can predispose to screw loosening. When a small bony fragment or bone graft is being lag-screwed onto a plate to bridge a bone defect, the increased torque associated with self-tapping screws may result in displacement and difficulties maintaining the position of the bone segment. Tapping has been shown to decrease insertional torque by 35%–40% (Hughes and Jordan 1972). If a screw must be reinserted into the same drill hole at surgery due to the cutting ability of the flutes, the risk of cross-threading is increased with self-tapping screws, leading to poor screw purchase. However, these potential disadvantages of the self-tapping system are far outweighed by its benefits in increased compressive forces in thin bone.

Recent in vivo studies on the biomechanics of the facial skeleton by Rudderman and Mullen have shown that treatment of structural defects of midface should be directed to the reconstruction of normal pretraumatic load paths (Rudderman and Mullen 1992). This is best performed by the reconstruction/reconstitution of normal buttresses.

Plates should be applied separately to the medial and lateral buttresses. Optimal placement of the lateral buttress plate is from the thick bone of the zygomatic body along the lateral aspect of the anterior maxilla where the bone is thickest. The medial buttress plate is best placed along the rim of the pyriform fossa. Placement of load-bearing plates across the thin bone of the anterior maxilla should be avoided as screw holding power is significantly decreased. Passive contouring of the plate to ensure a perfect fit to the underlying bone is important as attempts at in situ plate bending place undue stress on the bone leading to screw stripping and microfractures of the bone. Continuous irrigation when creating the drill hole is important to prevent bone necrosis and ring sequestra.

Care must also be taken to avoid inadvertent placement of screws into tooth roots. The position of the canine tooth root should be used to determine the superior extent of the tooth roots. On occasion a low lying fracture along the lateral buttress directly adjacent to the tooth roots prevents application of the plate; otherwise screwplacement between tooth roots. It is best to span the plate from the zygomatic body to the thick bone near the anterior nasal spine in these circumstances, in addition to the use of primary bone grafts. It has not been necessary to fix the posterior buttresses internally, however IMF can substitute for posterior buttress support.

Plates become the path for load distribution, and if placed abnormally, force distribution may place undue loads on plates and thus lead to high-stress concentrations. This may ultimately lead to screw fatigue and failure. Placement of multiple screws (at least two) on each side of fracture leads to a more even distribution of loading (load sharing between plate and bone). If biomechanics are not considered with regards to internal fixation, the incidence of infection, nonunion and tissue injury may increase.

In the edentulous maxilla, bone stock may be diminished, and for adequate fixation plates may be placed low on the buttress through residual alveolar bone. However, this may interfere with denture fitting, and the plates may have to be removed once bone healing is complete.

Bone Grafting. Primary bone grafting (iliac, split rib, or calvarium) has been advocated to reconstruct defects in the medial or lateral buttresses where bone has been lost or comminuted (Gruss and Mackinnon 1986; Gruss and Phillips 1992; Manson et al. 1985). The use of miniplate fixation has reduced the need for immediate bone grafting but the ability of plates to bridge bone gaps is location dependent (Gruss and Phillips 1992). Masticatory forces and cyclical loading on the maxilla can result in implant fatigue and failures if miniplates are used to span significant bone gaps without restoration of bony continuity using bone grafts.

Gaps in the maxillary buttresses greater than 5 mm should be replaced with bone grafts. Bone grafts may be lag-screwed under a miniplate used to span the bone gap or may be held in place directly onto the buttress using lag screws at either end (see Fig. 4.1.5, 4.2.8 c, and 4.2.13). Loss of the anterior wall of the maxilla may predispose to invagination of the overlying soft tissues into the

maxillary antrum, creating overlying contour defects. Bone grafts may be used to prevent this deformity.

The general principles of internal fixation should be applied to the use of bone grafts as this has been shown to prevent resorption and allow maintenance of volume in the presence of infection (Fialkov et al. 1993).

Although bone grafts may be harvested from several sites (ilium, rib, calvarium), split calvarial bone is the material of choice for buttress reconstruction. It is readily available in large quantities, accessible within the same operative field, tolerates being exposed to the open maxillary antrum when rigidly fixed, has minimal donor morbidity, provides for excellent screw purchase and fixation, and may be rigidly fixed to miniplates or lag-screwed onto underlying bone due to its high cortical component. In addition, it is strong enough to withstand the forces of soft-tissue contraction and mastication. The main disadvantage of calvarium is brittleness or the inability to shape and contour the bone due to its low modulus of elasticity as the bone tends to fragment when attemps are made to bend it.

Palatal Fractures. Sagittal fractures of the maxilla and palate are present in 15% of patients with Le Fort fractures (Manson et al. 1983) and are associated with increased instability due to rotation of dentoalveolar segments which may not respond to conventional forms of fixation. Fractures involving the palate commonly divide the palate longitudinally, adjacent to the midline as this represents a line of weak thinner bone (medial palatal split; see Fig. 4.2.6). The fracture usually exits anteriorly between the incisors or lateral incisor and canine tooth and results in buccal, anterior, and lateral displacement of the segment. Alternatively, palatal fractures may occur through the maxillary tuberosity (lateral palatal split), involving a dentoalveolar segment bearing the molar teeth. This fragment may displace superiorly, laterally and posteriorly. Both fracture patterns may coexist and are extremely difficult to treat. Rarely, coronal or transverse fractures of the palate may occur.

Conventional fixation techniques involving extensive plate and screw fixation along the pyriform aperture and anterior nasal spine have not consistently provided satisfactory accuracy or stability to correct the increased transverse maxillary arch dimension or changes in inclination of the dentoalveolar segments that occur with palatal fractures. Manson et al. have described techniques of transpalatal miniplate fixation through lacerations or incisions in the palatal mucosa supplemented by arch bar placement and fixation at the pyriform aperture, in addition to the usual fixation along the medial and lateral maxillary buttresses (Fig. 4.2.10, insets; Manson et al. 1983, 1990). Reduction and fixation of the palate is performed initially to restore proper width of the maxillary arch and is followed by buttress fixation. It is recommended to maintain mandibulomaxillary fixation for 3 weeks postoperatively followed by motion and soft diet. As bone healing tends to be slower following palatoalveolar fractures, it is recommended to watch for occlusal discrepancies and drift up to 4 months after fixation. Due to local symptoms hardware removal in the roof of the mouth may be required.

Alveolar Ridge. When alveolar ridge fractures occur in isolation, management consists of reduction of the dentoalveolar segment and fixation to stable adjacent maxillary segments using 26-gauge wire loops or arch bars. This is immobilized for 4 weeks, during which time the patient maintains a soft diet and regular oral hygiene.

If there are associated maxillary fractures, it becomes difficult to achieve stability in this fashion. The use of an acrylic wafer splint may provide some degree of stability, but open reduction and plate fixation is usually required. Mini- or microplate systems may be employed. An attempt at achieving two points of stabilization prevents rotation and tilting of the dentoalveolar segment, and care must be taken to avoid placing screws in the apices of the adjacent teeth. Screws should not be longer than 4 mm to avoid tooth root injury. Soft-tissue attachments must be maintained to the dentoalveolar segments. Loss of gingival tissue from these segments due to trauma or exposure may devascularize the teeth. If a segment becomes devascularized, stability of the fracture is improved by replacement and fixation. However, should it remain clearly nonviable, a tooth extraction or removal of the segment may be necessary.

4.2.2 Upper Midface (Le Fort II and III)

The rules described in Sect. 4.2.1 also apply for the reduction and fixation of fractures of the upper midface.

4.2.2.1 Anatomy

The upper midface includes both zygomatic bones, the orbits whose superior sections belong to the upper face, and the central nasoethmoidal region (see Fig. 4.1.1 c).

As it has been said before the classic fracture patterns II and III as described by Le Fort are rarely seen. These fractures are observed mostly in combination with skull base or cranial vault fractures as well as with Le Fort I and mandibular fractures. In these instances they are part of panfacial fractures.

4.2.2.2 Diagnosis

In addition to the clinical evaluation – which generally provides only a rough impression since swelling and the overlying soft tissues hide the underlying bony structures – X-ray evaluation via plain facial radiographs and 5 mm axial and, if possible, coronal CT images are the basis for a precise diagnosis and consequently the therapeutic approach.

4.2.2.3 Treatment

Midfacial fractures should be treated as early as possible, at least within the first week after the accident. As soon as the general condition of the patient allows it, definitive treatment should be undertaken. Fractures of the upper midface are generally quite extensive and include damage to the soft tissues. As noted by Manson (see Sect. 4.1), delayed treatment of midfacial fractures may mean a second injury to the already contused soft tissues. Edema should not be a reason to delay treatment since – on the contrary – we have observed that edema subsides faster when correct anatomic bone conditions have been achieved. This is especially true for orbital edema.

Intubation must not interfere with the ability to use mandibulomaxillary fixation during surgery. The original occlusion is one of the most important landmarks for correct reduction and fixation of midfacial fractures. Therefore either nasal, oral (behind the teeth, or if teeth are lacking), submental intubation, or an endoscopically placed tracheostoma is necessary.

In addition to the infraorbital approaches and the transconjunctival and upper blepharoplasty approach (see Figs. 2.1, and 2.5), the coronal incision is the most important approach. In recent years we have learned that extensive facial degloving is feasible, and via this exposure accurate skeletal reconstruction is possible. The coronal approach is mandatory especially for the correct reconstruction of the nasoethmoidal area and the correct placement of the zygomatic arch area. A hemicoronal incision should not be used. Eyebrow incisions and other routes via the nasal dorsum should be exceptions. A gingivobuccal incision is necessary for a correct fixation of the link between the upper and lower midface (Le Fort I area).

A very important precondition is a team approach. Since most of the upper midface fractures appear in combination with skull base fractures, the neurosurgeon in most areas is the most important partner. Depending on the special situation all specialties (oral-maxillofacial, plastic surgery, neurosurgery, ENT, and ophthalmology) should be involved at the same time in the treatment of panfacial fractures.

It is also important to visualize all fractures first before any fracture is stabilized. In severely comminuted fracture situations a preliminary approximation may be performed with wire before definite fixation with plates and screws is undertaken.

Upper midface fractures are located between the cranial vault and the occlusal unit.

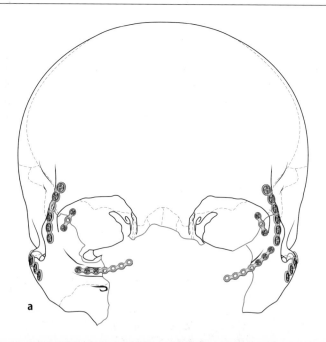

a

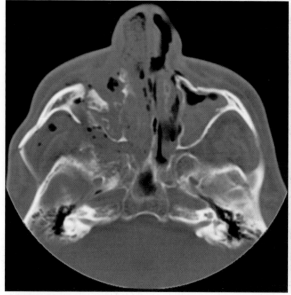

b

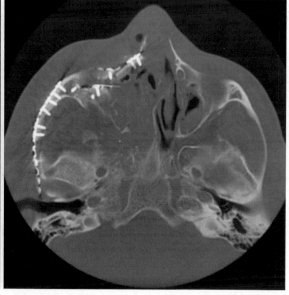

c

Fig. 4.2.12 a–c

a Diagram showing reconstruction and fixation of outer facial frame, consisting mainly of correct positioning of zygomatic bones to the cranial vault and posterior root of zygoma. This may be the first step in an outside to inside management.

b CT scan, axial view. Severe fracture of left zygoma with considerable displacement of the zygomatic arch, necessitating exposure via coronal approach.

c CT scan, axial view. Repair of zygomatic arch with 2.0 miniplates after exposure of both zygomatic arches for comparison reasons.

Although establishment of the correct occlusion is absolutely mandatory as a guideline, for correct reduction of upper midfacial fractures it may be misleading. Formerly, when we used wire for fixation together with craniofacial suspension, we often observed a considerable amount of telescoping in the Le Fort II and III areas with facial deformation although the occlusion was correct.

Gruss (1986) stressed the importance of the correct reconstruction of the outer facial frame (Fig. 4.2.12 a) for proper reestablishment of the facial dimensions. The fixation of both zygomas in the correct position in relation to the cranial vault guaranties correct facial width and

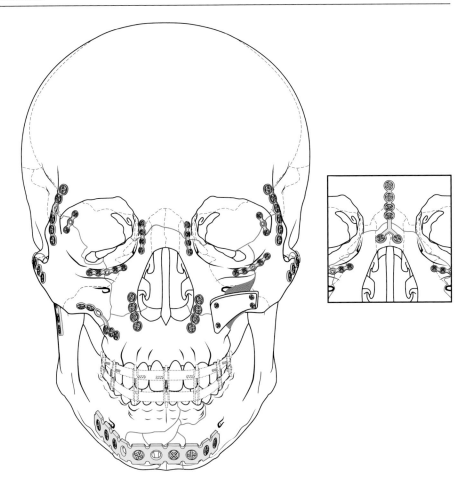

Fig. 4.2.13

Fixation of central midface to the outer facial frame and to the frontal bar within the nasal ridge with the 1.3 system. *Inset*: Fixation at the nasal ridge area with one 2.0 plate as an other option. The vertical buttresses are stabilized with the 2.0 system or a bone graft. Intermaxillary fixation is kept only during surgery.

helps to find the correct position for the nasoethmoidal complex. Therefore it is also a key area for reestablishing the correct facial projection and facial length. This is part of the presently advocated concept of an "outside to inside" management. Even in unilateral upper midface fractures it may be necessary to use a coronal approach since it may be important to compare the position of the unfractured zygomatic arch with the reduced arch (Fig. 4.2.12 b, c). Reconstruction of the central part of the upper midface – the nasoethmoidal complex – is extensively described in Sect. 4.3.

Reestablishment of the correct intercanthal distance by means of correctly placed transnasal wires is a very important step (see Figs. 4.1.5, 4.3.3 b, 4.3.4 b). Securing the links between central and lateral upper midface in the area of the inferior orbital rim, as well as fixation to the frontal bar and along the medial buttress, follows thereafter (Fig. 4.2.13). After the complete reconstruction of the orbital frame the orbit itself is reconstructed (see Sect. 4.5). Thereafter the occlusal unit with correct mandibulomaxillary fixation is fixed with plates and and screws at the buttress zones (medial and lateral) to the upper midface.

In extensive midface fracture situations (panfacial fractures) the vertical buttresses should be stabilized with the 2.0 system. The links to the cranial vault at the zygomaticofrontal sutures should also be stabilized with the 2.0 system in these instances. If fixation in the nasal root area is performed with one plate, it should preferably be a 2.0 plate (Fig. 4.2.13, inset), while in the situation of fixation with two plates the 1.3 system could be used (Fig. 4.2.13). The horizontal buttresses in the zygomatic arch area are fixed preferably with the 2.0 system (see Figs. 4.2.5 b, and 4.2.12 c) while stabilization in the orbital rim area is adequate with 1.3 plates (Figs. 4.2.12, 4.2.13).

Figure 4.2.14 presents a further example of a typically dislocated Le Fort III fracture with a zygomatic fracture

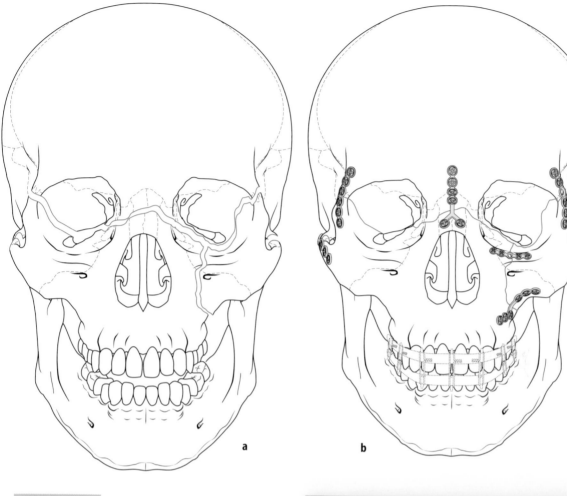

Fig. 4.2.14 a, b

a Diagram of a Le Fort III fracture with zygomatic fracture on the left and typical dislocation.
b Diagram showing fixation of fracture shown in **a**, using the 2.0 and 1.3 system.

on the right and its stabilization. Figure 4.2.15 demonstrates adequate fixation of a Le Fort III fracture on the left in combination with an orbital fracture on the left and a Le Fort II fracture on the right on a water's view.

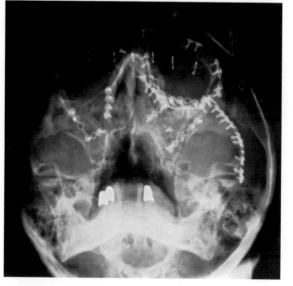

Fig. 4.2.15

X-ray (water's view) after fixation of a Le Fort II fracture on the right, and a severe orbitozygomatic fracture on the left. The patient was edentulous in the maxillary area.

References and Suggested Reading

Adams WM (1942) Internal wiring fixation of facial fractures. Surgery 12:523–540

Bechtol CO, Ferguson AB, Laing PG (1959) Metals and engineering in bone and joint surgery. Williams and Wilkins, Baltimore

Ciaburro H, Dupont C, Prevost Y, Cloutier GE (1973) Forward traction in the correction of the retrodisplaced maxilla. Can Med Assoc J 108:1511

Danis A (1949) Theorie et pratique de l'osteosynthèse. Masar, Paris

Diehl K, Hanser U, Hort W, Mittelmeier H (1974) Biomechanische Untersuchungen über die maximalen Vorspannkräfte der Knochenschrauben in verschiedenen Knochenabschnitten. Arch Orthop Unfall Chir 80:89

Ferraro JW, Berggren RB (1973) Treatment of complex facial fractures. J Trauma 13:783–787

Fialkov JA, Phillips JH, Walmsley SL (1994) The effect of infection and lag screw rigid fixation on the union of membranous bone grafts in a rabbit mode. Plast Reconstr Surg 93:574–581

Gentry LR, Manor WF, Turski PA, Strogher CM (1983) High-resolution CT analysis of facial struts in trauma: normal anatomy. Am J Radiol 140:523

Gruss JS, Mackinnon SE (1986) Complex maxillary fractures: role of buttress reconstruction and immediate bone grafts. Plast Reconstr Surg 78:9–22

Gruss JS, Phillips JH (1992) Rigid fixation of Le Fort maxillary fractures in rigid fixation of the craniomaxillofacial skeleton. Butterworth-Heinemann, London

Hughes AN, Jordan BA (1972) The mechanical properties of surgical bone screws and some aspects of insertion practice. Injury 4:25–38

Klotch DW, Gilland R (1987) Internal fixation vs conventional therapy in midface fractures. J Trauma 27:1136–1148

Kuepper RC, Harrigan WF (1977) Treatment of midfacial fractures at Bellevue Hospital Centre, 1955–1976. J Oral Surg 35:420–422

Kuhn A, McIff T, Cordey FW et al (1995) Bone deformtion by thread-cutting and thread-forming cortex screws. Injury 26 [Suppl]1:12–21

Le Fort R (1901) Etude experimentale sur les fractures de la machoire inferieure. I, II, III. Rev Chir Paris 23:208, 360, 479

Luce EA, Tubbs TD, Moore AM (1979) Review of 1000 major facial fractures and associated injuries. Plast Reconstr Surg 63:26–30

Manson PN (1986) Some thoughts on the classification and treatment of Le Fort fractures. Ann Plast Surg 17:356–363

Manson PN, Crawley WA, Yaremchuk MJ et al (1985) Midface fractures: advantages of immediate extended open reduction and bone grafting. Plast Reconstr Surg 76:1–10

Manson PN, Glassman D, Vander Kolk C et al (1990) Rigid stabilization of sagittal fractures of the maxilla and palate. Plast Reconstr Surg 85:711–717

Manson PN, Hoopes JE, Su CT (1980) Structural pillars of the facial skeleton: an approach to the management of Le Fort fractures. Plast Reconstr Surg 66:54–61

Manson PN, Shack RB, Leonard LG et al (1983) Sagittal fractures of the maxilla and palate. Plast Reconstr Surg 72:484–488

Phillips JH, Rahn BA (1989) Comparison of compression and torque measurements of self-tapping and pretapped screws. Plast Reconstr Surg 83:447–456

Rudderman RH, Mullen RL (1992) Biomechanics of facial skeleton. Clin Plast Surg 19:11–29

Schilli W, Ewers R, Niederdellmann H (1981) Bone fixation with screws and plates in the maxillo-facial region. Int J Oral Surg 10 [Suppl]1:329

Sicher H, DeBrul EL (1970) Oral anatomy, 5th edn. St. Louis

4.3 Naso-Orbital-Ethmoid Fractures

Contributors: Beat Hammer
             Joachim Prein

4.3.1 Definition

The term naso-orbito-ethmoid (NOE) fractures is
employed for injuries involving the area of confluence of
the nose, orbits, and ethmoids (Gruss 1985; Paskert et al.
1988). A number of delicate structures are involved in
these fractures: the nose, medial and lower orbits, frontal sinus and anterior skull base, and the pyriform rim.
Managing all these structures and reconstructing the
complex three-dimensional architecture of the NOE
area are among the most difficult problems in treating
facial trauma.

4.3.2 Anatomy

The main structural buttress of the NOE area is the frontal process of the maxilla, which articulates cranially to
the internal angular process of the frontal bone. This
buttress contains the insertion of the medial canthal ligament (Fig. 4.3.1) and extends superiorly beyond it. The
canthal bearing area is also referred to as a "central fragment" (Markowitz et al. 1991), which shows typical fracture patterns (see below). The thin and easily comminuted lamina papyracea of the ethmoids is located posterior to the central fragment. Cranially the internal
angular process of the frontal bone is anterior and
superior to the anterior wall of the frontonasal duct.
Patency of the frontonasal duct may be lost in highly
comminuted NOE fractures, and obliteration of the
frontal sinus is then necessary (Stanley 1979).

Between the two central fragments the nasal bones
arch to form the proximal nasal skeleton. These small
and fragile bones often have multiple fractures. However, skeletal support and projection of the nose
depends proximally on the support of the nasal pyramid
and distally on the cartilaginous septum. The need for

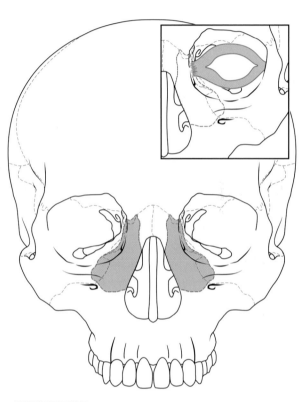

Fig. 4.3.1

The frontal process of the maxilla is the main structural buttress of the naso-orbital-ethmoid area, containing the insertion of the medial canthal ligament (*inset*). It is refered to as the
"central fragment."

dorsal nasal bone grafting is determined by the degree
of comminution to these structures.

4.3.3 Fracture Patterns

Three typical fracture patterns can be distinguished
(Markowitz et al. 1991), which occur either unilaterally
or bilaterally. The fracture patterns differ in the degree
of displacement and comminution of the canthal ligament bearing "central" fragment.

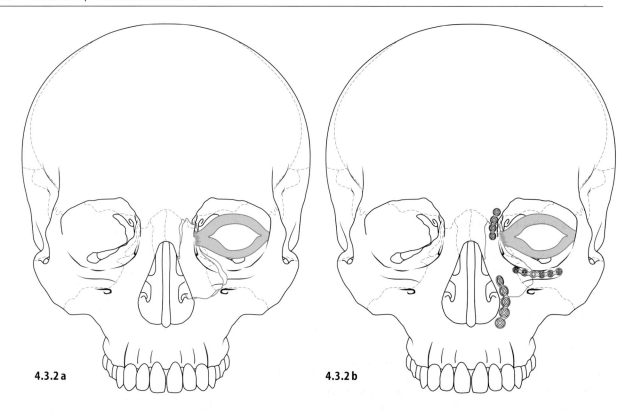

4.3.2 a   **4.3.2 b**

Type 1 (Fig. 4.3.2). In Type I fractures there is a single large fragment bearing the canthal ligament. This fragment is easily stabilized with miniplates or the 1.3 system. Type I injuries may be either complete or incomplete (greenstick fracture at the internal angular process of the frontal bone and may be uni- or bilateral).

Type II (Fig. 4.3.3). Here there is some degree of comminution of the central fragment, but the canthal ligament is attached to a fragment large enough to be stabilized with wires or the 1.3 plate and screw system. The comminution is external to the canthal ligament insertion.

Type III (Fig. 4.3.4). In Type III fractures comminution extends beneath the insertion of the canthal ligament. Canthal detachment is required to achieve the bone reduction. Direct canthopexy is necessary, with attention to construction of the canthal insertion point which should be posterior and superior to the lacrimal fossa.

Fig. 4.3.2 a, b

a NOE fracture, type I. There is a single large fragment containing the insertion of the medial canthal ligament.
b Stabilization of a NOE fracture, type I. The 2.0 and 1.3 systems are used. Remark: under certain circumstances, stabilization can be carried out without the plate at the frontonasal juncture, e.g., in fractures undislocated at the internal angular process of the frontal bone.

Fig. 4.3.3 a, b

a In NOE fractures type II there is some degree of fragmentation of the central fragment. However, the fragment containing the insertion of the canthal ligament is large enough to be stabilized with a plate. ▶
b Stabilization is achieved with a combination of 1.3 plates and a transnasal wire. The wire is inserted through the ligament-bearing fragment and should prevent outward rotation of this fragment.

Fig. 4.3.4 a, b

a NOE fracture type III. There are multiple small fragments. The fragment containing the insertion of the canthal ligament is too small to be stabilized. There may even be avulsion of the canthal ligament. ▶
b Stabilization of a NOE fracture type III. The small bone fragments are aligned and stabilized with 1.3 mini- or 1.0 microplates. To reconstruct the canthal ligament insertion, a direct transnasal canthopexy is necessary. The insertion point is created posterior and superior to the lacrimal fossa. If the bone in this area is missing, the insertion point may be created with a bone graft or a 2.0 plate as shown in the figure. The most common error is to insert the ligament too far anteriorly.

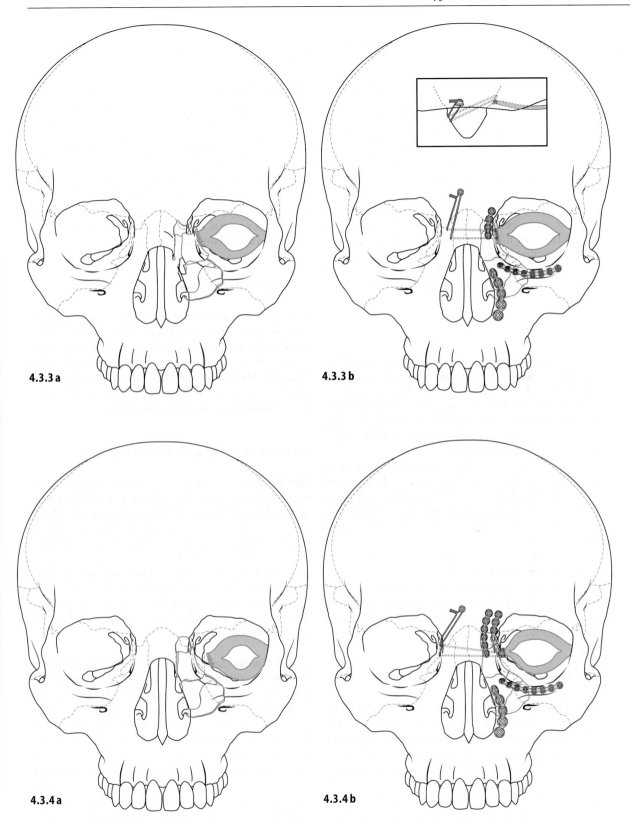

4.3.3 a

4.3.3 b

4.3.4 a

4.3.4 b

4.3.4 Plates Used for Internal Fixation of NOE Fractures

Plates from the midface sets 1.0 (micro) and 1.3/1.5 (miniplates) are used to stabilize NOE fractures. Microplates are especially helpful in putting the very small fragments of the nasal root together. They also may be used to link a large central fragment to the frontal bone. Miniplates are indicated when increased mechanical stability is required. Because of their relative thickness *they should not be employed anterior to the lacrimal crest.*

NOE fractures are the only type of injury in which stainless steel wires are still used for transnasal reduction and fixation. In type II or III injuries transnasal wiring of the central fragment or/and direct transnasal canthopexy is used to reduce the intercanthal distance, or distance between the frontal process of the maxilla.

4.3.5 Exposure

A combination of coronal, lower eyelid, and upper buccal sulcus incisions is usually employed. The coronal flap is reflected to expose the nose. In most cases dissection of at least two-thirds of the orbital circumference is necessary. Stripping of the canthal ligament from the bone is avoided, except in type III injuries where the fractures extend beneath the canthal insertion.

If there are fractures of the posterior frontal sinus wall or anterior skull base, cranial base exploration and dural repair may be required. If the anterior wall of the frontal sinus is fractured, all fragments are temporarily removed, which exposes the interior of the sinus and the nasofrontal duct.

The orbital floor and the infraorbital rim are exposed through a lower eyelid incision.

Type I fractures undisplaced at the internal angular process of the frontal bone do not require exposure with a coronal incision but only the lower eyelid and gingival buccal sulcus.

4.3.6 Diagnosis

Clinical Examination. Every injury to the central midface is suspicious for a NOE fracture. The clinical examination should include mobility and comminution of the central fragment and loss of septal support for the nose. Severe nasal fractures may be misdiagnosed as NOE injuries, but more frequently NOE fractures are misdiagnosed as nasal fractures. An accurate diagnosis can be made with bimanual examination. Furtheron motion of the canthal-bearing segment can be detected between finger and clamp, placing the clamp internally and the finger externally. Gentle pressure on the nasal dorsum

(Paskert et al. 1988;) allows examination of septal support for the nose, thereby assessing the need for dorsal bone grafting.

Computed Tomography. While the NOE injury itself is evaluated clinically, CT scans are indispensable in the diagnosis of associated injuries (orbits, frontal sinus, skull base) and to confirm the pattern of the NOE fracture. Details for the other fractures are given in the sections dealing with these injuries.

The NOE fracture diagnosis requires (at a minimum) fractures surrounding the "central fragment"; these include fractures of the nose, orbit, medial orbital wall, and inferior orbital rim. Fractures of the internal orbit (floor and medial orbital wall) are routine.

4.3.7 Operative Treatment

Operative treatment should be undertaken as early as possible. This consists of graded exposures with anatomic reduction and rigid fixation of bone fragments. Special attention must be paid to the medial canthal ligament. The fracture usually extends into the nasomaxillary or zygomaticomaxillary buttress, and therefore a buccal sulcus incision is necessary.

4.3.7.1 Management of the Central Fragment

Type I Injuries (see Fig. 4.3.2). A large canthal ligament bearing fragment may be reduced and stabilized with plates alone. In this case plates at the infraorbital rim and pyriform aperture stabilize the fragment. Before placing the plate at the infraorbital rim the articulation of the fragment with the nasal process of the frontal bone must be ensured to avoid malrotation. This fracture is stabilized by a 1.3-mm plate at the inferior orbital rim and a 2.0-mm plate at the pyriform aperture. Microplates are not sufficient to stabilize the fragment against rotation.

Type II Injuries (see Fig. 4.3.3). The ligament bearing fragment is isolated without stripping the ligamentous insertion. Temporary alignment of the bone fragments with wires may facilitate reduction. Two 0.3-mm (28-gauge) transnasal wires are passed through drill holes in the central fragment. The wires must be placed posterior and superior to the lacrimal fossa. The task of this wire is to secure the correct rotational position of the central fragment and maintain the correct intercanthal distance. Miniplates, 1.3, or microplates are employed to stabilize the multiple small fragments of the nose (Fig. 4.3.5b), or, interfragmental wires can be used.

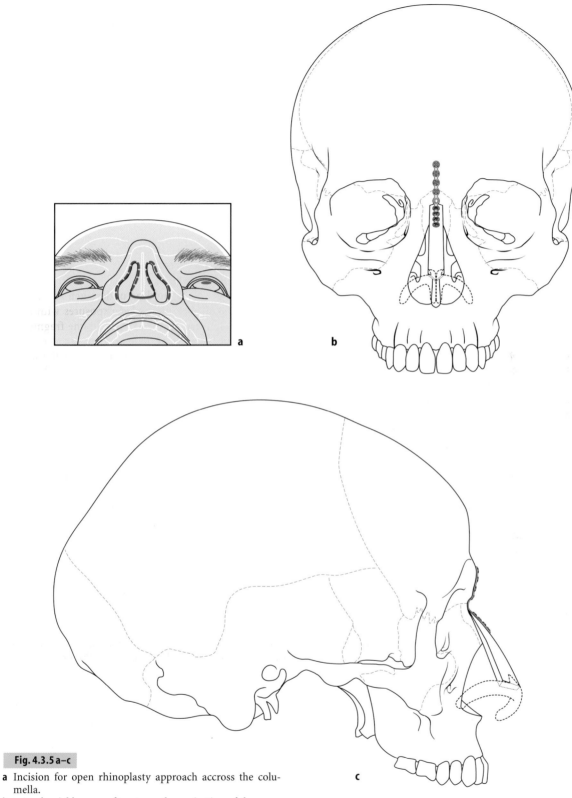

Fig. 4.3.5 a–c

a Incision for open rhinoplasty approach accross the columella.

b, c A calvarial bone graft restores the projection of the nose. The bone graft is cantilevered to the frontal bone with a 2.0 miniplate. The tip of the graft is placed between the two crura of the alar cartilages.

Type III Injuries (Figs. 4.3.4). In Type III injuries the central fragment is too small to be used for canthopexy, or fractures extend beneath the canthal insertion. There may also be even avulsion of the medial canthal ligament, although this is a rare event. Reconstruction of these fractures requires a direct transnasal canthopexy after bone reconstruction. Initially the canthal ligament is completely detached. If a bone fragment is left attached to the canthal ligament, it may interfere with direct canthopexy. Small bone fragments may be aligned and fixed with 1.3 or microplates.

4.3.7.2 Transnasal Canthopexy

There are two important steps in canthopexy: First the ligament is identified and transfixed with a suture. This is done through a small transverse external incision medial to the palpebral fissure (Stanley 1979). This suture is passed directly to the internal aspect of the coronal incision and to a separate set of transnasal wires. The second step involves choosing the insertion point for the transnasal wire. It should be chosen posterior and superior to the lacrimal fossa. In some cases, the fragile bone of this area is comminuted. The insertion point of the transnasal wire must then be constructed. This can be done with a bone graft fixed with a miniplate placed along the medial orbital wall. The wire is then passed through the bone graft, or one of the holes of the miniplate (see Fig. 4.3.4b) (Hammer 1995). The bone graft must be positioned with a miniplate to be stable.

4.3.7.3 Nasal Reconstruction

The nasal bones are reduced and stabilized with mini-, microplates or wires, and the glabella and frontal sinus are reconstructed by bone reassembly. If there is lack of septal support, dorsal nasal bone grafting is necessary to reestablish the height and anterior projection of the nose. Cranial bone grafts or rib are the choices. To allow precise placement of a rib graft and provide columella support an open rhinoplasty approach is preferred (Fig. 4.3.5a). Placement of the dorsal nasal bone graft and fixation to the nasal root with a miniplate are shown in Fig. 4.3.5b,c and see Fig. 4.2.5b,d. Nonabsorbable sutures suspend the cartilaginous septum to the dorsal graft. The tip of the graft is placed underneath and between the domes of the alar cartilages. In this way a naturally appearing, smooth nasal tip can be obtained.

4.3.8 NOE Fracture-Related Problems

4.3.8.1 Lacrimal Duct Injuries

Lacrimal duct injuries resulting in obstruction are present in less than 10% of fractures involving this area. Primary exploration of the lacrimal apparatus is generally not recommended unless an open laceration has divided the lacrimal system.

4.3.8.2 Frontal Sinus

The management of frontal sinus injuries is discussed in Sect. 4.6.

4.3.8.3 Skull Base Injuries

Associated skull base injuries may be repaired transcranially. For skull base injuries localized to the anterior cranial fossa, "subcranial" management (a minicraniotomy) is often another option providing limited exposure.

4.3.8.4 Orbital Reconstruction

Section 4.5 deals with the management of internal orbital fractures.

References and Suggested Reading

Gruss JS (1985) Naso-ethmoid-orbital fractures: classification and role of primary bone grafting. Plast Reconstr Surg 75 (3):303–315

Hammer B (1995) Orbital fractures. Diagnosis, operative treatment, secondary corrections. Hogrefe-Huber, Bern, pp 52–54

Markowitz BL, Manson PN, Sargent L, Vander Kolk CA, Yaremchuk M, Glassman D, Crawley WA (1991) Management of the medial canthal tendon in nasoethmoid orbitae fractures: the importance of the central fragment in classification and treatment. Plast Reconstr Surg 87 (5):843–853

Paskert JP, Manson PN, Iliff NT (1988) Nasoethmoidal and orbital fractures. Chir Plast Surg 15 (2):209–223

Stanley RB Jr (1979) Fractures of the frontal sinus. Clin Plast Surg 16 (1):115–123

4.4 Zygomatic Complex Fractures

Contributors: Bernard L. Markowitz
              Paul N. Manson

4.4.1 Definition

Zygomatic fractures include any injury which disrupts the five articulations of the zygoma with the adjacent craniofacial skeleton (Fig. 4.4.1): the zygomaticofrontal suture, infraorbital rim, zygomaticomaxillary buttress, zygomatic arch, and zygomaticosphenoid suture. The degree to which the sutures are involved depends on the direction and magnitude of the fracturing force. Dis-

Fig. 4.4.1

The five articulations of the zygoma with the craniofacial skeleton are visualized. Any of the multiple zygomatic fracture sites may be exposed either to confirm alignment or to provide fixation.

The best areas to determine reduction are the internal surface of the orbit ❺, and the zygomaticomaxillary buttress ❸, inferior orbital rim ❷, and the zygomatic arch ❹ (the multiple articulations of the zygoma).

Inset: The placement of bone hook underneath malar eminence allowing reduction of the fracture in an anterolateral direction.

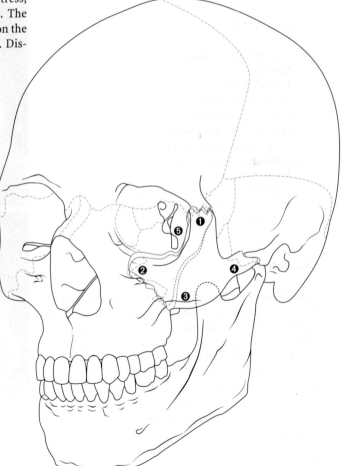

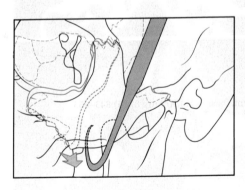

placement is parallel to the direction and force of the injury and the action of the masseter muscle. Regional, monoarticular fractures (isolated zygomatic arch, etc.) are also seen.

4.4.2 Treatment

Displaced or unstable zygomatic fractures benefit from open reduction. The extent of open reduction is determined by displacement and comminution of the five articulations. There are two reasons to explore any of the multiple zygomatic fracture sites: to confirm alignment and to provide fixation. Operative exposure may be used for one or both purposes. In many zygomatic fractures the degree of stability and the minimal displacement do not justify open reduction. The majority of displaced zygomatic fractures (type I; Fig. 4.4.2) may be managed with inferior exposures and stabilization. Fractures which exhibit lateral displacement of the zygomatic arch (type II) (Figs. 4.4.3) require superior exposures in addition to inferior approaches (see Figs. 2.1, 2.5).

4.4.3 Exposure

For details see Chap. 2.

- Inferior orbital exposure
  - Subciliary
  - Extended subciliary
  - Transconjunctival
  - Lateral canthotomy
- Inferior maxillary exposure
  - Gingival buccal sulcus incision
- Superior orbital exposure
  - Brow
  - Lateral limb of upper blepharoplasty
  - Canthal detachment with lower eyelid incision
  - Coronal

4.4.4 Reduction

Reduction of zygomatic fractures is performed through a combination of incisions as explained in Chap. 2. Exposure of the fracture site provides an opportunity to confirm alignment and provide fixation. As a general principle, alignment of the zygoma must be confirmed in at least three areas and fixation in at least two. An anterolateral and superior reduction force, directed from underneath the medial aspect of the malar eminence, is usually necessary to reposition the displaced zygoma.

One way to achieve this is via a bone hook, which is introduced underneath the malar eminence through a

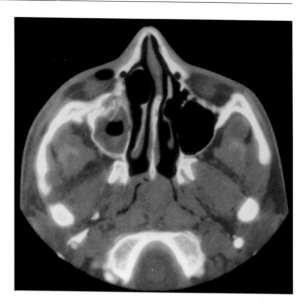

Fig. 4.4.2

Low energy zygoma fracture. No lateral displacement of the arch. In this case anterior approach.

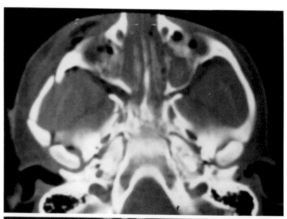

a

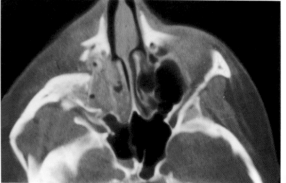

b

Fig. 4.4.3 a, b

High-energy zygoma fracture. Considerable lateral displacement of the zygomatic arch and displacement of body. Coronal approach required.

small 3 mm incision in the skin of the cheek (Fig. 4.4.1, inset). Further access is achieved through either the mouth, the upper sulcus incision, or the external incisions by dividing the deep temporal fascia above the zygomatic arch, near the zygomaticofrontal suture, exposing the temporalis muscle, and then placing a blunt elevator (such as Dingman) behind the malar eminence. A force opposing that of the injury is generated, and the fracture is reduced.

For intraoral reduction the zygomaticomaxillary buttress is followed superiorly to its junction with the malar eminence. At times fibers of the masseter need to be elevated. A blunt elevator is positioned beneath the eminence or within the lateral aspect of the maxillary sinus and an appropriate reduction force produced by delivering force to the malar eminence. Movement of the displaced bone into anatomic alignment is sometimes appreciated by a "click" and confirmed by inspecting each buttress articulation. Minor adjustments in position are performed with Brown forceps prior to fixation.

The zygomaticosphenoid suture is a commonly overlooked determinant of anatomic alignment (see Fig. 4.4.1). Considerable experience is required to appreciate the use of this area as an isolated fracture alignment site. The zygomaticomaxillary buttress is an excellent determinant, the infraorbital rim is a good determinant, and the zygomaticofrontal suture is a poor determinant of proper reduction. Zygomatic arch reductions sets midfacial width and, reciprocally, malar eminence projection (Table 4.1).

4.4.5 Stabilization

The "stability" of the reduction (determined by the degree of comminution within the zygomatic complex and at its articulations) determines the type and number of fixation devices to be used. Frequently 1.3 and miniplating systems (1.5 and 2.0) are used in combination. Low-profile 1.3-mm plates are less conspicuous in areas where devices may be visible and palpable (infraorbital rim), but they may not be sufficient to ensure rigidity at the zygomaticofrontal suture. The stronger but larger 2.0 miniplates are best reserved for areas covered by adequate soft tissue (zygomaticomaxillary buttress, zygomatic arch, and in some cases zygomaticofrontal suture; Figs. 4.4.4–4.4.6; see also Table 4.1).

The zygomaticofrontal suture contains the strongest bone for stabilization; the zygomaticomaxillary buttress is a good location for stabilization. The inferior orbital rim and zygomatic arch are fair areas for stabilization (Figs. 4.4.4–4.4.6).

Type I Fractures. Numerous plating schemes are successfully employed for the stabilization of zygomatic fractures. Fracture stability must be considered carefully

Table 4.1. Fracture sites as points of alignment and strength of fixation as suture sites

Value of fracture sites as points of alignment (↑ Increasing value)	Strength of fixation as suture sites (↑ Increased strength)
Zygomatic arch–orbit (greater wing sphenoid)	Z-F suture
Inferior orbital rim	Z-M buttress
Z-M buttress	Zygomatic arch
Z-F suture	Inferior rim

after the initial reduction maneuver, and appropriate plates chosen for fixation. Fractures that "snap" back into place and are stable have different fixation requirements (Fig. 4.4.4) than injuries that are comminuted and require positioning placement, such as temporary interosseous wires, or constant reduction force to maintain the position prior to rigid fixation (Figs. 4.4.5, 4.4.6; Pearl 1990).

For most type I zygoma fractures stabilization of the inferior orbital rim, zygomaticomaxillary buttress, and zygomaticofrontal suture are routinely advised (see Fig. 4.4.5). Stable injuries may have two plate fixations (see Fig. 4.4.4). The initial fixation is provided by at least a miniplate at the zygomaticofrontal suture or the zygomaticomaxillary buttress while the remainder of the fracture sites may then be managed with 1.3 plates. When the buttress is comminuted, or the fracture pattern is not conducive to microplating, miniplates should be placed at the zygomaticofrontal suture and zygomaticomaxillary buttress. Microplates or 1.3 system plates are placed at the inferior orbital rim.

The 90° or 110° L or Y miniplate is best suited for the zygomaticomaxillary buttress (see Fig. 4.4.5). The low profile mini-DC plate or the 2.0, 1.5 or 1.3 system is used at the zygomaticofrontal suture (Fig. 4.4.6, insets 1–3). Screw holes must be directed away from tooth roots near the maxillary alveolus. A single 1.3 plate usually suffices at the inferior rim.

Type II Fractures. For type II fractures (Fig. 4.4.3), in addition to the described anterior points of fixation, the zygomatic arch is exposed, reduced, and stabilized. Zygomatic arch fixation is the initial step in the stabilization of type II fractures after eventual placement of positioning wires at the Z-F suture and the infraorbital rim. The anterior articulations are then stabilized as described above.

The key to correct zygomatic arch reduction and stabilization is the appreciation of its normal anatomy. The zygomatic arch is not a true arch but is straight in its middle portion. It is best stabilized with an adaption miniplate of the 2.0 system, fashioned by "overflattening" the central zone and then securing the reduction with 2.0 screws (see Fig. 4.4.6). At times an oblique sagittal fracture at the posterior aspect of the arch may be

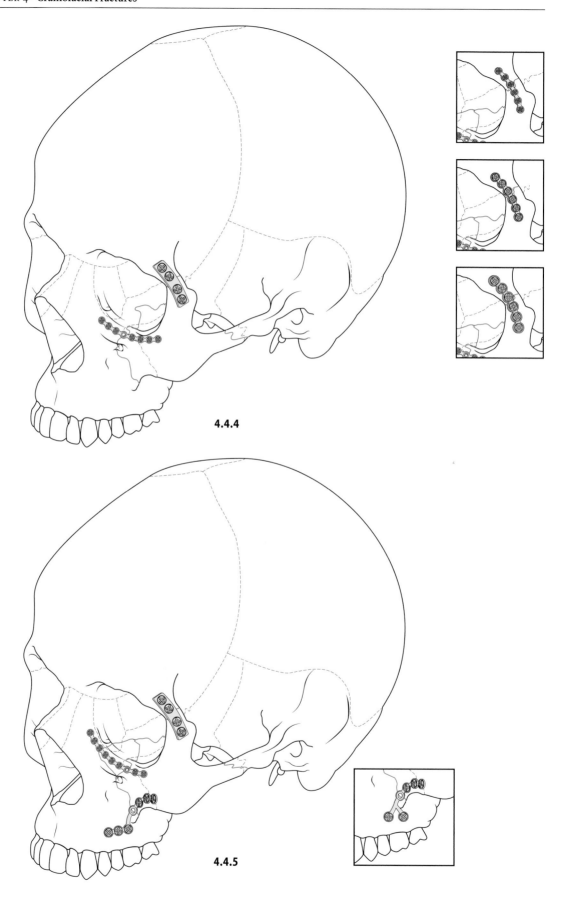

4.4.4

4.4.5

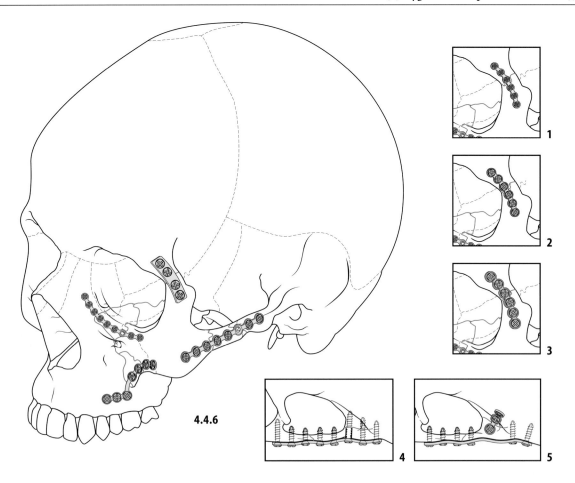

4.4.6

Fig. 4.4.4

◀ Two-plate fixation of the zygoma. Miniplate (1.3) fixation at the inferior orbital rim and miniplate (2.0) fixation at the zygomatico-frontal suture. The three *insets* show the various options in between 1.3 and 2.0 adaption plates at the lateral orbital rim.

Fig. 4.4.5

◀ Miniplate fixation in a comminuted fracture at three anterior fracture sites. Miniplate fixation at the zygomaticofrontal suture and zygomaticomaxillary buttress and 1.3-mm plate fixation at the orbital rim. The limbs of the L or Y miniplate in the zygomaticomaxillary buttress must be bent around tooth roots.

A longer L or Y miniplate is best suited for the comminuted zygomaticomaxillary buttress. The separate buttress fragment is lag-screwed to the plate.

Fig. 4.4.6

Miniplate fixation in a comminuted fracture of the lateral upper midface. In addition to the fixation type in Fig. 4.4.5 fixation of the zygomatic arch is performed with a 2.0 miniadaptation plate. *Inset 4*, lag screw fixation for a sagittal fracture at the posterior aspect of the arch. *Inset 5*, plate fixation for the roof of the glenoid fossa. *Insets 1–3* show the various options for fixation at the zygomatico-frontal suture.

managed with a lag screw (1.5 or 2.0 mm; see Fig. 4.4.6, inset 2). Screws should be diverted away from the temporomandibular joint. Plating the roof of the glenoid fossa may be required prior to arch plating (see Fig. 4.4.6, inset 3). A lag screw may be placed through one of the posterior holes of the plate.

4.4.6 Internal Orbit

Once the external orbital rim is stabilized, the internal orbit is evaluated and its continuity assessed. If a defect exceeding 5 mm is present, it must be entirely exposed and stable ledges identified for graft stabilization. Orbital wall defects larger than 1–2 cm are grafted with split (outer table) calvarial bone grafts or alloplast (Medpor 1.5 mm or polyvynil sheets). Titanium plates alone are used for small or large defects (see Fig. 4.5.6). Skull outer table or split rib grafts are used for larger defects. Grafts must be placed accurately to restore orbital volume. Globe position, because of edema, is frequently an imprecise guide to adequate restoration of orbital volume. Once grafts are placed, globe motility (forced duction) examinations are assessed and compared to pre- and postdissection ductions. The grafts are then anchored with lag or tandem screws. If complex (three or four wall fractures) are present, internal mesh or stable fixation should be used to provide a platform for orbital volume correction (see Sect. 4.5).

4.4.7 Soft-Tissue Closure

Strict attention must be given to layered closure which includes resuspension of the soft tissue. Lateral canthal reattachment is performed if the canthus has been detached (see Fig. 4.1.9). The lateral canthus is isolated and a 3-0 nonabsorbable suture is passed through the canthus and hooked through a plate hole at the zygomaticofrontal suture. When an extended transconjunctival incision is used, the divided canthus is carefully reapproximated. The malar fat pad is resuspended to an orbital rim plate with a 4-0 Prolene prior to closing the periosteal incisions in the lateral orbit and inferior orbital rim. The lower eyelid incision is closed with a Vicryl muscle suture. The skin is closed with interrupted 6-0 plain gut sutures.

The coronal incision is closed in two layers, the galea with 2-0 Vicryl and the scalp with staples. The superficial layer of the deep temporal fascia is repaired with 2-0 Vicryl as is the periosteum over the zygomaticofrontal suture.

Avoiding Complications. Problems associated with zygomatic fracture treatment can often be avoided by precise diagnosis, careful dissection for exposure, anatomic reduction by direct observation, stable fixation, the appropriate use of bone grafts, and soft-tissue closure.

References and Suggested Reading

Jackson IT (1989) Classification and treatment of orbito-zygomatic and orbitoethmoid fractures – the place of bone grafting and plate fixation. Clin Plast Surg 16:77–91

Larsen OD, Thomsen M (1976) Zygomatic fractures. Scan J Plast Reconstr Surg 12:59–63

Lundin K, Ridell A, Sanberg N, Ohman A (1973) One thousand maxillofacial and related fractures at the EENT Clinic in Gothenburg: a two year prospective study. Acta Otolaryngol 75:359

Manson PN, Ruas E, Iliff N et al (1987) Single eyelid incision for exposure of the zygomatic bone and orbital reconstruction. Plast Reconstr Surg 79:120–126

Matsunaga RS, Simpson W, Toffel PH (1988) Simplified protocol for treatment of malar complex fractures. Facial Plast Surg 5:269

Pearl RM (1990) Prevention of enophthalmos: a hypothesis. Ann Plast Surg 25:132–133

Stanley RB Jr (1989) The zygomatic arch as a guide to reconstruction of comminuted malar fractures. Otolaryngol Head Neck Surg 115:1459–1462

Tajima S (1977) Malar bone fractures: experimental fractures on the dried skull and clinical sensory disturbances. J Maxillofac Surg 5:150–156

Watumull D, Rohrich RJ (1991) Zygoma fracture fixation: a graduated approach to management based on recent clinical and biomechnaical studies. In: Manson PN (ed) Problems in plastic and reconstructive surgery. Lippincott, Philadelphia

Yanigasiwa E (1973) Pitfalls in the management of zygomatic fractures. Laryngoscope 83:527–543

4.5 Orbital Fractures

Contributor: Paul N. Manson

4.5.1 Definition

Fractures involving the orbit are common injuries that involve multiple surgical specialties. The magnitude of fractures within the orbit varies considerably. Simple fractures may involve only a portion of the internal bone area of the orbit, the common "blow-out" fracture. More commonly, multiple portions of the orbit are fractured with the orbital rim and several internal orbital walls therefore injured simultaneously. Most fractures of the orbit therefore require stabilization of both the rim and the internal portions of the orbit (Fig. 4.5.1). The regional approaches for stabilizing fractures of the rim are discussed in the Sect. 4.4 and Chap. 2 but are reviewed again here in the context of a broad reconstructive perspective for fractures of the orbit.

As a general principle the orbital rim is reconstructed by aligning its fractured parts with adjacent stabilized or intact structures. Simultaneously visualizing multiple areas of alignment increases the accuracy of the reduction. Initially, interfragment wiring or loose "two screw" fixation in a plate provides temporary but adjustable positioning of rim segments. Stable fixation then stabilizes the position while final adjustment is provided by manual positioning.

The bony orbit may be conceptualized in anterior, middle, and posterior sections (see Fig. 4.5.1): The anterior third of the orbit is the thick bony orbital rim. The middle section of the orbit is thin and often breaks before the rim, absorbing fracture forces. The posterior section of the orbit is thick and is thus protected from fracture by the dislocation of the anterior and middle orbital segments.

The orbital rim is divided into three segments: superiorly, the supraorbital section; medially, the nasoethmoidal section; laterally and inferiorly, the zygomatic section. The supraorbital region consists of the frontal bone laterally and the frontal sinus medially; the section

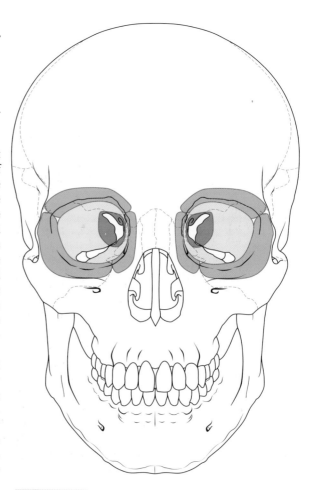

Fig. 4.5.1

The orbit consists of the rim and the internal orbit. The internal orbit is conceptualized in anterior, middle, and posterior sections. The anterior third of the orbit consists of the thick bony orbital rim which is divided into three sections. The rim has three components, supraorbital section, nasoethmoidal area, and zygomatic section. The middle section of the orbit is thin, often breaking before the rim and consists of four sections. The posterior portion of the orbit is thick and contains the superior and inferior orbital fissures and the optic foramen.

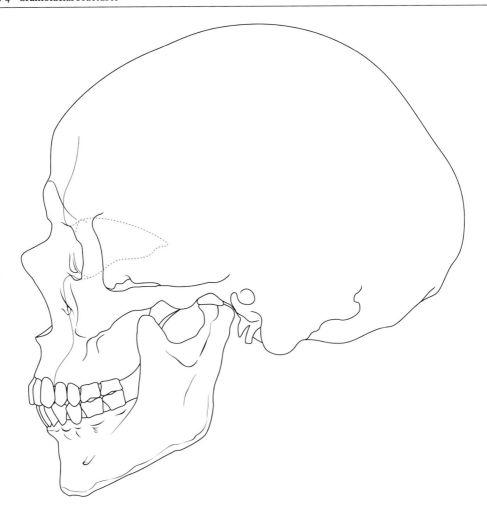

begins medially at the frontomaxillary suture (the junction of the internal angular process of the frontal bone with the frontal process of the maxilla). The supraorbital area extends laterally to the zygomaticofrontal suture and the external angular process of the frontal bone. The lateral and inferior portions of the orbital rim are formed by the zygomatic bone. The lower two-thirds of the medial orbital rim represents the nasoethmoidal area; the important characteristic here is the attachment of the medial canthus with the medial horn of the levator palpebrae superioris, and the medial attachment of Lockwood's ligament around the superior aspect of the lacrimal fossa.

Whitnall's tubercle is located on the inner aspect of the lateral orbital rim, 10 mm below the zygomaticofrontal suture and 2–4 mm posterior to the anterior margin of the lateral orbital rim. This provides attachment to the lateral canthal complex, consisting of the lateral canthal tendon, the lateral extension of the levator tendon, and Lockwood's suspensory ligament. Three foramina perforate the superior and inferior orbital rims. These are the supraorbital foramen (either a fora-

Fig. 4.5.2

The roof is bowed anteroposteriorly and mediolaterally. The floor inclines at a 30° angle from anterior to posterior. The floor of the orbit contains a postbulbar constriction. The optic foramen is located posterior and superior to the usually intact section of the orbital floor, 35–38 mm behind the rim.

men or notch) located in the supraorbital rim at the limbus of the cornea in straight forward gaze, and the infraorbital foramen, located 8–10 mm below the inferior orbital rim, parallel to the limbus of the cornea when the eye is in straight forward gaze. The third foramen is the zygomaticofacial foramen located in the lateral section of the malar eminence. Because these openings weaken the bone, fractures commonly occur in these areas and bruise the nerves and produce symptoms of anesthesia or hypesthesia in the nerve distribution.

The middle third of the orbit is thin and is composed of four sections: the roof, medial wall, floor, and lateral wall. The roof is a portion of the frontal bone and separates the anterior cranial fossa from the orbital cavity. It is a thin extension of the supraorbital rim and is arched

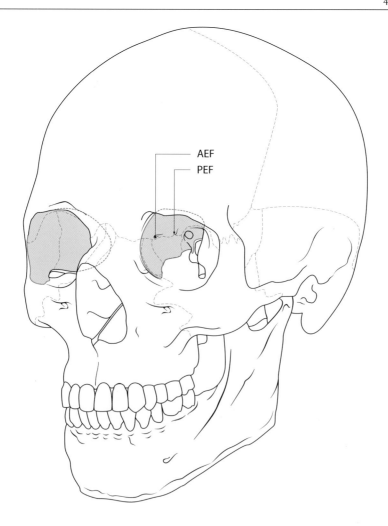

AEF
PEF

The medial wall separates the orbit from the ethmoid sinuses and nasal cavity. There is a postbulbar constriction of the orbit behind the globe in the medial wall and floor. The medial wall is directly in line with the optic foramen posteriorly. *AEF*, anterior ethmoidal foramen. *PEF*, posterior ethmoidal foramen. The lateral orbit is formed by the greater wing of the sphenoid. The anterior lip of the sphenoid is usually fractured in high-energy orbital fractures. Alignment of the lateral orbit forms one of the most accurate guides to volume restoration.

superiorly, anteroposteriorly, and mediolaterally. It is important to reconstruct the contour of the roof and floor (Fig. 4.5.2) in accordance to its curving structures, extending backward from the supraorbital rim, permitting a space for the globe in its proper position. The roof, from anterior to posterior, first inclines upward, then posteriorly, then finally inferiorly near the orbit apex.

The medial wall of the orbit consists of the thin orbital plate of the ethmoid bone which separates the orbit from the ethmoid sinuses and nasal cavity (Fig. 4.5.3). The medial wall of the orbit is formed by the thin orbital plate of the ethmoid bone but gains strength from

multiple partitions through the ethmoid sinuses. Anteriorly the lacrimal bone and its crest articulate with the frontal process of the maxilla. The anterior and posterior ethmoidal foramina in the medial wall of the orbit are at the same vertical level as the optic canal. The ethmoid foramina are located 24 and 35 mm, respectively, from the anterior lacrimal crest and serve as guides to the optic nerve located 40–45 mm from this bony landmark and 5–8 mm posterior to the posterior ethmoid foramen.

The floor of the orbit separates the orbit from the maxillary sinus. The orbital floor has an initial shallow convex section behind the rim, then inclines upward behind the globe, and inclines to meet the medial wall, creating a distinct bulge behind the globe (see Fig. 4.5.2). These convex curves of the medial wall and floor create a "postbulbar constriction" of the orbital cavity (see Figs. 4.5.2 and 4.5.3), which must be reconstructed when the orbit is rebuilt following fractures. Generally floor fractures first involve the floor medial to the infraorbital nerve groove or canal and then extend to the lower half of the medial wall of the orbit.

The lateral portion of the orbit (see Figs. 4.5.1, 4.5.3) is formed by the greater wing of the sphenoid, which articulates with the orbital process of the zygoma. The zygoma and the anterior half of the greater wing of the sphenoid are commonly fractured simultaneously. Achieving alignment of the entire lateral orbit is one of the most critical components of orbital volume restoration.

The posterior third of the orbit is constructed of thicker bone and incorporates the superior and inferior orbital fissures and the optic foramen (see Fig. 4.5.1). The superior orbital fissure is surrounded by the greater and lesser wings of the sphenoid bone. Important structures passing through this fissure include the third, fourth, and sixth cranial nerves and the ophthalmic division of the trigeminal nerve. The inferior orbital fissure separates the orbital floor from the lateral orbital wall. The infraorbital division of the maxillary portion of the trigeminal nerve, the zygomaticofacial nerve, and the infraorbital artery all pass through this fissure posteriorly. Anteriorly the inferior orbital fissure contains ligamentous structures, fat, and veins. The optic foramen is contained within the roots of the lesser wing of the sphenoid bone and transmits the optic nerve and ophthalmic artery. It is located 40–45 mm from the inferior orbital rim and is distinctly higher than the orbital floor, which serves to protect it in dissection.

4.5.2 Diagnosis

Fractures of the orbit are diagnosed both by physical examination and computed tomography (CT; Fig. 4.5.4a). CT scans are obtained in the axial and coronal planes with both bone and soft-tissue windows for each orientation. A thorough physical and radiographic examination is requisite to a satisfactory plan for reconstruction. This should consist of a visual inspection, palpation, assessment of visual acuity, visual fields, fundoscopy, and assessment of intraocular pressure. Duction evaluations are indicated when there is diplopia. The most common physical signs of an orbital fracture are periorbital ecchymosis and subconjuctival hematoma. Three-dimensional CT scans, while sometimes providing additional perspective, are not required.

4.5.3 Treatment

Isolated middle section (internal) orbital fractures (small fractures of the internal portion of the orbit) are best treated by bone grafting (Fig. 4.5.4b, c) or the use of an alloplastic implant, as desired. Autogenous tissues are generally preferred. The bone graft or alloplastic implant should be anchored behind the internal orbital rim with the "lag" or "tandem" screw technique or a

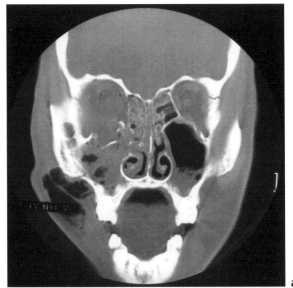

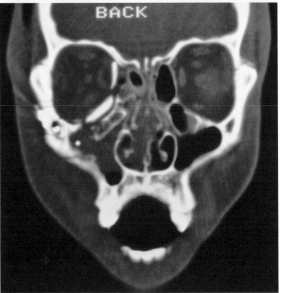

plate. This prevents displacement or migration of the implant; further, the use of stable fixation improves bone survival. Ductions are assessed before dissection, after dissection, and after insertion of the implant or graft to access freedom of the muscular apparatus.

It is important in dissecting a fracture defect inside the orbit to identify intact bone on all sides of the fracture. The posterior portion of intact bone forms a guide to internal orbital reconstruction and represents the intact bone "ledge." Posteriorly this intact "ledge" is often referred to as the "posterior ledge" and is usually located some 35–38 mm behind the orbital rim. The new orbital floor should be positioned to incline from just behind the reconstructed rim to reach this intact "ledge." Recent studies emphasize the importance of

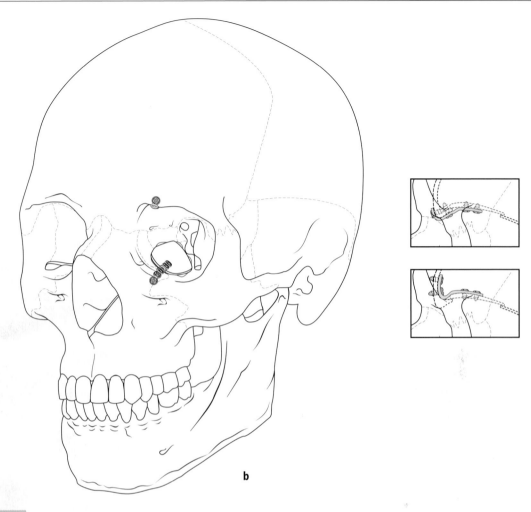

b

Fig. 4.5.4 a–c

a CT scan, coronal view. Fracture of medial orbital wall and orbital floor with considerable enlargement of the orbit.

b Small fractures of the floor or medial portion of the orbit are best treated by on-lay bone grafting or alloplastic material. The bone grafts or alloplastic material may be anchored either with a microplate or with a lag screw. Stabilization of larger superior and inferior orbit grafts requires stable fixation to the rims.

Insets: Orbital roof reconstruction either with extracranial or intracranial plating and bone grafts performed prior to frontal bone replacement.

c Reconstruction of orbital floor and medial orbital wall with autogenous bone grafts, securing the correct orbital volume.

ligament system by the bone graft material. Reconstruction of floor and roof defects from a lateral perspective is seen in the insets of Fig. 4.5.4 b.

4.5.4 Reconstruction of Ethmoid Defects

Ethmoid or medial orbital wall fractures are commonly a portion of a multiple wall orbital injury. Symmetric compression of the ethmoid air cells is frequently seen. Restoration of bony orbital volume requires bone grafting to reduce effective orbital volume. Several layers of bone graft should be placed at the ethmoid area to provide a thickness equal to that of the normal ethmoid region (Fig. 4.5.5). When simultaneous defects of the floor and the medial orbital wall are present, a strut of stable fixation material may be required to provide positioning support for other grafts (Fig. 4.5.6). A universal orbital floor plate (see Fig. 1.20 and Fig. 4.5.6 b) should be cut to the minimum size required. The use of a template may be appropriate for contouring.

It should be emphasized that all internal orbital plates require contouring, trimming of redundant

anatomic reconstruction of the bone defect rather than globe position at surgery as the best guide to volume restoration. Duction tests should be performed following the placement of either bone or alloplastic material. These are compared to duction examinations performed *before* the surgical dissection and *after* the surgical dissection. In this manner stiff duction examinations from muscle contusion or edema can be distinguished from impingement of the musculofibrous

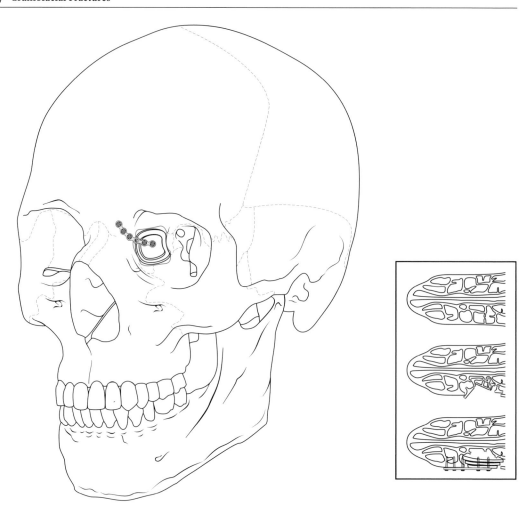

Fig. 4.5.5

Enlargement of medial orbital wall is seen by comparison of the width of the ethmoid cells in a CT scan. Several layers of bone grafts are placed in the medial orbit area through a coronal incision to provide thickness equal to that of the normal ethmoid region contralaterally.

Fig. 4.5.6 a, b

When extensive defects of both the floor and medial orbital ▶ wall exist simultaneously, a strut of stable fixation material such as an orbital wall plate (**a**) or an orbital floor plate (**b**) may be required for stable positioning of the grafts. Alternately, a graft can be linked to the orbital rim with a small plate which allows supervision of position of the remainder of the grafts (**a**).

wings, and anchoring tabs. All the wings cannot be left intact; most of the anchoring tabs should be trimmed except the exact minimum fixaton points desired. The use of titanium implants or plastic sheets in large orbital defects exposed to the maxillary and ethmoid sinuses permits the possibility of a late infection. With titanium plates the first infections were observed more than 1 year after implantation. Therefore the use of autogenous bone alone is preferred where possible as late infection is rare. Metallic implants cannot be considered a routine substitute for the use of autogenous material unless no other solution is possible.

There are two varieties of internal orbital plates. One is used for medial wall defects (see Fig. 1.20, 4.5.6a) and one for inferior wall defects (see Fig. 1.20, 4.5.6b).

4.5.5 Zygomatic (Lateral and Inferior Wall) Injuries

Zygomatic fractures involve injuries to the lateral and inferior portion of the orbital rim. The zygoma must be stabilized accurately by aligning it with all of its neighboring bones. A small increase in the size in the orbital rim diameter produces a dramatic increase in orbital volume; stabilizing the dimensions of the orbital rim controls orbital volume. Therefore it is important to achieve an exact zygomatic reduction which stabilizes the orbital volume.

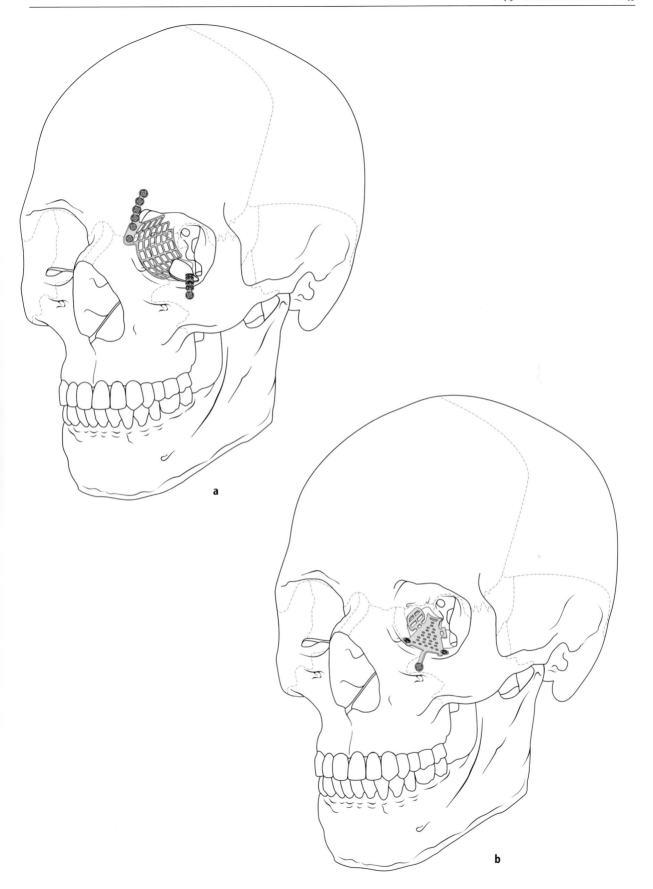

a

b

Generally the lower and lateral portions of the orbit are exposed with a lower lid incision. Either a skin-muscle flap, or a transconjunctival incision with a lateral canthotomy are preferred to incisions lower in the lid. Both the lower and lateral orbit can be explored through this incision.

The superior and upper medial portion of the orbit must be approached with a coronal incision. Anterior approaches alone may suffice for noncomminuted and medially displaced zygomatic fractures (a subciliary skin-muscle flap and a gingivobuccal sulcus incison). The lateral canthus may be detached to allow inspection of the lateral orbit for a comparison of alignment of the orbital process of the zygoma with the greater wing of the sphenoid. Conceptually, for grossly displaced and comminuted fractures, four articulations are visualized for a zygomatic open reduction: the zygomaticofrontal suture, inferior orbital rim, lateral wall of the orbit, and maxillary buttress (through a gingival buccal sulcus incision). The lateral canthus should be reattached at the close of the procedure. The exploration of the lateral and inferior portions of the internal orbit is a component of every zygomatic fracture reduction.

If a coronal incision is not used, the zygomatic arch may require a separate temporal (Gillies') reduction maneuver if medially displaced. No direct open reduction is required for medially displaced arch fractures. When the zygomatic arch is laterally displaced, a coronal incision (see Fig. 2.5) is required. The coronal incision allows exposure for stable fixation of the zygomatic arch. Placing a bone hook (see Fig. 4.4.1, inset) beneath the malar eminence permits strong anterior traction on the zygomatic body to achieve reduction. The arch, if opened, should be reduced as flat as possible. Indeed, it is not an arch, as it is flat in its middle portion. Achieving the proper straight reduction of the zygomatic arch reduces midface width and improves the anterior projection of the zygoma.

4.5.6 Naso-Orbital-Ethmoid Fractures

The complex anatomy of nasoethmoidal orbital fracture reduction makes this one of the most difficult of facial fractures to manage (see also Sect. 4.3). The simplest nasoethmoid injury is fracture of the medial orbital rim. The frontal process of the maxilla is therefore dislocated. The simplest fractures show dislocation only at the inferior orbital rim and pyriform aperture. In these injuries the junction of the frontal process of the maxilla with the internal angular process of the frontal bone is undisplaced; therefore the areas requiring open reduction are visualized by subciliary and gingival buccal sulcus incisions.

If the medial orbital rim is dislocated at all its articulations, reduction is achieved by coronal and inferior approaches (see Fig. 2.5). Nasoethmoid fractures may be either unilateral or bilateral. The injury is managed by first dislocating the canthal bearing fragment laterally and anteriorly (the attached canthal ligament should not be stripped in the reduction). Holes are drilled to link this area loosely by interfragment wires to adjacent bone. The most important maneuver is to place two wires posterior and superior to the lacrimal fossa for use as a transnasal reduction. This is the most important step in stabilizing a nasoethmoidal orbital fracture, as the transnasal reduction of the medial orbital rims stabilizes the intercanthal distance (see Fig. 4.3.3b). Once all the nasal and medial orbital bones are linked to one another and linked transnasally, the wires are tightened, and the entire assembled segment of fractures is then stabilized to adjacent bones with "junctional" rigid fixation. Practically, it is impossible to overcorrect bony intercanthal distance.

4.5.7 Superior Orbital Rim and Roof Fractures

Fractures in the area of the frontal bone and orbital roof are less common than zygomatic and nasoethmoidal fractures. They are frequently seen in children. They may involve the frontal sinus or portions of the frontal bone. Neurosurgical exploration requires bone removal. Bone segments should be marked in sequence as they are removed as a guide to their reassembly. Frontal bone segments can be harvested for bone graft by section of the internal table. These procedures can be performed on a back table while neurosurgery is in progress. Once the neurosurgeons have completed dural repair, the segments, reassembled on a back table and stabilized either with wires or plates and screws, are placed into the defect. Remnants of frontal sinus mucosa are removed and intra sinus bone grafts placed to reconstitute the anterior cranial floor. The frontal bone fragments are replaced following orbital roof reconstruction. The roof is stabilized by rigidly fixing a bone graft to the frontal bar. The orbital roof should not be reconstructed by placing bone graft within the orbit, but by placing bone graft targent to the normal position of the roof. The precise reconstruction of each internal orbital wall is related directly to proper globe position.

References and Suggested Reading

Antonyshyn O, Gruss JS, Galbraith DJ et al (1989) Complex orbital fractures. A critical analysis of immediate bone graft reconstruction. Ann Plast Surg 22:220–233

Glassman RD, Manson PN, Vander Kolk CA et al (1990) Rigid fixation of internal orbital fractures. Plast Reconstr Surg 86:1103–1104

Hammer B (1995) Orbital fractures. Diagnosis, operative treatment, secondery corrections. Hogreve & Huber, Bern

Manson PN, Clifford CM, Su CT et al (1986) Mechanism of global support and posttraumatic enophthalmos. I. The anatomy of the ligament sling and its relation to intramuscular cone orbital fat. Plast Reconstr Surg 77:193–214

Markowitz BL, Manson PN, Sargent L et al (1991) Management of the medial canthal tendon in nasothmoidal fractures: the importance of the central fragment in classificaiton and treatment. Plast Reconstr Surg 87:843–853

Mathog RH, Hillstrom RP, Nesi FA (1989) Surgical correction of enophthalmos and diplopia. A report of 38 cases. Arch Otolaryngol Head Neck Surg 115:169

Pearl RM (1987) Surgical management of volumetric changes in the bony orbit. Ann Plast Surg 19:349–358

Phillips JG, Gruss JS, Wells MD, Chollet A (1991) Periosteal suspension of the lower eyelid and cheek following subciliary exposure of facial fractures. Plast Reconstr Surg 88:145–148

Romano JJ, Wellisz T, Manson PN et al (1993) Experience with porous density polyethylene implants in 97 patients with facial fractures. J Craniofac Surg 4:142–147

Sullivan WG (1991) Displaced orbital roof fractures: presentation and treatment. Plast Reconstr Surg 87:658–661

Wolfe SA (1982) Application of craniofacial surgical precepts in orbital reconstruction following trauma and tumor removal. J Maxillofac Surg 10:212–213

4.6 Cranial Vault

Contributors: Patrick Sullivan
               Paul N. Manson

4.6.1 Frontal Sinus and Frontal Bone

The frontal sinus is a respiratory epithelial-lined cavity situated superior to the bony orbits and anterior to the frontal lobes (Fig. 4.6.1 a). It is irregular in shape, asymmetric, and is divided in the midline and often laterally by irregular sinus septae. The sinus has been postulated to serve a protective role for the ocular globes and the frontal lobes. The location of the sinus adjacent to the cranial cavity makes inadequately treated injury to the frontal sinus have grave consequences (Newman and Travis 1973).

Frontal sinus fractures can be classified by the anatomic involvement of the anterior table, posterior table, and nasofrontal duct. Fractures are either displaced or nondisplaced for each location (Fig. 4.6.1 b). These injuries occur as isolated entities or in any combination with other fractures. Clinical signs and pattern of injuries to the anterior and posterior tables and nasofrontal duct, visualized in radiological studies, are used to determine appropriate treatment, operative or nonoperative (Stanley and Becker 1987), and type of operation.

4.6.2 Special Conditions Influencing Open Reduction and Internal Fixation

There have been multiple attempts to establish a correlation of radiological findings with intraoperative findings and the degree of injury in order to develop (Stanley 1989) protocols for the various types of frontal sinus fractures. Classification systems usually divide frontal sinus fractures into the following categories:

- Anterior table, displaced or nondisplaced
- Posterior table, displaced or nondisplaced
- Anterior and posterior table, displaced or nondisplaced

Fig. 4.6.1 a, b

a Anterior view of frontal sinus. The two sides are asymmetric, and the sinus may be also divided by lateral septae. The nasal frontal duct orifice usually empties into the nose by a short, funnel-shaped channel.
b Classification of frontal sinus fractures is by involvement of the anterior table (*Inset 1*), posterior table (*Inset 2*) and nasal frontal duct (*Inset 3*). Fractures are either nondisplaced or displaced for each location.

Any of these fractures may have nasofrontal duct injury (Hoffman and Krause 1991), and if so, operative intervention is preferred as sinus function following duct injury is not predictable.

4.6.3 Sinus Function and Operative Treatment

There is general agreement that isolated nondisplaced anterior table fractures can be managed nonoperatively without significant sequelae. Displaced anterior table fractures are usually explored and the displaced fragments elevated with minimal manipulation of mucosa. Sinus function may be preserved in these injuries in the absence of nasofrontal duct injury. Injury to nasofrontal duct or orifice is determined by radiographic characteristics of the fractures, by the presence of fluid in the sinus (which implies absence of ductual function), and by visual inspection of the duct at surgery. Dye, saline, or contrast studies may be used intraoperatively to assess duct patency. None of these criteria are absolute as far as predictability of duct function. The correlation of these tests with clinical function has yet to be established.

4.6.4 Types of Fixation

Fragmentation of the anterior table is reconstructed either with 1.0 microplates or the 1.3 system (Fig. 4.6.2), depending on the strength required, to provide the best cosmetic result. If the anterior wall is excessively fragmented, the bone pieces may be discarded and replaced with a bone graft (Fig. 4.6.3).

There is significant disagreement on management strategy in the presence of posterior table fractures. The

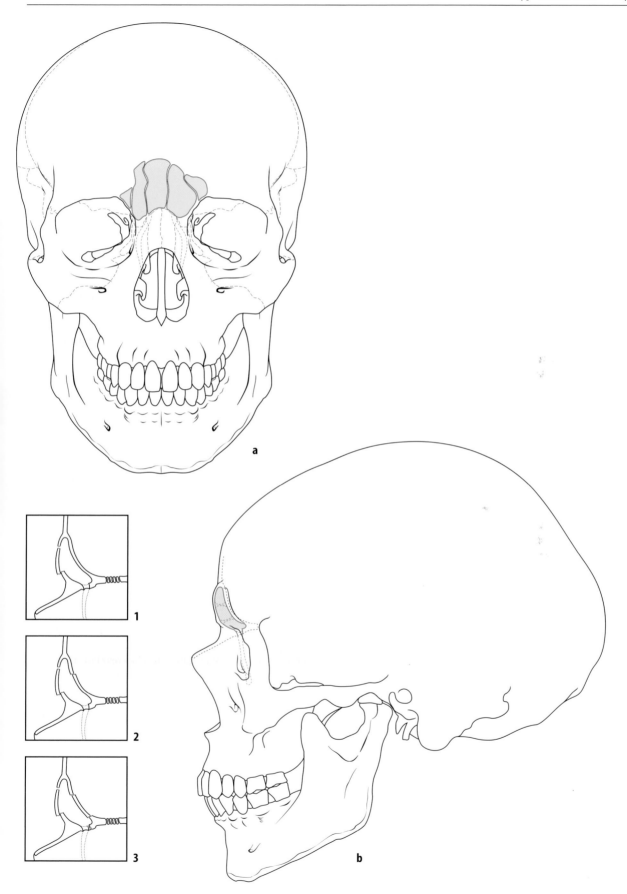

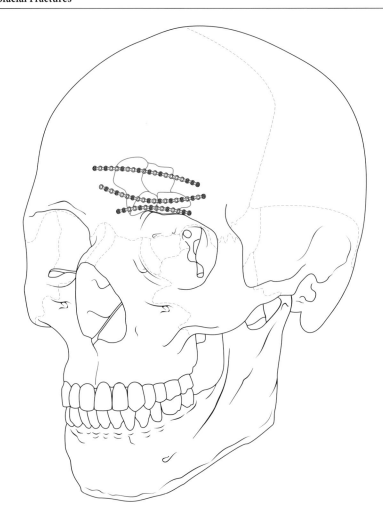

degree of posterior wall displacement is evaluated on preoperative radiological studies, and the need for sinus exploration is determined by experience and the probability of damage to the dura and the possibility of sinus obstruction.

The thickness of the posterior table has been used as the limit of acceptable posterior wall displacement in which nonoperative management may be considered (Rohrich and Hollier 1992). Some authors, however, believe that the presence of posterior table fractures, regardless of amount of displacement, requires an exploration of the sinus to rule out associated injury to the nasofrontal duct and dura which are difficult to appreciate on radiographic studies (Fig. 4.6.4; Donald 1986). Sinus infection or obstruction may lead to meningitis or intracerebral abscess and may result in serious morbidity if a nasofrontal duct injury is not appreciated and managed. These considerations are cited as reasons for operative inspection of any posterior table frontal sinus fracture.

A CSF leak in a displaced fracture is a clear indication

Fig. 4.6.2

The contour of the frontal bone may be templated on the non-fractured side; bone fragments are stabilized with plate and screw fixation. Better contour and projection are established by stable fixation than by wires because the bone fragments may be expanded and elevated to ensure proper contour. Reconstruction of frontal sinus fractures with 1.3 plates. The plates should be bent to reproduce the convex contour.

for operative exploration. The dural tear is directly closed. When the dural closure is weak, the closure is buttressed by a fascial graft and fibrin glue (Levine et al. 1986). In frontal sinus fractures with associated craniofacial injuries the approach has been to manage the sinus simultaneously with other craniofacial injuries. The technique of cranialization is preferred. The resistance of the frontal sinus to fracture is several times greater than in midfacial areas of the craniofacial skeleton but less than that of the surrounding frontal bone. This implies that there is a significant chance of associated injuries when injury to the frontal sinus is identified.

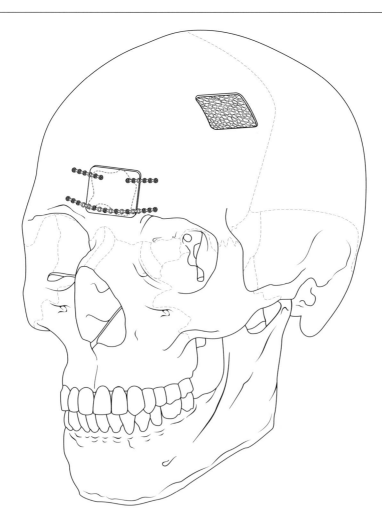

Fig. 4.6.3

When the anterior table is excessively comminuted, the esthetic result is improved by use of a bone graft to reconstruct the entire anterior sinus wall. It is stabilized with either the 1.3 or microsystem.

ity in combined extensive fractures of the midface and frontal cranium (Fig. 4.6.5). If the bone is comminuted, bone grafts are used to fill in the defects and are stabilized with screw fixation to the plates (Fig. 4.6.5). Final contouring is then performed with a shaping burr.

4.6.5 Esthetics

The normal forehead and cranial vault shapes are easily reconstructed with plate and screw fixation, especially when compared to wires. Better contours and projections are established (see Fig. 4.6.2); bone gaps may be established when expanding the bone vault to its proper contour. Bone grafts may be used to replace comminuted bone segments.

One can bend 1.3 plates to recreate the shape of the normal forehead (see Fig. 4.6.2). Microplates are less visible beneath the soft-tissue cover of the forehead. The thicker miniplates are occasionally necessary for stabil-

4.6.6 Osteotomy

Fractures which are very significantly impacted, or which have already begun to heal may be freed and mobilized by craniotome following access incisions with burr holes.

Bone flaps are often required to provide exposure for dural intracranial injury management. Plate and screw fixation proves helpful in stabilizing these bone flaps to promote rapid healing and provide optimal esthetic results.

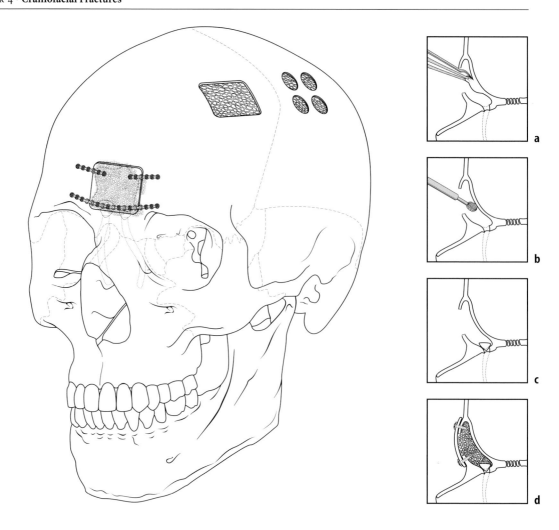

4.6.7 Exposure

The coronal incision (see Fig. 2.5) gives excellent exposure and is optimal for access to the nasofrontal duct, posterior table, and intracranial region. Exploration of the frontal sinus may also be performed via several other approaches. In very limited fractures the sinus can be accessed through a laceration or a local incision. Local approaches permit only limited visualization (sometimes of an ipsilateral sinus) and may not allow bilateral assessment of nasofrontal duct injury. Dye studies can be used to determine duct patency by the appearance of the contrast material in the nose. In cases of bilateral frontal sinus fractures and in all severe injuries the preferred approach employs a coronal incision with removal of at least the anterior table.

Sinus obliteration is indicated when nasofrontal duct injury or wall displacement implies sinus nonfunction, or when anterior and posterior table sinus fractures pre-

---

Fig. 4.6.4

Technique of sinus obliteration is demonstrated on insets.
Inset a: The sinus mucosa is removed.
Inset b: The intra sinus bone cortex is removed with a high speed burr. The posterior table is inspected for fracture and dural integrity confirmed. Rigid fixation may stabilize posterior wall or bone graft segments.
Inset c: The nasal frontal duct is occluded with a bone graft.
Inset d: The sinus cavity is filled with particulate bone, taken from the calvarium with a neurosurgical perforator. The sinus is fully packed with particulate cancellous bone material. The anterior table is reassembled with stable fixation.

---

dict that the probability of duct function is low. Sinus obliteration (see Fig. 4.6.4) requires:

1. Removal of all sinus mucosa
2. Removal of inner sinus bone cortex by high speed burr
3. Reapproximation of the displaced posterior table elements and fixation, or removal

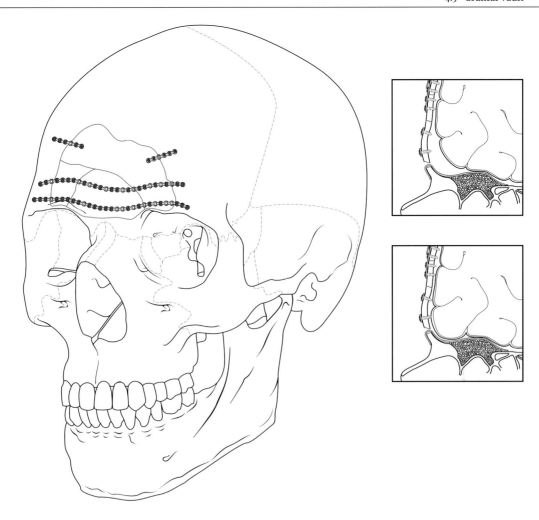

Fig. 4.6.5

Cranialization of a frontal sinus fracture requires removal of the mucosa, removal or replacement of the posterior wall, and reconstruction of the anterior wall. Occasionally a galeal-frontalis flap is used to improve the seal between the nose and the intracranial cavity. The floor of the frontal sinus and the floor of the anterior cranial fossa must be extensively bone grafted with layers of "formed to fit" calvarial bone grafts. The brain is slowly able to expand to fill the defect.

4. Occlusion of the nasofrontal duct with a "formed to fit" calvarial bone graft
5. Filling of the sinus cavity with particulate bone, packing the sinus fully to allow osteogenesis to occur
6. Replacement of the anterior table with stable fixation

It is sometimes maintained that in cases of duct injury the duct can be reconstructed (via the Sewal-Boyden mucosal flap) to maintain patency or by stint duct intubation (Prolo and Duvall III 1986; Luce 1987); however, the procedures (as in any duct reconstruction techniques) are unpredictable. If extensive comminuted fractures of the posterior table prevent adequate reconstruction of the posterior table, the frontal sinus may be cranialized by removal of the posterior table to permit expansion of the frontal lobes into the new space, a process which takes several months (see Fig. 4.6.5).

The diagnostic and treatment strategies for frontal sinus fractures have undergone significant evolution. Short- and long-term complications suggest that the more aggressive management strategy produces the best results. The lack of large, well-controlled studies allows the selection of one treatment plan over another to be based more on personal preference than on scientific findings.

References and Suggested Reading

Donald PJ (1986) Frontal sinus fracture. In: Cummings CW, Fedrickson JM, Harker LA, Krause CJ, Schuller DE (eds) Otolaryngology – head and neck surgery. Mosby, St. Louis. pp 901–921

Hoffman HT, Krause CJ (1991) Traumatic injuries to the frontal sinus. In Fonseca RJ, Walker RV (eds) Oral and maxillofacial trauma, vol 1. Saunders, Philadelphia, pp 576–599

Levine SB, Rowe LD, Keane WM et al (1986) Evaluation and treatment of frontal sinus fractures. Otolaryngol Head Neck Surg 95(1):19–22

Luce LA (1987) Frontal sinus fractures: guidelines to management. Plast Reconstr Surg 80(4):500–508

Newman MH, Travis LW (1973) Frontal sinus fractures. Laryngoscope 83:1281–1292

Prolo DP, Duvall III AJ (1986) Long-term results with nasofrontal duct reconstruction. Laryngoscope 96:858–862

Rohrich RJ, Hollier lH (1992) Management of frontal sinus fracture – changing concepts. Clin Plast Surg 19:219–232

Stanley RB (1989) Fractures of the frontal sinus. Clin Plast Surg 16:115–123

Stanley RB, Becker TS (1987) Injuries of the nasofrontal orifices in frontal sinus fractures. Laryngoscope 97:728–731

CHAPTER 5

Reconstructive Tumor Surgery in the Mandible

5

Chapter Author: Douglas W. Klotch
Contributors: Douglas W. Klotch
Christian Lindqvist
Mark A. Schusterman
Joachim Prein

5.1 Diagnosis

Aside from benign and malignant odontogenic and osseous lesions of the mandible, tumors involving the mandible are usually squamous cell cancers arising from the oral mucosa. The majority of patients presenting with these cancers to the head and neck surgeon have an extensive lesion which is identifiable on the head and neck examination. Generally confirmation of the pathology is readily obtained with biopsy and routine pathological examination. Primary tumors of the mandible are less common. Both these and metastatic lesions may require more extensive open biopsy to confirm the diagnosis. Benign tumors of the mandible are either found incidentally by routine dental radiography or present as a palpable mass with or without dental complaints. Loss of inferior alveolar nerve function is seldom seen even with larger tumors, unless there is extensive mandibular involvement.

When oral cancer is suspected, a routine head and neck examination to evaluate the oral cavity, oropharynx, nasopharynx, hypopharynx and larynx, and neck is indicated. Careful assessment of cranial nerve function is mandated, specifically loss of function of the inferior alveolar nerve (V3). Loss of lingual nerve, facial nerve, or hypoglossal nerve function is usually found only with more advanced primary oral cancers. Lesions which involve the mandible are by definition T4, stage IV oral cancers, and radiographic examination should include the chest. One can argue the merits of including computed tomography (CT) of the chest and mediastinum for advanced disease; however, a minimum of a chest X-ray is required to examine the chest for potential metastatic disease or synchronous primary disease. Generally a panorex view of the mandible is adequate to assess mandibular disease. CT examination with bone windows may help to clarify more subtle mandible involvement but is generally not needed. Bone scans are very sensitive, but not specific to determine bone involvement and as a rule are not ordered. Magnetic resonance imaging (MRI) gives very good soft tissue images, however disease within the bone is not well demonstrated.

5.2 Patient Selection

Benign mandibular tumors or tumorlike lesions are generally discovered in the younger population with dentition. Therefore discussion of patient selection is more relevant to the cancer patient. The mandible supports the lower dental arch, the tongue and floor of mouth structures, and the muscles for position and function of the lower lip. It therefore functions to provide mastication and maintain support of the oral cavity and oral pharyngeal airway, and it is necessary for the insertion of the tongue and floor of the mouth musculature required for the initiation of swallowing and articulation of speech. Mastication is a complex function which requires the interaction of synergistic and non-synergistic muscle function. The muscle function varies through the full range of motion which is provided by the temporomandibular joint. The temporomandibular joint allows deviation, translocation, and hingelike opening. Maintenance of condylar positioning is essential for pain-free mandibular motion and function.

The mandible is a conduit for the third-division sensory branch of the fifth cranial nerve which provides sensation to the lower dental arch and the skin above the chin. In proximity in the surrounding soft tissues are the motor branches for mastication (V3), the sensory branches to the floor of the mouth and the anterior tongue, the mimetic muscles of the lower face, and the hypoglossal nerve supply to the tongue. Violation of these neural structures and the soft tissues and muscles which they supply is generally more important in determining function following tumor ablation than is bone loss alone. If the anterior mandible is not removed, the oral function may be adequate regardless of the size of the bony defect as long as motor and sensory function is not significantly altered. The anterior mandible, however, is essential to provide support for the lip, floor of the mouth, and tongue. Failure to provide this support produces an oral cripple with speech, swallowing, and cosmetic disability characterized by the "Andy Gump" deformity.

The pathological process and extent of disease determines the amount of bone and soft tissue to be resected.

Once this is determined, the treatment including adjuvant therapy can be planned. Generally patient selection becomes a problem only when extensive resection for malignancy is anticipated. Although osseous free flaps ultimately promise the best functional result, their increased operating time adds to the potential morbidity and mortality in high-risk patients. The surgeon may choose to provide only soft-tissue closure for lateral defects if the patient's general health is poor. Anterior defects pose a different problem. Higher incidence of plate extrusion and wound complications are certainly anticipated if immediate vascularized bone repair and appropriate soft-tissue cover is not performed. The surgeon may have to accept this problem in high-risk patients to avoid potential severe morbidity or mortality.

Patients who have significant pulmonary disease, cardiac disease, or nutritional deficiency should be medically maximized before attempting extensive resection. Generally patients who can walk a flight of stairs without discomfort can tolerate surgery. Rapid attention to nutritional support is mandated, and since many patients require extensive postoperative radiotherapy a PEG tube may be considered in extreme cases. Extreme substance abuse and psychosocial dysfunction must frequently be addressed. Such patients are often complicated by poor nutrition, poor dental care, poor generalized health, and alcohol and tobacco abuse and require team support to optimize care. Aggressive dental care is mandated for all patients requiring radiotherapy. Following this careful assessment of the tumor the patient's general condition and preoperative function and the discussion of the surgery and rehabilitation, the surgeon may proceed with the treatment plan. This usually includes a family consultation to allow optimal care for the patient.

Most surgeons choose a course of antibiotic therapy for patients undergoing mandible resection. For less extensive benign cases a prophylactic course given on call to surgery and for the first postoperative day is sufficient. When more extensive resection with elaborate reconstruction is performed, most surgeons use a therapeutic course of the same antibiotics. This regimen provides an on-call dose with at least a 5-day postoperative antibiotic coverage.

A general anesthetic is required. Generally patients can be intubated via either an orotracheal or nasotracheal route. The preference should be discussed between the surgeon and the anesthesiologist. The nasotracheal route provides the most exposure without interference in the operative site. This is more time consuming to deliver and may be difficult if there are extensive septal deformities. Epistaxis can be an annoying complication of nasotracheal intubation. It is preferable not to have the patient paralyzed when operating to allow observation of the motor nerve function (i.e., VII, XII). The surgeon should communicate his preference to the anesthesiologist. Tracheostomy is mandated for patients with poor pulmonary status. It is generally required for dissections that extend to the posterior oral cavity or oropharynx and is more commonly needed when extensive bilateral neck dissection is required. It is never wrong to perform a tracheostomy, and if there is any doubt about the patient's airway or pulmonary status, it is safer for the patient to opt for tracheostomy.

5.3 Description of Procedures

5.3.1 Mandibular Osteotomy

Performing an osteotomy within the mandible may be required to obtain surgical access either for the tumor or for the reconstruction. Access to the lateral skull base and the lateral nasopharyngeal region may require displacement or condyle removal to facilitate exposure. Lateral mandibulotomies can improve access to the parapharyngeal space. Midline or paramedian mandibulotomies enhance exposure to the oropharynx, anterior medial skull base, and the parapharyngeal space. The selection of the surgical approach is frequently related to the tumor type, location, and the physician's preference. Certain guidelines are essential to minimize complications with these approaches since the osteotomy site cannot be equated with a fracture.

Anterior midline or paramedian (anterior to mental foramen) mandibulotomy is usually performed in conjunction with a lip-splitting incision. Although this can be achieved without splitting the lip, a more extensive denuding of the mandible is required to displace the superior visor flap adequately to allow the osteotomy to improve the exposure. Some microvascular surgeons prefer the anterior mandibulotomy approach to facilitate soft-tissue free-flap placement in patients not requiring mandibular resection. Osteotomies are generally made between the central incisors or between canine and first premolar. This preserves sensory function of the inferior alveolar nerve. The anterior surface of the mandible is dissected to allow placement of a seven- or eight-hole bridging plate (a reconstruction plate, either a THORP or UniLOCK, may be used). It is helpful to remove the inferior projection of the mental process with a cutting burr (see inset Fig. 5.1a). This greatly simplifies plate bending and does not interfere with the stability of the fixation since the bone in this region is dense and thick.

A template is contoured to the anterior inferior surface of the mandible to allow precise plate bending without overmanipulating the plate. The plate is positioned inferior to the mental nerve and should be contoured to precisely fit the mandible. Although plates such as the THORP and the UniLOCK plate do not require compres-

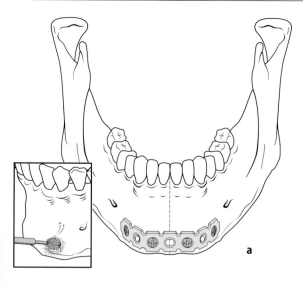

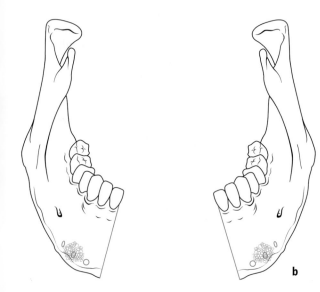

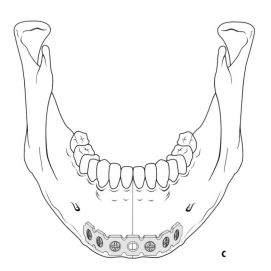

Fig. 5.1 a–c

a Placement and fixation of a seven-hole reconstruction plate prior to performing the ostotomy.
Inset: Removal of inferior bony projection at the mental process with a burr to simplify plate application in this area.

b Mandible after midline osteotomy. On both sides of the osteotomy three provisionally placed screw holes are visible.

c Fixation of the osteotomized mandible with a seven-hole reconstruction plate, fixed with three screws on each side. The innermost screws are placed well away from the osteotomy.

sion of the plate against the bone surface to provide stability, they still require reasonably precise bending. If there is a significant gap between the plate and bone at several areas, it is possible to distort the ends of the mandible with resultant malocclusion as the THORP screws are tightened. The UniLOCK system uses no compression between screwhead and plate hole. The locking mechanism is achieved through a second thread under the screwhead which engages in the plate hole. Nearly perfect contouring of the standard reconstruction plate is required to avoid malpositioning of the mandible by screw placement since screws without locking mechanism press the plate against the surface of the bone (see also Fig. 1.28 b–d).

Two bone screws are initially placed in either end of the mandibular plate to prevent its displacement during the drilling process (Fig. 5.1 a). The residual screw holes are drilled and tapped (if necessary), having premeasured and recorded all screw lengths. The screws are then removed, marking the end of the plate with a suture to ensure correct orientation for plate reapplication. All screws and hole lengths are properly marked on a diagram. Care must be taken when self-tapping screws are used. If possible they should only be placed once. If they are placed a second time, careful insertion along the same axis of the previous placement is necessary in order not to distort the existing threaded bone hole. The osteotomy and surgical resection are performed (Fig. 5.1 b).

If radiotherapy is planned postoperatively, and an incisor tooth root is exposed or lost, the tooth should be removed to prevent subsequent infection which may lead to osteoradionecrosis. It is helpful to keep the inner screw holes empty using only the outer three screw holes for radiated patients to decrease screw complications. This is an individual judgement based on the proximity of the hole to the osteotomy and the character of the bone in combination with the quality of the soft-tissue closure. Screws should be placed in all remaining screw holes (Fig. 5.1 c). If using the reconstruction plate, the screws are placed in the neutral position. The osteotomy site should not be placed under compression as malocclusion and mandibular distortion may result. If screws are not secure in the bone, they should be removed.

Emergency screws may be positioned in these holes if the plate system offers this option. Although the THORP and UniLOCK plates are more forgiving of small bending errors, even they can distort the mandibular repair if bent unprecisely. If this is noticed, the plate should be removed and correctly bent to normalize the occlusal relationship and condylar position.

Lateral osteotomies may be performed without lip-splitting incisions. Plate application follows the same principles as for medial mandibulotomies. It is important not to apply compression to these osteotomies since occlusal disturbances result. In the case of radiated patients compression is also not advised since bone integrity is essential for plate stability, and bone density is diminished secondary to the diminished vascular supply of the mandible from the surgical approach and radiotherapy. Lateral osteotomies are more susceptible to failure when bridging plates are not used since the vascular supply (facial artery) to the periosteum and the nutrient vessel supply are normally interrupted. There is also less muscle vascularity to revascularize the body of the mandible than in the region of the chin. The THORP and UniLOCK plate systems do not produce compression and simplify this application process.

5.3.2 Stabilization of Curetted Mandibular Defects

A variety of benign disease processes such as dentigerous cysts (Fig. 5.2a), giant cell granulomas, and fibro-osseous lesions may be adequately treated by curettage and cleaning with a burr or by partial resection without segmental resection of the mandible. Extensive cortical thinning by the disease process or its removal may produce instability of the mandible. Large defects may be grafted primarily with autogenous cortical and cancellous bone which is frequently taken from the iliac crest. However, this does not provide immediate stability for the weakened mandible. If a fracture of the mandible appears during the procedure, or there is suspected instability of the mandible, a bridging plate may be used to protect or stabilize the area of the lesion. If the fracture occurs at the time of the procedure, the patient may be placed into intermaxillary fixation and the bridging plate applied without compression in the same manner in which one would fix a fracture with bone loss or comminution. If a reconstruction plate is used to repair this defect, a minimum of three or preferably four screws are fixed at each segment (Fig. 5.2b–d). If one selects the THORP or the UniLOCK plate to repair this defect, only three screws are required at each mandibular end to achieve adequate stability.

When the procedure is planned in an atrophic mandible or extensive curettage is anticipated, it is preferable to prebend the plate to the mandible contour prior to the removal of the lesion or the tumor. Evaluation of the radiographs prior to removal generally allows adequate plate length selection. A template is prebent to the contour of the mandible, planning an adequate number of screw holes in each stump. It is preferable to plan the first screw to be placed at least 1 cm away from the tumor margin. This allows some leeway to account for possible miscalculation of the tumor size when selecting the plate length. If the benign tumor extends anteriorly, the anterior cortex may be burred away to allow the plate to be adapted to the mandible. It is better to plan for additional plate length when selecting the plate since it is far easier to shorten a plate than to reapply a new plate because the one selected was too short.

Once the plate is adapted, the plate is held in place with the plate-bone holding forceps. Holes are drilled, and the screw lengths are measured and recorded on a diagram. After the placement of the plate it can generally be left in place during the removal of the lesion. If plate placement interferes with adequate removal, it is removed. The orientation of the plate may be marked with a suture and then the lesion adequately curetted or resected. If the mandible is fractured during removal, the patient does not have to be placed in intermaxillary fixation since the prebent plate has reestablished the correct mandibular position, which is maintained once the plate is secured into position. (This procedure is comparable to that described in the following section; see Fig. 5.3a–c). Cancellous bone may be used to fill the bone defect either prior to or after plate application (Fig. 5.2c,d). If there is an incidental fracture, the bone graft is best applied after the plate is positioned, and the mandibular contour and length is reestablished.

If the surgical approach was extraoral, prophylactic antibiotic therapy is adequate since subsequent infection by intraoral contamination is unlikely. If an intraoral approach was used, a therapeutic course of antibiotics is preferred since intraoral contamination is present. Successful bone grafting via an intraoral approach depends on a reliable closure of the oral mucosa.

Patients are placed on a blenderized diet for 2 weeks. Fastidious oral care is mandated for intraoral approaches to prevent wound breakdown and subsequent infection. If patients are noncompliant, it may be necessary to use a nasogastric feeding tube to ensure proper wound healing.

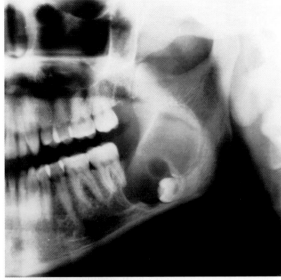

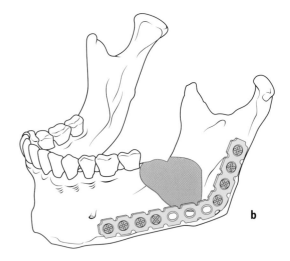

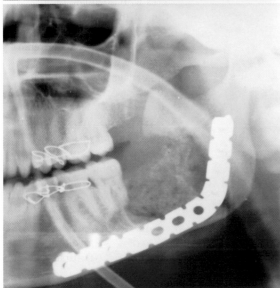

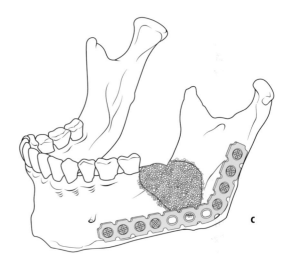

Fig. 5.2 a–d

a Cystic lesion in a left mandible, appearing like a follicular cyst. Within the cyst wall, however, an ameloblastoma was found.
b The cyst had thinned the cortical walls and weakened the mandible so that the reconstruction plate was fixed prior to the removal of the lesion.
c After removal of the leasion, the bone defect was filled with cancellous bone taken from the iliac crest.
d Same situation as in Fig. 5.2 c on X-ray. Note fixation of the reconstruction plate with four screws on each side. The plate should be removed only on special request.

5.3.3 Segmental Resection for Benign Tumors

Benign tumors or tumorlike lesions, such as ameloblastoma, giant cell granuloma, keratocysts, and myxomas may require segmental resection of the mandible. Resection of these tumors usually does not require sacrifice of the mucosa unless the tumor occurs in the tooth row or in the soft tissues. Likewise, patients do not require adjuvant radiotherapy. Both these factors allow optimal conditions for bone and soft-tissue healing. The surgeon may choose the option of using primary nonvascularized bone to repair these defects with an expected success rate exceeding 90%.

Appropriate planning prior to resection is essential to avoid selection of a plate that is too short to stabilize the

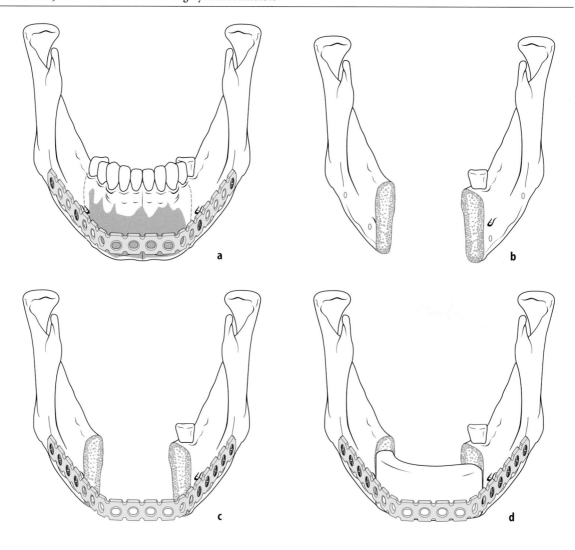

defect. Depending on the local situation a UniLOCK or THORP plate can be used. The preoperative radiographs (panorex) provide adequate information to determine the extent of the resection. Sometimes the lesion extends further than anticipated and requires additional bone removal. If one plans to place the first screw 1 cm from the planned osteotomy with at least four screws in each segment, incorrect plate selection is unlikely. Exposure is obtained with an upper cervical incision carefully preserving the mandibular branch of the facial nerve. The buccal periosteum is elevated, exposing the mandible surface. A template is used to select the correct plate length and to facilitate plate bending. If the plate is to be bent over the mental region, shaving down the inferior projection of the mental process with a cutting burr helps to simplify plate application (see inset of Fig. 5.1a). This should not be performed with tumors extending into this area.

The correctly adapted plate is fixed with at least two screws in each segment to ensure proper placement of

Fig. 5.3 a–e

a Placement and provisional fixation of the reconstruction plate prior to resection of the chin area.
b Situation after removal of the chin area. Two screw holes within each lateral segment are visible.
c Reapplication of the reconstruction plate after removal of the tumor and fixation with five or four screws on each side.
d Same defect as in **c** after insertion of a nonvascularized corticocancellous bone graft of the iliac crest.
e Same situation as in **d**. After resection of an anteriorly located ameloblastoma primary reconstruction with a nonvascularized bone graft was performed. Note that there is no screw fixation for the bone graft. On the left side the first screw was placed too close to the osteotomy line.

the residual screw holes. The remaining screw holes may be drilled before or after removal of the tumor (Fig. 5.3a). The plate is removed and labeled for reapplication following the tumor resection (Fig. 5.3b). Care is taken to free the mucosa and periosteum along the alveolar surface to avoid entering the oral cavity if pos-

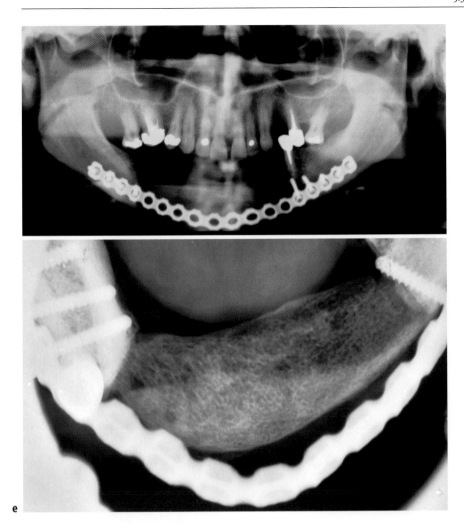

e

sible. When the resection is within the row of teeth, entry into the oral cavity is unavoidable. Following the resection the plate is replaced in the correct location to anatomically repair the defect (Fig. 5.3c). Precise plate bending and handling of the plate guarantees correct positioning of the mandibular stumps. Significant distortion would require placing dentate patients in IMF and recontouring the plate to precisely position the mandible. The plate is replaced and IMF is removed. The occlusion and mandibular position are rechecked. The mandible is put through a range of motion to ensure that there is no deviation or dislocation of the condyle, and that the occlusion continues to remain correct. When correct, the IMF may be released and the arch bars removed.

The placement of a free nonvascularized bone graft immediately after resecting the tumor is acceptable only under the conditions that closure of the oral mucosa is easy, and that no dehiscence is to be expected (Fig. 5.3d,e). Most free bone grafts are lost if the oral mucosa opens up postoperatively. If bone grafting is successful, a titanium plate need not be removed if it does not disturb the patient. After full incorporation of the bone graft and therefore closure of the bony defects because of the continuous bone remodeling, the plate is neutralized and does not cause any stress protection.

5.3.4 Plate Application for Tumors with Extension Through the Anterior Buccal Cortex

Benign tumors occasionally extend anteriorly through the buccal cortex. This prevents accurate prebending of the plate to the mandibular contour without violating the tumor. There are several possible ways to solve this problem. The patient may be placed in IMF prior to resection. If the resection is within the row of teeth, replacing the patient's IMF following resection aligns the mandible for correct plate bending and application. If the resection extends proximal to the teeth, precise

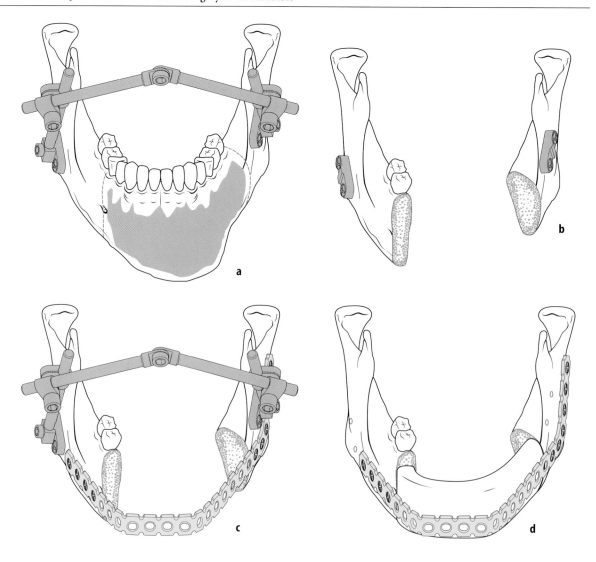

positioning of the condyle cannot be achieved by this method alone. A Mandible Fix Bridge (Fig. 5.4) or mandibulomaxillary fixation with miniplates (2.0; Fig. 5.5) or a reconstruction plate (Fig. 5.6) can be placed to bypass this anterior tumor extension to allow tumor resection with secondary contouring to the bridging plate which subsequently recontours the mandibular defect.

5.3.4.1 Plate Application for Anterior Tumor Extension Using the Mandible Fix Bridge Device

Two base plates with attachment pins are positioned inferiorly or superiorly on the mandible at least 1 cm from the planned osteotomy sites. The base plates fit 2.4 self-tapping screws and are readily applied to the mandibular surface. The bridging bow is then adjusted by its universal joints to couple with the attachment pins of

Fig. 5.4 a–d

a Placement of a fixation device prior to resection of the anterior part of the mandible.
b Situation after resection. Note: the fixation devices are placed in different posiltions. On the right side inferiorly and on the left side on the superior aspect of the mandible.
c For the correct reconstruction of the mandible the previously used bridging bow is reapplied. After that the reconstruction plate can be bent according to the positioning of the mandibular stumps, followed by fixation with 2.4-mm screws.
d After bridging the defect with the plate, the gap may be filled with a bone graft.

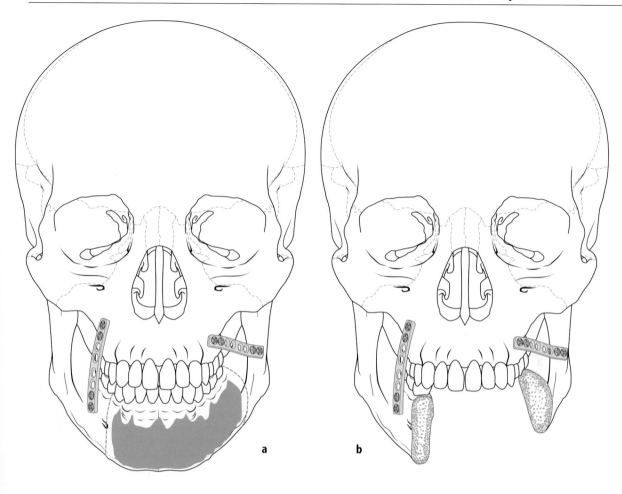

the base plate. Once final adjustments are made, the bow's universal joints are rigidly tightened to ensure maintenance of the bow position (see Fig. 5.4a). The clamps are then loosened from the attachment pins. The bridging bow is removed. The resection of the mandibular tumor is unhindered by the positioning device (Fig. 5.4b). Following the resection the bow is then reattached to the base plate. The bridging bow reestablishes the original position of the residual mandibular segments with return of normal condylar orientation. A bridging plate (UniLOCK or THORP) can then be bent precisely to the contour of the mandible to provide projection at the anterior border of the mandible and stabilization of the mandibular segments (see Fig. 5.4c). The surgeon may use an alloplastic model to help in the preliminary contouring of the plate. Experienced surgeons can generally achieve this freehand. The Mandible Fix Bridge is removed once the reconstruction plate is fit precisely to recontour the defect (see Fig. 5.4d). If the

Fig. 5.5 a–d

a Intermaxillary fixation of the mandible to the maxilla with miniplates.
b After resection of the tumor the mandibular segments are kept in intermaxillary relation.
c, d (see page 164)

condylar fixation device is not available, any external fixator of the appropriate size may be used to achieve the same function.

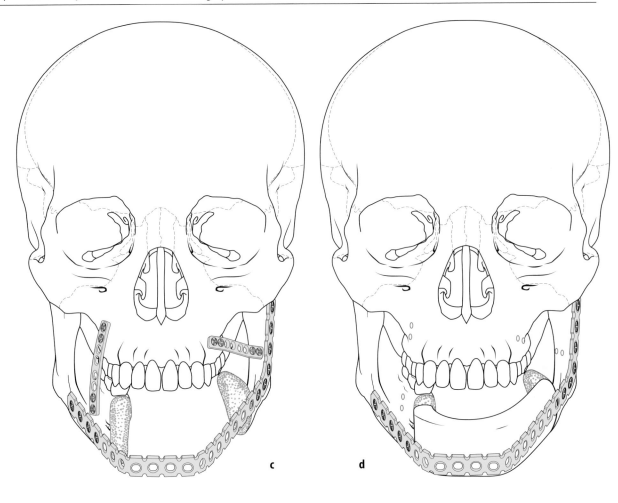

Fig. 5.5 c, d

c Bridging of the defect with a reconstruction plate (UniLOCK or THORP).
d Filling of the bony defect with an autogenous bone graft and removal of the miniplates.

5.3.4.2 Fixation With Miniplates

Further means for establishing an original positioning of the mandibular bone stumps are an intermaxillary fixation with miniplates from mandible to maxilla (see Fig. 5.5).

5.3.4.3 Fixation With a Reconstruction Plate

If one uses a plate to solve this problem, a previously used sterilized reconstruction plate may be bent into an omega shape such that the legs of the omega attach to the normal portion of the mandible, and the curved portion of the omega is either superiorly or inferiorly located to avoid the bulging tumor mass (see Fig. 5.6 a, c). The plate is adapted precisely so that the legs of the plate correspond to the mandible contour and thus ensure stable positioning of the mandibular ends following resection. Two screws are sufficient to fix each leg into the uninvolved mandible. The plate is then appropriately tagged and removed. The tumor is resected, clearing all the margins. The positioning plate is reapplied in the previously drilled screw holes. This reestablishes the normal anatomic relationships of the mandible. Since this positioning plate is usually placed at the superior margin of the mandible, a template can be bent in the middle portion of the mandible, assuring that at least three and preferably four screw holes are available for each mandibular stump for plate fixation.

After bending a template the reconstruction plate (THORP or UniLOCK) is accordingly bent and adapted

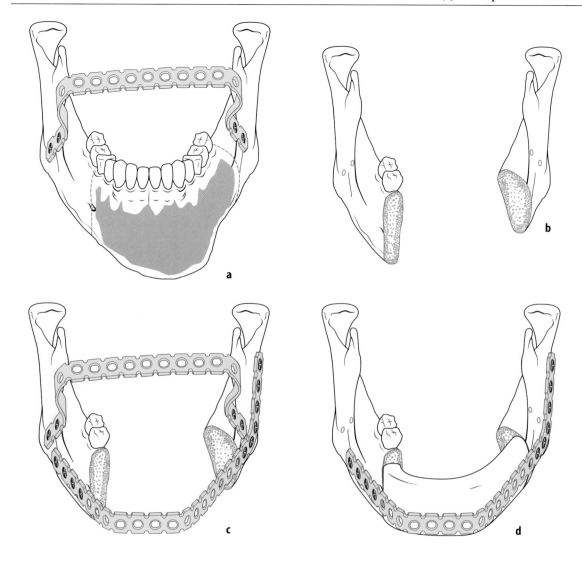

Fig. 5.6 a–d

a Positioning of an Omega-like bent used reconstruction plate for temporary alignment of the mandibular stumps.
b For the time of tumor resection the positioning plate may also be removed.
c Replacement of the positioning plate and adaptation and fixation of the reconstruction plate which bridges the defect.
d After removal of the positioning plate and fixation of the bone stumps with a bridging plate, a bone graft of either type may be brought in.

to fit the mandible contour (see Fig. 5.6). Screw holes are drilled using copious irrigation. Hole length is measured, and if the system requires, holes are tapped prior to placing appropriate length screws. Once the mandibular bridging plate has been securely screwed, the positioning plate is removed from the inferior surface of the mandible. Range of motion of the mandible, condylar position, and occlusal relationships should be checked, and readjustment must be made prior to closure.

5.3.4.4 Three-Dimensional Computer Modeling

A three-dimensional computer generated model may be used to preshape the plate in the laboratory. This is an elegant, but expensive, means of achieving appropriate plate contouring. Such models are not immediately available and are useful only when significant time and resources are available to provide this service.

5.3.5 Application of Bone Grafts Following Bridging Plate Stabilization

Once the bone defect has been stabilized precisely with a bridging plate (UniLOCK, THORP), primary or secondary grafting can be considered. If the mucosa is intact or can be reliably closed, immediate nonvascularized bone grafts may be used, with excellent results. Very large defects may be reconstructed with microvascular

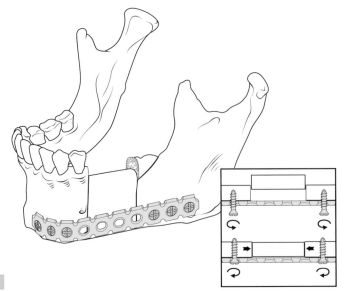

Fig. 5.7

Fixation of a nonvascularized graft in the lateral mandible by compressing the graft between the mandibular stumps. *Inset*, the technique.

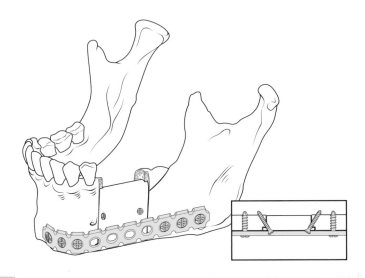

Fig. 5.8

In this case after bridging the defect with a reconstruction plate, the nonvascularized bone graft is fixed to the mandibular segments via a lag screw technique.

grafts (see Fig. 5.10). Smaller defects may be repaired with cancellous bone obtained from the iliac crest. This highly cellular graft is extremely reliable even for previously infected cases. However, a substantial loss of mineral bulk of the graft is expected. Corticocancellous grafts are preferred for larger defects. Cancellous bone grafts require some means of stabilization, possibly with resorbable meshes. The means of fixation of the graft is determined by the bridging plate selected for mandibular stabilization.

Fixation of bone grafts together with reconstruction plates can be carried out by one of several means. If the screws can be locked within the hole of the plate (as in UniLOCK or THORP), it is safe to fix the grafts with these screws. If the screws cannot be locked, however, grafts should not be fixed with these screws since the

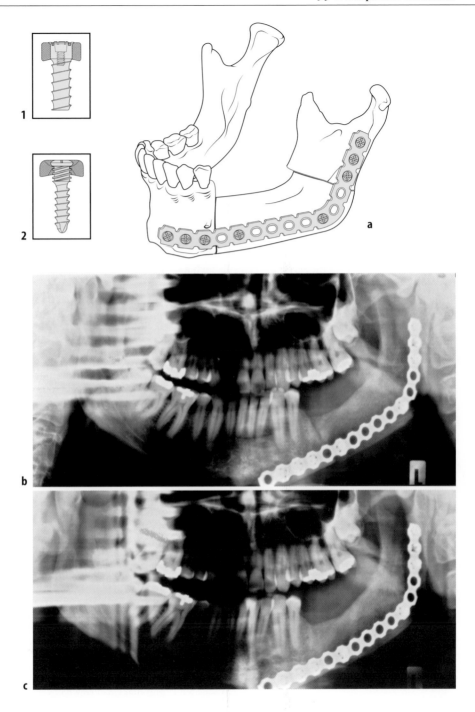

Fig. 5.9 a–c

a Fixation of a nonvascularized bone graft with screws is feasable when locking of the screws into the plate hole is possible (*inset* 1, THORP; *inset* 2, UniLOCK).

b After resecting the angular area of the left mandible, the defect was bridged with a THORP plate and filled with a nonvascularized bone graft fixed with two locking screws.

c Same situation as in **b** 4 months later, showing a complete incorporation without much resorption of the graft.

screws may loosen during the process of revitalization of the bone graft and promote infection.

One possibility for stabilizing a nonvascularized graft is to use the advantage of bidirectional screw holes of the reconstruction plate, allowing for compression. If the inner screws are loosened, a slightly oversized graft (approximately 2 mm larger than the defect) may be wedged between the mandible edges (Fig. 5.7). When the screws are tightened (inset in Fig. 5.7), the graft is compressed between the mandible edges stabilizing the graft.

Another technique uses a mortise joint to fix the graft to the mandible with lag screws. An oversized graft is harvested. A step incision is cut into the ends of the graft so that the measurement from the inner bone edge is the exact dimension of the mandibular defect. The outer flange of the bone graft overlaps the mandibular ends. It is preferable to cut back the outer cortex of the mandible at both mandibular ends to precisely fit the flange of the bone graft. Lag screws may then be placed to fix the bone graft securely in place (inset in Fig. 5.8). The bridging plate provides temporary stability for functional loading (Fig. 5.8). Eventually, after completion of the healing process, the bone graft takes over the functional forces.

Plate designs that lock the screw to the plate such as the UniLOCK and THORP allow screws to be placed through the plate hole to fix the graft (Fig. 5.9). This can greatly facilitate the speed of repair. It does not negate the benefits of lag screw fixation of the graft. With each of these techniques it is recommended to pack cancellous bone liberally around the graft-mandibular joints to ensure more predictable bone healing at the osteotomy sites.

Primary, nonvascularized bone grafting is recommended only when there are no mucosal defects and in the occasional instances in which the mucosa can be closed securely. Most studies predict significant bone loss if nonvascularized bone grafts are attempted for cases where there are mucosal defects. In fact, a dehiscence above the graft almost always causes the loss of a nonvascularized free graft. It is usually best to wait approximately 2 months or until adequate healing has occurred to provide secondary bone repair. The plates allow immediate function without bone being present. They are subject to breaking if the bone is not replaced. This generally occurs, depending on the loading situation, after months or years.

Dental implants may be placed secondarily in cortical cancellous bone grafts. A high rate of success can be expected with this application. Primary implantation of dental implants within nonvascularized bone is not recommended.

5.3.6 Reconstruction of Tumor Defects With Vascularized Bone Grafts and Their Fixation With Plates

Vascularized tissue transfer provides optimal bone and soft tissue for major defect reconstruction. Nonvascularized bone heals by creeping substitution and remodeling. The revitalization of the bone depends upon the vascularity of the surrounding tissue. Vascularized flaps introduce viable bone and soft tissue to initiate repair.

Vascularized bone grafts heal similarly to fractures, and stabilization can mimic techniques for fracture repair.

Free vascularized composite bone grafts have become the treatment of choice for repair of large segmental mandibular and soft-tissue defects. The vascularized bone and soft-tissue flaps tolerate radiotherapy with minimal complications of osteoradionecrosis, wound breakdown, plate extrusion, and screw or plate loss. Dental implants may be placed primarily to accelerate the dental restoration process.

The choice of fixation of the vascularized bone flap includes regular fracture plates (2.4), lag screws, miniplates, Universal Fracture plates (microvascular plate) and reconstruction plates (UniLOCK, THORP). The goal of the fixation is to provide adequate stability to allow bone healing without distortion of the occlusion or temporomandibular joint function. Longer grafts require segmental osteotomies for correct contouring of the graft. Intuitively, this simulates segmental fractures. One could predict better control of maxillomandibular and condylar positioning using load bearing bridging plates. Regardless, the different schools of surgeons advocate a variety of fixation methods, with similarly good results. Bridging plates have another advantage in not requiring patients to be placed in IMF to secure occlusal relationships. With tumors lacking anterior cortical extension the plate can be prebent to the mandibular contour prior to resection of the mandible. This provides precise recontouring of the mandibular defect, and osteotomies within the graft can be planned according to the plate shape (see Sect. 5.3.3; Fig. 5.3).

As mentioned in the sequence on three-dimensional computer modeling, it may be helpful to prebend a plate on the basis of a three-dimensional model. This may be too expensive for consideration as a regular procedure.

5.3.7 Repair of the Anterior Defect Using a Microvascular Free Bone Flap and Fixation With Universal Fracture Plates (Microvascular Plates), UniLOCK, or Mini Plates

Selection of bone donor site depends upon the size and location of the bone defect, the amount of soft tissue resected, and the preference of the surgeon. Both fibula and iliac crest free flaps contain excellent bone. The iliac crest is usually required when more soft-tissue repair is needed. The scapula free flap may also be used. This has the advantage of excellent independent soft-tissue flaps. The bone, however, has a periosteal blood supply and has substantially less volume. The decreased bone generally requires a bridging plate (UniLOCK or THORP) to guarantee mandibular form and function, while iliac crest and fibula flaps can be fixed with miniplates as well. The radial forearm flap with bone is rarely used in our groups. Since the amount of bone is small, this would require a reconstruction plate for fixation.

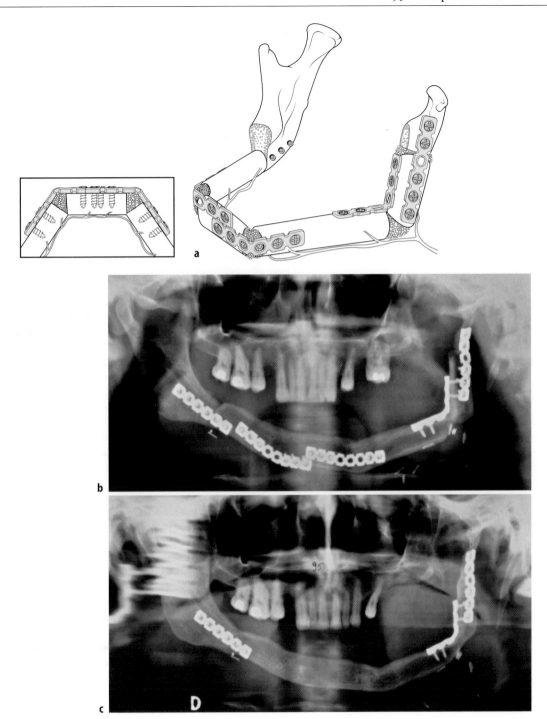

Fig. 5.10 a–c

a Reconstruction of the complete horizontal part of the mandible, including the ramus on the left side with a microvascular free fibula bone graft. In this case fixation of the graft and the anterior osteotomies was performed with Universal Fracture plates. Small bony gaps were filled with cancellous bone taken from the iliac crest. *Inset*: monocortical screw fixation to avoid injury to vessels.

b Clinical situation shown on X-ray, alike the situation in **a**.

c Situation as in **a** after removal of the anterior plates used for the fixation of the osteotomies within the graft. This allows for the placement of dental implants.

The anterior surface of the mandible is widely exposed, and the osteotomy sites are marked with a bone saw. A template is prebent to the contour of the mandible. The template also can guide the selection of plate length. The plate is measured so that the first screw is placed about 1 cm from the osteotomy, and at least four screws should be planned for each side. Extensive anterior projection of the inferior border of the mental process may be removed with a cutting burr if the tumor does not extend into this region (see inset of Fig. 5.1). This facilitates plate bending and decreases overprojection of the repair. The plate is contoured precisely to the anterior surface of the mandible. The plate is positioned, and at least two screws are placed in each side to ensure that the remaining screw holes are placed correctly without plate displacement (see Fig. 5.3a,d). Sharp drills, correct drill guides, and copious irrigation is required to prevent screw failure. Either pretapped or nonpretapped holes are required depending on the kind of screws for fixing the reconstruction plate. Screw length is measured before tapping to avoid potential damage to the tapped bone threads. All screw holes are drilled, measured, and tapped (if required), and a diagram of the plate and screw orientation is recorded. Special care must be taken when replacing self-tapping screws (2.4 UniLOCK) to avoid stripping previously cut threads. It is preferable not to place all screws prior to resection to avoid this potential problem. This is less likely to occur with pretapped holes (2.7 and THORP screws). The plate is removed and the surgical resection completed.

The plate may be taken to the donor site to shape and fix the bone to the plate in situ before transacting the vascular pedicle to decrease ischemic time. This applies to the fibula free flap and is a matter of surgeon's preference. Screws are placed monocortically in the graft to decrease potential injury to the vessels behind the opposite cortex (see inset to Fig. 5.10a). The plate bone unit may then be fitted to the mandibular defect and the plate secured to the mandible. Vascular anastomosis is then completed, followed by wound closure (Schusterman).

An alternative is to fix the vascularized free flap with Universal Fracture plates (Fig. 5.10b,c) or miniplates. In these instances it is essential to have adequate bone in order to guarantee form and function of the mandible and then sustain the soft tissues. The osteotomy defects should be filled with cancellous bone (inset to Fig. 5.10a).

In another variation the bridging plate is placed first to restore the mandibular defect. The graft must be fixed with a reconstruction plate only if it is taken from the scapula (see Fig. 5.11b). After harvesting the grafts, osteotomies are performed in the bone graft to precisely fit the mandibular defect and plate contour. The bone is secured to the plate. Intraoral soft-tissue closure is completed, followed by the microvascular anastomosis. This technique is generally employed when using the iliac crest or scapula free flap with skin for intraoral lining.

5.3.8 Repair of Tumor Defects With Anterior Soft-Tissue Extension With Microvascular Free Bone Flap and Bridging Plate

The method of supervising mandibular and condylar position for tumors extending anteriorly is decribed above (see Figs. 5.4–5.6). Dentate patients may be placed in IMF to supervise maxillomandibular relationships. The method of using an oversized positioning device is also described above.

An alternative method uses the condylar positioning device which provides an excellent unobstructed resection of the tumor. Base plates applied proximal to the planned mandibular osteotomies secure the positioning bow. The bow is removed and the tumor is resected. The mandible is repositioned by reattaching the positioning bow to the mandibular base plates. A bridging plate can be contoured to the mandible to maintain the mandibular position. The bridging plate is applied, and the Mandible Fix Bridge base plates are removed (see Fig. 5.4b,d). The free flap can be harvested and shaped and fixed to the plate as previously described (Fig. 5.11b,c).

5.3.9 Reconstruction of the Condyle: General Remarks

Reconstructing the temporomandibular joint (TMJ) articulation is one of the most demanding challenges in facial surgery. Restoration must address the complex function of the joint while restoring occlusion, facial symmetry, and projection and maintaining normal mastication. Many of the problems of joint reconstruction have been addressed in the literature in relation to repair of the ankylosed joint. Efforts to provide repair with alloplastic condylar prostheses have been associated with the complications of malpositioning, infection, glenoid fossa erosion, heterotropic bone formation, and even erosion into the skull (middle cranial fossa; see also sections 5.3.11 and 5.3.12).

These problems are even more apparent with patients requiring tumor ablation and repair, especially when combined with high-dose radiation therapy. Lindqvist et al. (1992a) reported 3 of 11 condylar prosthesis used for tumor repair required removal secondary to infection. One patient aged 11 years had a plate fracture necessitating plate removal. Four of the patients' condyles were displaced out of the fossa. Reconstruction of the TMJ with an alloplastic condyle after radical removal of the joint with planned postoperative radiotherapy is probably contraindicated because of the high probability of failure and the poten-

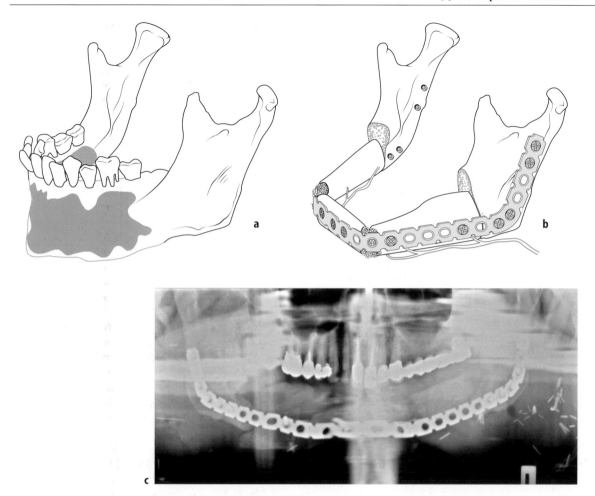

Fig. 5.11 a–c

a Extensive invasion of the horizontal part of the mandible by a malignant tumor necessitating an almost complete resection of the horizontal mandible.

b Reconstruction of the horizontal branch of the mandible with a microvascular anastomosed scapular graft with two soft-tissue flaps. In this case it is necessary to use a reconstruction plate (UniLOCK or THORP) for stabilization of the mandibular segments and fixation of the graft. While screw placement within the mandibular stumps is bicortically, fixation of the bone graft is carried out monocortically.

c Clinical situation as described in **a, b**, shown on the Orthopan tomogram.

tial erosion of the condyle into the middle cranial fossa. Prosthetic reconstruction of the TMJ has largely been abandoned in the United States due to legal ramifications relating to other artificial joint devices. None such device is presently approved by the Food and Drug Administration.

5.3.10 Joint Repair With Costochondral Grafts

Repair of the condyle with costochondral cartilage is an accepted modality for reconstructing the resected condyle following the removal of benign lesions or ankylotic joints. Other indications include dysplasias and osteomyelitis. The goal of reconstructing the TMJ is not only to rehabilitate the complex mechanism of the normal joint but also to restore facial symmetry, occlusion, and mastication. Alleviation of pain is of great importance, especially in the surgical treatment of degenerative joint disease. Mandibular growth imposes additional constraints on the reconstructive procedure in children.

Because of a number of biological and anatomic similarities to the mandibular condyle costochondral grafts have been considered to be among the most acceptable tissues for TMJ reconstruction. Primary nonvascularized cartilage grafts are not recommended for patients receiving planned postoperative radiotherapy. Benign tumors involving the ascending ramus and condyle of the mandible are amenable to reconstruction with costal

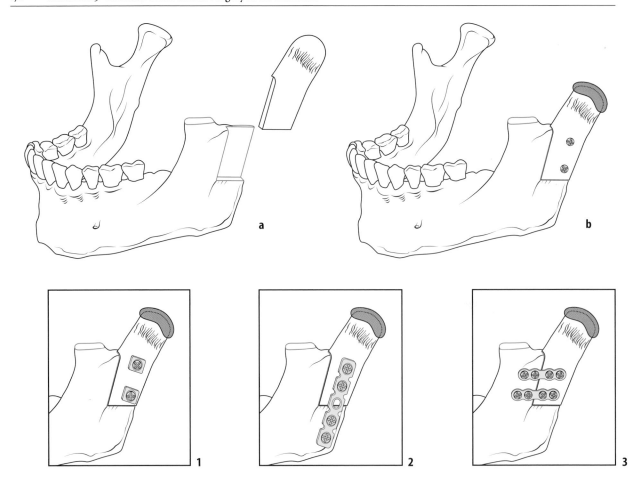

chondral grafts in order to reconstitute the mandibular and condylar defect. In ankylotic cases coronoidectomy must also be performed. Great care must be taken to preserve the neurovascular bundle of the mandible.

Exposure is achieved through the submandibular incision (see Figs. 2.1, 2.3), usually in combination with a preauricular incision followed by the resection of the condylar head and the ascending ramus segment. If possible, the meniscus is preserved as well as the joint capsule. The length of the resection is measured.

The rib may be harvested, including about 5–10 mm of cartilage. The fifth, sixth, or seventh ribs are suitable for this purpose. Care must be taken not to tear the parietal pleura during the resection of the rib. Small pleural rents may be checked by inflating the lung with positive pressure, with water in the wound looking for air leaks. If no air bubbles are detected after the lung is fully reinflated, the pleura may be closed without inserting chest tubes.

The cartilage end of the costal chondral rib graft is shaped to approximate the original condyle and to fit within the condylar fossa (Fig. 5.12a). Sufficient rib should be harvested to allow fixation with a minimum of

Fig. 5.12 a–d

a Situation after the resection of the left condylar and subcondylar area, as well as the coronoid process. An osteochondral graft is shaped. A groove is carved into the remaining part of the ascending ramus to receive the graft.
b Fixation of the osteochondral graft with two 2.0 lag screws.
Inset 1: Fixation with lag screws with washers.
Inset 2: Fixation with Universal Fracture plate.
Inset 3: Fixation with 2 horizontally placed miniplates.
c Situation as in **b**, *inset* 3, shown radiographically.
d Situation as in **b**, *inset* 1, shown radiographically.

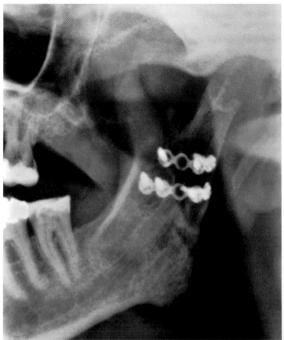

c

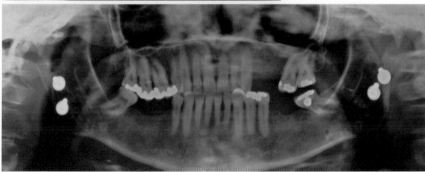

d

two or three lag screws. If the rib is soft, washers made from cut portions of 2.0 adaptation plates are helpful to prevent screws from splitting or pulling through the bone. Screws of 2.4 mm are particularly well suited for this procedure (see Fig. 5.12, inset 1). The graft may also be applied to the mandible by fixation with miniplates (see Fig. 5.12, inset 3). Lindqvist et al. (1992a,b) have demonstrated success with this technique. However, stability is not adequate to allow patients to function immediately. Depending on the situation, 10 days–2 weeks of immobilization in IMF is recommended.

Other possibilities are to use the 2.0 mandibular plate (six hole) or the 2.4 Universal Fracture plate (see Fig. 5.12, inset 2). Two holes are placed with lag screws fixing the graft (through the plate) to the mandible. Two or three additional holes provide additional stability to the graft. This repair is also best protected with 10 days of intermaxillary fixation.

5.3.11 Alloplastic Replacement of the Condylar Process

There are only few indications for using a condylar implant in TMJ arthroplasties. If an autogenous transplantation is contraindicated for any reason, such as the general condition of the patient, massive ankylotic structures, and reankylosis after autogenous arthroplasty, an allogenic joint prostheses may be the best method for primary reconstruction. The same is true in traumatic cases in which the condyle is lost or fractured into several pieces, and primary restoration of mandible and joint function by osteosynthesis is impossible (Fig. 5.13b). As noted above, this prosthesis in not approved by the United States Food and Drug Administration.

A combined preauricular and sub- or retromandibular approach is advisable (see Figs. 2.1, 2.3). After substantial removal of ankylotic masses a new fossa is

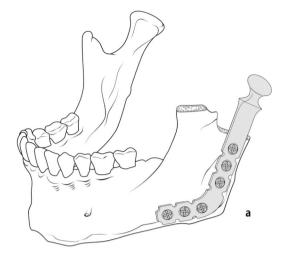

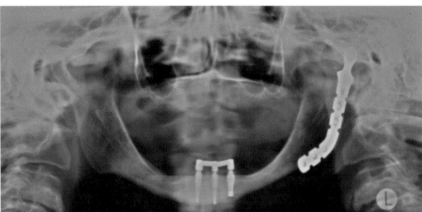

created in the region of the damaged mandibular condyle. In nontumor cases, however, no attempt should be made to remove the distroyed condylar process totally (Fig. 5.13 b). On the contrary, it may be advisable to leave some of this bone as a precaution against penetration of the condylar head into the temporal fossa. Coronoidectomy is always performed in cases of ankylosis. After removing the desired amount of bone the correctly sized prosthesis (three different sizes) is chosen after evaluating the defect with a template. The goal is to choose a prosthesis that is placed at the posterior aspect of the ramus engaging with its most posterior hole into the mandibular angle (Fig. 5.13). These prostheses are currently made of stainless steel, and they should be fixed with the 2.7 screws in a bicortical manner. Since these prostheses are rarely used, they will probably remain available only on special request and with the 2.7 screws.

IMF is always used intraoperatively. In edentulous patients the fixation is with the patient's total dentures, which are then fixed to the maxilla and mandible by screws or wires. The mandible is thus immobilized during plate bending and insertion. In these cases effort is taken to remove the condyle carefully in order to pre-

Fig. 5.13 a, b

a Schematic drawing with coronoidectomy because of an ankylosis.
b Replacement of the mandibular condyle and subcondylar area with a joint prosthesis in an edentulous patient after traumatic loss of condyle.

serve the disc intact in the fossa, if possible, unless a temporary muscle flap including the fascia can be used to line the fossa. This can prevent to some extent the formation of ectopic bone and the possible erosion of the joint head in the fossa. IMF is relieved before the patient is extubated.

It may be difficult to place the condylar head correctly in the glenoid fossa. Lindqvist et al. (1992 a,b) report that in 23 instances in which a joint prosthesis was used only 16 were initially found to be situated correctly in the glenoid fossa. In one out of these 23 a perforation to the skull base occurred 10 months after the insertion of the implant. In Basel we have had experience with 23 condylar prostheses over an average follow-up time of 101 months in 17 patients; no erosion of the glenoid fossa has yet been observed (Prein 1998).

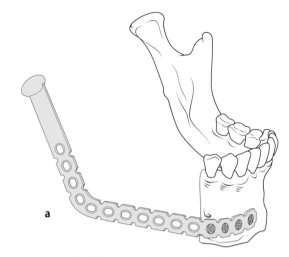

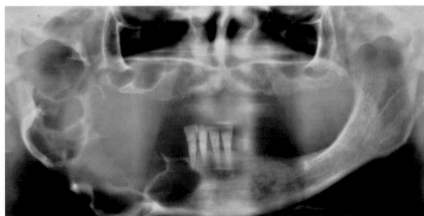

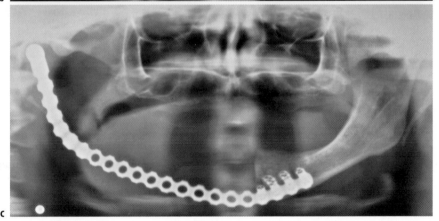

5.3.12 Condylar Prosthesis for Lateromandibular Defects Including the Joint

Condylar head prosthesis for replacing the lateral mandible including the ascending ramus currently uses the 2.7 reconstruction angled plate. Long and short, left and right plates are available by special order in countries other than the United States (see Fig. 1.26c,d). This

Fig. 5.14 a–c

a Reconstruction plate with condylar head bridging the right hemimandibular defect.
b Orthopan tomogram showing a recurrent ameloblastoma in the right mandible.
c Orthopan tomogram showing a THORP plate with condylar head, bridging a complete right hemimandibular defect.

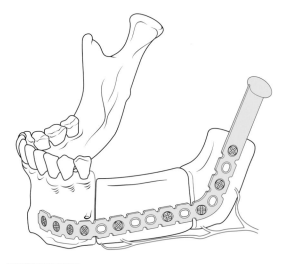

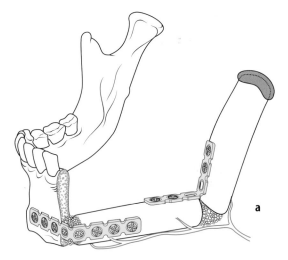

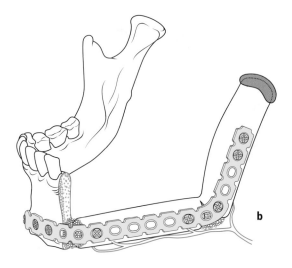

Fig. 5.15

Fixation of a microvascular anastomized bone graft to a reconstruction plate with condyle. Since this is a vital bone graft, fixation can well be performed with screws.

system uses the 2.7 screw, which has a hexagonal head
and requires pretapping. When patients require resection of the mandible but not the meniscus or joint capsule, this plate may temporize to maintain mandibular
relationships until bone repair is feasible (Fig. 5.14).

Its use requires that the patient be placed in stable
occlusion with arch bars. Ameloblastoma and extensive
keratocysts are the most common pathology involving
the ascending ramus and condyle (Fig. 5.14b). The
tumor can frequently be removed using an external incision with the dissection remaining extraorally. This
approach is helpful in decreasing wound infection. Care
is taken to assess the extent of the disease on the radiographs. The area of resection is carefully marked to
allow complete removal of the tumor. It is beneficial to
plan for at least an additional 1 cm of bone removal
when sizing the plate so as not to lack sufficient plate
length. Since the condyle cannot be removed from the
fossa to allow precise adaptation of the plate to the glenoid fossa, precise bending is not possible until the tumor
is resected. The template is prebent to the anterior lateral
surface of the mandible from inferior joint capsule to a
point allowing at least five screws to be placed in the
remaining mandible. Following the resection the patient
is placed in IMF, reestablishing the normal occlusion.
The plate is then positioned. Care is taken to place the
condyle within the joint space without forcing the condyle to the posterior position. Further bending adjustments are made with the bending irons. The plate is
secured to the mandible with at least four screws placed
in the neutral position. Screw holes are drilled to 2.0 mm
using copious irrigation. The screw length is measured
with a depth gauge before tapping the holes. The 2.7

screws are placed firmly bicortically to ensure adequate
stabilization of the plate. Fig. 5.14c shows this situation
with the THORP system.

Adequate joint capsule usually remains for suturing
the tissue around the neck of the prosthesis. Likewise, a
heavy 2-0 nonabsorbable suture is used to secure the
most superior plate hole segment to the joint capsule. If
inadequate tissue remains, one can secure the plate to
the temporal fascia or zygoma superiorly. This helps to
prevent the condyle from dislocating out of the glenoid
fossa postoperatively. IMF is removed following soft-tissue closure. The arch bars are left in place in case the surgeon wishes to apply loose elastics to help train the
occlusion, or if there is concern about possible condylar
displacement. This is usually not necessary if plate
bending has been precise.

The condylar head prosthesis plate should be considered only a temporary repair. There is a tendency for
plate fracture and for plate erosion into the temporal
bone. Bone grafts may be attached to this plate to pro-

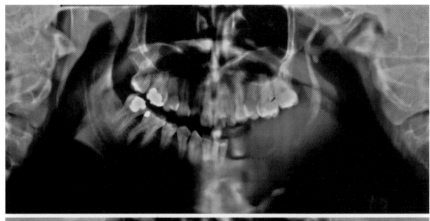
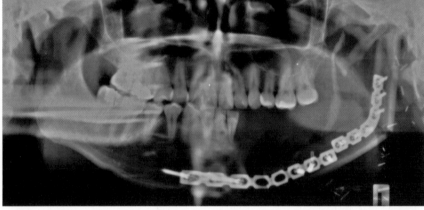

c

Fig. 5.16 a–c

◄ **a** Fixation of a microvascular free fibular graft replacing corpus and ramus, including the condylar head, on the left side.
Fixation of graft and osteotomy (angle) with Universal Fracture plates. Bone gaps are filled with cancellous bone.
b Fixation of a microvascular free fibular graft with a reconstruction plate. Note the joint area is replaced by bone only,
no condylar head of the plate.
c Pre- and postoperative X-ray showing the defect of the left
corpus and ramus of the mandible and the reconstruction of
this area with a microvascular anastomosed fibular graft
fixed with Universal Fracture plates. Situation corresponds
with **a**.

vide more stability (Fig. 5.15). However, this resolves
only the problem of potential plate fracture. Most surgeons would recommend replacing this plate with bone
graft if the patient remains free of disease. Microvascular free flaps are certainly considered a better choice for
young patients who can expect long-term survival. Fixation of these grafts is performed with either Universal
Fracture plates (Fig. 5.16a) or bridging plates
(Fig. 5.16b,c).

Care must be taken to size the new condyle free end
of the graft adequately and to position it within the glen-

oid fossa (see Fig. 5.16c). Failure to position the graft
adequately and to supervise it may lead to malpositioning the graft into the temporal fossa, which impairs correct functioning of the mandible.

5.3.13 Management of Mandibular Resection Including the Condyle Using Microvascular Bone Flaps and Various Plates for Fixation

Fortunately, malignancies rarely involve the TMJ. This
may be due to the limited lymphatics in this region, or to
the lack of interconnections of the ascending ramus to
the condyle with either a common canal or a blood supply. When malignancies involve this region, they usually
also invade the joint capsule and the meniscus and
require resection of these structures followed by high-
dose radiotherapy. These extensive tumors frequently
involve the lateral skull base and require skull base
approaches with resection of the floor of the middle cranial fossa which limits the ability for primary mandibular reconstruction. Microvascular osseous free flaps may
be used for mandibular repair, including the condyle, if
no significant defect has been created in the skull base.
The fossa may be covered with a temporalis flap. The

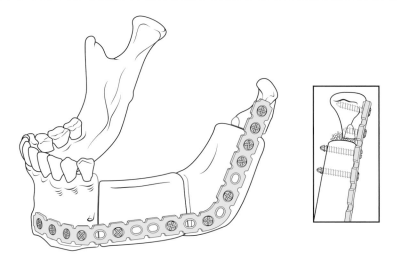

Fig. 5.17

Reconstruction of the left mandible. The unaffected condyle was left in place and used for fixation of the reconstruction plate with two screws, one in the head and one in the subcondylar area. In this situation a free nonvascularized bone graft was used. Therefore stabilization must be performed with a reconstruction plate.

free end of the bone flap is carefully shaped to fit the glenoid fossa (see Fig. 5.16).

Careful osteotomies need to be planned with precise adaption of the graft to provide width, projection, and height of the mandible. There is a slight tendency of these grafts to migrate into the temporal fossa. Therefore fixation of the graft to the residual mandible is generally best achieved with a bridging plate such as the UniLOCK or THORP to prevent mandibular deviation (see Fig. 5.16b). These plates are more difficult to adapt but provide the stability to maintain condylar and mandibular positioning during functional load. The joint capsule should be secured around the condyle if possible to help prevent dislocation from the glenoid fossa. If occlusal relationships are questionable, a period of IMF is mandated. If occlusal relationships cannot be achieved after graft placement, careful readaptation of the plate and graft are required prior to closure to prevent mandibular dysfunction.

Positioning of the graft in relationship to the remaining mandible is difficult. It is beneficial to place the dentate patient into arch bars. The patient is placed in IMF prior to final adaptation and fixation of the graft and plate.

Another option is to position the mandible in relationship to the maxilla. A variety of techniques may be used to achieve this positioning. The patient may have a fracture plate placed between the noninvolved mandible and the maxilla (see Fig. 5.5a). This is placed when the patient is in the normal closed occlusal position. The plate can be removed to facilitate the resection. Once the resection is completed, the plate can be replaced, reestablishing normal mandibular position for the adaptation of the graft and plate. This may also be achieved by the use of the Synthes Mandible Fix Bridge (see Fig. 5.4a). The base plates are attached to the maxilla and the mandible. The mandible is placed in normal closed occlusal position, and the fixation bow is adjusted to

attach to the base plates. The position is fixed using the locking universal clamps. The fixation bow is removed from the base plates allowing free access to the oral cavity during tumor resection. Reapplication of the fixation bow allows precise repositioning of the mandible for the adaptation of the plate and the bone graft. Base plates are removed at the end of the procedure. The advantage of installing arch bars over other techniques is that it allows the surgeon to maintain or reapply IMF more easily in the postoperative period if desired. It is helpful to maintain patients in IMF with elastics for 2 weeks postoperatively to train the occlusion. Dentures or appropriate splints may be used in edentulous patients to help restore normal position and function.

Several techniques have evolved for repairing the lateral mandibular defect including the condyle. These include using an osseous free flap in combination with a reconstruction plate with a condylar head (see Fig. 5.15). Osseous free flaps may also have the proximal end of the bone contoured into a neo condyle (see Fig. 5.16a–c).

Hidalgo suggests removing the residual unaffected condyle and using it as a free graft attached to the osseous free flap. Adequate length of the condyle neck generally remains to be attached with two or three screws to the bridging plate, which is necessary if no vascularized grafts are transplanted (Fig. 5.17, 5.19a) or other stabilization plates in combination with microvascular grafts (Fig. 5.18). This is preferable to producing a free condylar graft, which ultimately undergoes significant resorption and remodeling over time. Of course, the

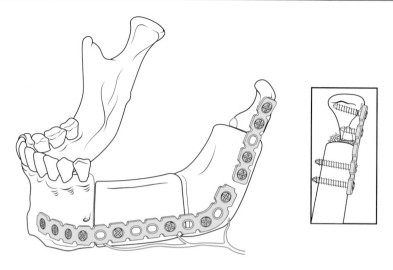

Fig. 5.18

In this situation the same defect as in Fig. 5.17 was recon-structed with a vascularized bone graft. Therefore individual Universal Fracture plates can be used for fixation.

latter condition and repair is not comparable to the situation in which the tumor involves the joint, with obligatory resection of the entire joint to ensure tumor supervision.

5.3.14 Repair of the Lateral Mandible Including the Condyle: Osseous Free Flap and Bridging Plate

The approach to the mandible is similar to that described above. The choice of whether to obtain the free flap from the fibula or the iliac crest depends upon the amount of soft tissue required, the total bone length, and the preference of the surgeon. The iliac free flap provides adequate bone for the hemimandible reconstruction. The ipsilateral hip places the vascular pedicle posteriorly and is not recommended if contralateral donor vessels are to be used.

A temporalis flap may be used to cover the glenoid fossa if extensive soft-tissue dissection is required at the skull base. The proximal end of the bone flap should be contoured to approximate the size of the residual patient's condyle. A template contoured to the mandible prior to the resection helps to shape the bridging plate. The plate is bent according to the template and positioned such that the proximal screw is in the region of the neo condylar neck. The plate should not extend to the joint. Four screws should fix the plate to the residual mandible. Prior to securing the plate to the mandible, an osteotomy should be made to fit the graft in the para-

symphyseal area. The plate is fastened to the proximal mandible. The patient is maintained in IMF during the final contouring and positioning of the plate. In situ bending of the plate may ensure correct graft positioning. The graft is situated with the preshaped neocondyle placed in the glenoid fossa (see Fig. 5.16b). Residual soft tissue at the joint should be sewn to make a cuff around the condyle. The tissue cuff may be attached laterally to the proximal screw in the plate. Patients are maintained in IMF for 1–2 weeks.

These extensive resections tend to be plagued by decreased function, and some mandibular deviation usually occurs postoperatively. The functional results are worse if postoperative radiotherapy is required. Postoperative mandibular rehabilitation is mandated for all patients to optimize function.

5.3.15 Repair of the Lateral Mandible and Condyle: Microvascular Free Flap and Reconstruction Plate With Condylar Prosthesis (Schusterman)

This repair (see Figs. 5.13, 5.14) is technically feasible but poses significant problems. The condylar head prosthesis is not approved by the Food and Drug Administration and is not available in the United States. Long-term use of the condylar head prosthesis within a heavily radiated field increases the possibility of skull base erosion by the prosthesis, with potential dislocation of the condyle into the middle cranial fossa. Therefore the use of this technique is guarded.

The patient should be placed in arch bars if dentate. If the patient is edentulous, a dental splint or dentures may be fixed to the mandible and maxilla with 2.0 lag screws. It is helpful to trim the denture to be slightly smaller than the planned osteotomy to facilitate tumor removal. Once the resection is completed, the patient is placed in IMF. The appropriately sized condylar head

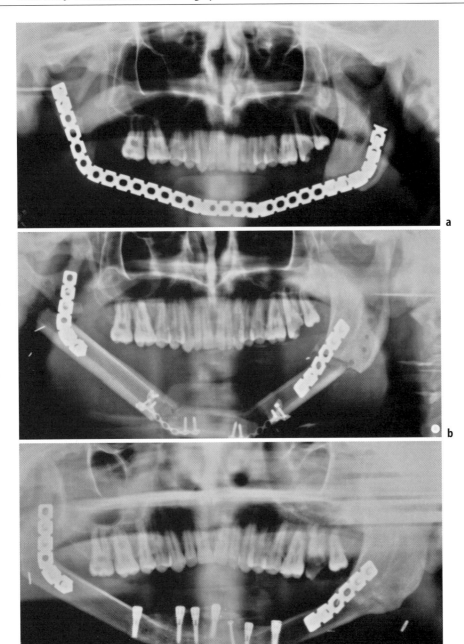

Fig. 5.19 a–c

a Situation after resection of the horizontal part of the mandible including the ascending ramus on the right side because of osteosarcoma. A small part of the condyle remains in place and was used for fixation on the bridging plate with two screws.

b Patient remained free of disease and reconstruction of the mandible was performed with a free vascularized bone graft

from the fibula. In this case the previously used reconstruction plate was removed, and fixation carried out with Universal Fracture plates to the mandibular stumps and miniplates for fixation of the osteotomies in the chin area.

c Situation after removal of the miniplates in the chin area. Additional bone graft in the chin area and placement of dental implants.

reconstruction prosthesis is chosen and bent to reestablish the mandible contour. It is helpful to prebend a template prior to resection of the mandible. This helps in recontouring the plate more closely to the mandible. Stay sutures placed in the lateral, medial, anterior, and posterior joint capsules aid in assuring correct condylar placement within the joint space. Care must be taken not to force the prosthesis into the posterior superior joint position since this produces a canted open bite occlusion at the side of the repair. Once contoured, the plate should be fixed to the mandible with at least four bicortical 2.7 pretapped screws. Small adjustments of the plate may be made in situ. It is desirable to remove IMF temporarily to ensure normal occlusion, joint function, and range of motion. This also facilitates the placement of the free flap. The plate is generally removed and the free bone flap osteotomized and contoured to fit the plate. The final sizing of the graft may require adjustment once the prosthesis is secured in its previous established position (see Fig. 5.15).

5.3.16 Condylar Reconstruction: Condylar Transplant and Vascularized Bone Flap Reconstruction

If a planned resection includes disarticulation of the condyle and a small condyle and neck remnant is found to be free of tumor, the condyle may be transplanted to a vascularized free flap (Hidalgo). Another option is to leave the condylar head in place and attach it to the shaped bone flap (Figs 5.17, 5.18). Proponents of this procedure are concerned with poor results achieved by using vascularized free flaps to create the neocondyle. Few patients with oral cancers are amenable to this procedure since lesions extending to the proximal mandible and TMJ usually have extensive involvement to the tissues of the skull base. The majority of tumors allow preservation of substantial condylar neck and posterior ramus to fasten securely a reconstruction plate (Fig. 5.19a). Although transplanted condyles have shown resorption apparent short-term function is reported to be better than other bone reconstructions even when patients receive radiotherapy.

Exposure is described above. The free or microvascular flap may be secured to the residual mandible with either a reconstruction plate, Universal Fracture plate, or miniplates (Fig. 5.19).

In the case of a condyle transplanted or left in place fixation to the microvascular bone flap is carried out with miniplates or Universal Fracture plates. Two or three screws, if possible, should be placed in the transplanted condyle. The screws must not protrude into the articular surface. If screws are to be placed in the condyle, they should not be placed bicortically (see Fig. 5.17 inset, 5.18). A screw 2 mm shorter than the measured

transcondylar screw hole length is chosen to avoid screw protrusion.

Patients are recommended to remain in IMF for 2 weeks to ensure correct positioning and to allow preliminary bone and soft-tissue healing. Functional rehabilitation is advised to achieve maximal results.

5.4 Complications

Complications occurring from reconstruction of tumor defects are related to technical errors, screw failure, soft-tissue failure, joint failure, bone failure, and material failure.

Many problems are obviously intrinsic to the healing process and are unavoidable. The use of microvascular bone flaps has greatly reduced the rate of soft-tissue and plate failures compared to that when repairs relied only upon the plate providing mandibular integrity. Other considerations involve patient selection, cost containment, and objective assessment of reconstruction benefits for patients with these aggressive tumors.

5.5 Technical Errors

Technical errors involve inappropriate selection and application of stabilization. Likewise, appropriate contouring, application, screw placement and vessel repair are imperative when free flaps are applied, but discussion of these issues are not within the scope of this textbook.

There remains some variance in the choice of fixation of free flaps for mandibular repair. Some authors select "miniplates" to position and stabilize osteotomy sites. Ease of application and less potential interference with the graft and its vascular pedicle are the advantages of this method of fixation. Although larger bridging plates are more difficult to bend, they allow more precise contouring and supervision. They may also be helpful in providing increased stability for thinner bone flaps such as the scapula. Regardless of the surgeon's choice the stabilization must overcome the forces of mastication and allow bone healing with maintenance of normal mandibular and joint relationships. Failure to position the mandible anatomically results in a rigidly fixed mistake. Patients should be taken out of IMF (if used) to test the functional range of motion and maxillomandibular position before accepting the repair. Then, if the repair and surgeon's preference mandate, the patient may be placed in IMF for a short time. A period of IMF is generally not required when bridging plates are used to stabilize the defect. The only exception is the repair of large bone defects, including the condyle.

5.5.1 Plate Failure

Plate fracture is possible when any plate bears the entire functional load for extended periods. The surgeon must accept that the bridging plate ideally is only a temporary repair for tumor defects. Ultimately bone is required to allow total functional rehabilitation.

Several technical errors can contribute to plate failure. Overbending must be avoided. It is important to use prebent plates in the region of the angle to avoid overbending and metal fatigue when attempting to create the contour of the angle. The use of templates helps to simplify the number of bends required to achieve the desired shape. Correct bending pliers help to prevent bends that are too acute.

5.5.2 Screw Failure

The correct drill guides and the correct sharp drill bits and taps (when required) should be selected for each system. A general rule is to discard a drill bit after each use. This is far preferable to destroying a screw hole by burning through the bone and destroying the adjacent bone which is required to maintain screw anchoring. Copious irrigation is also required to cool the bone and remove debris during the drilling process. This is more important with screws of larger diameter as for their holes more heat is produced during drilling. High-speed drills are not recommended since they tend to produce more heat during the drilling process.

There has been a misconception in the literature that screw design is the factor determining osseous integration. Osseous integration is a characteristic of the material. Commercially pure titanium is essentially biologically inert and allows osseous integration without a fibrous capsule surrounding the implant. Therefore all of the AO titanium screws are capable of osseous integration. Some designs allow more surface area or potential bone apposition (i.e., THORP).

Urken et al (1992) have reported that the THORP screw entails fewer screw failures than the 2.7 screw of the older reconstruction plate. This was attributed to the unique screw design and locking feature of the plate to the screw. This may also be related to the screw dimension. If one considers the surface of the screw to be πDL, the surface of the 2.7 screw is 77% of that of the 3.5-mm screw. Likewise, the 2.4 screw is 69% of that of the 3.5 screw. Four 2.7 screws are therefore required for the same bone surface contact as three 3.5 screws. This fact is more important in bone that is more osteoporotic or demineralized as seen with radiotherapy. It is essential to prepare for three-screw holes for the UniLOCK or THORP screw and preferably at least four screws if locking screws are not used.

Care must be taken to place screws in viable bone. It is safer to keep the screws about 1 cm from the osteotomy site. One can conveniently plan to keep the one segment hole nearest the osteotomy without a screw. Care must be taken to replace screws along the previously formed thread axis. It is potentially easier to recut or damage a thread when reinserting self-tapping screws.

5.5.3 Soft-Tissue Failure

Adequate vascularized soft tissue must be available to close the wounds without tension. Small lateral defects may be closed primarily if patients are not to receive radiotherapy. Pectoralis major myocutaneous flaps may provide excellent closure if flaps are not fatty, and the random portion is not over the plate. These tend to be far better for nonradiated patients. The pectoralis major flap tends to separate from the mucosa for anterior defects. Once significant flap dehiscence occurs, plate exposure usually follows. Free vascularized bone flaps provide vascularized bone to which the deep tissues adhere. Plate exposures and small wound separations tend to heal without secondary repair when free vascularized flaps are used. This is unlike the case when a bridging plate alone is used to span the mandibular defect. When the soft-tissue closure separates and exposes the plate, the deep tissues tend to tear away from the plate and require extensive secondary procedures to attempt repair.

5.5.4 Joint Failure

A mobile pain-free TMJ is required to optimize oral rehabilitation. Installing correct occlusion and stabilizing the correct proximal mandibular position are mandated to achieve this goal. Unfortunately, procedures which attempt joint repair frequently produce joint dysfunction. The surgeon must realize that procedures which involve the joint require rapid mobilization to rehabilitate function. Long periods of IMF are contraindicated. Aggressive functional rehabilitation is required during the healing process and is mandated through radiotherapy. Radiation induces fibrosis and extraosseous calcification which lead to ankylosis and diminished joint function. The role of agents which increase oxygen transport or scavenge free radicals is still unanswered but may help to diminish joint dysfunction in the future.

Careful maintenance of the joint offers the best possible repair. Whether the condyle can be transplanted and maintained in long-term function is less predictable. What is clear is that radiotherapy is the single most critical factor in decreasing joint function when technical errors are avoided.

5.5.5 Bone Failure

The residual mandible may be subject to failure by acute infection, secondary infection (usually of dental origin), or osteoradionecrosis. It is imperative to restore good dental hygiene in the remaining mandible if one anticipates the bone to tolerate extensive operative restoration especially in the field of radiotherapy. The incidence of osteoradionecrosis exceeds 5 % and increases if fastidious dental care is not provided. Patients should have dental consultation prior to planned surgery and radiotherapy.

Screws that loosen are generally associated with infection. These should be removed to prevent extensive soft tissue and bone destruction. The plate length needs to be planned for the placement of an adequate number of screws to secure the plate. Exposed plates seldom lead to bone loss unless the plate is inadequately fixed to the bone.

The use of vascularized bone flaps has decreased localized bone failure. Immediate bone repair produces rapid bone healing, which decreases the functional load on the plate system. This decrease in local soft-tissue and screw failures reduces potential bone loss. Microvascular iliac crest, fibula, or scapula free flaps have a better blood supply than the denuded mandible, which frequently has alveolar artery and facial artery injury. These grafts are relatively tolerant to radiation. It will be interesting to determine whether there is an increase in bone loss in patients receiving immediate implants and postoperative radiotherapy. A higher incidence of implant failure has certainly been observed in view of radiotherapy.

It has been well documented that plates do not significantly interfere with the delivery of standard radiotherapy. Back scatter and shielding are not significant at distances greater than 1 mm from the implant when opposed ports are used. Therefore bone complications are more likely due to the extensive devascularization required by the surgical approach than to the interface of the implant and bone.

References and Suggested Reading

Adamo A, Szal RJ (1979) Timing, results and complications of mandibular reconstructive surgery: report of 32 cases. J Oral Surg 37:755–763

Anthony JP, Rawnsley JD, Benhalm P et al (1995) Donor leg morbidity and function after fibula free flap mandible reconstruction. Plast Reconstr Surg 96(1):146–152

Blackwell KE, Buchbinder D, Urken ML (1996) Lateral mandibular reconstruction using soft-tissue free flaps and plates. Arch Otolaryngol Head Neck Surg 122(6):672–678

Boyd B, Mulholland S, Gullane P et al (1994) Reinnervated lateral antebrachial cutaneous neurosome flaps in oral reconstruction: are we making sense? Plast Reconstr Surg 92(1):1266–1275, 93(7):1350–1359

Daniel RK (1978) Mandibular reconstruction with free tissue transfers. Ann Plast Surg 1:346–371

Durkin JF, Heeley JD, Irving JT (1973) The cartilage of the mandibular condyle. Oral Sci Rev 2:29

Figueroa AA, Gans RJ, Pruzansky S (1984) Longterm follow-up of mandibular costochondral graft. Oral Surg 58:257–268

Futran ND, Urken ML, Buchbinder D et al (1995) Rigid fixation of vascularized bone grafts in mandibular reconstruction. Arch Otolaryngol Head Neck Surg 121(1):70–76

Gullane PJ (1991) Primary mandibular reconstruction: analysis of 64 cases and evaluation of interface radiation dosimetry on bridging plates. Larangoscope 101 [Suppl 54]:1–24

Gullane PJ, Holms H (1986) Mandibular reconstruction: new concepts. Arch Otolaryngol Head Neck Surg 112:714–719

Hoffman HT, Harrison N, Sullivan MJ et al (1991) Mandible reconstruction with vascularized bone grafts. Arch Otolaryngol Head Neck Surg 117:917–925

Klotch DW, Futran N (1996) Considerations for reconstruction of the head and neck oncologic patient. Springer, Berlin Heidelberg New York

Klotch DW, Prein J (1987) Mandibular reconstruction using AO plates. Am J Surg 154:384–388

Klotch DW, Gumps J, Kuhn L (1990) Reconstruction of mandibular defects in irradiated patients. Am J Surg 160:396–398

Klotch DW, Ganey T, Greenburg H, Slater-Haase A (1997) Effects of radiation therapy on reconstruction of mandibular defects with a titanium reconstruction plate. Otolaryngol Head Neck Surg 114(4):620–627

Komisar A, Shapiro BM, Danziger E (1985) The use of osteosynthesis in immediate and delayed mandibular reconstruction. Laryngoscope 95:1363–1366

Komisar A, Warman S, Danziger E (1989) A critical analysis of immediate and delayed mandibular reconstruction using AO plates. Arch Otolaryngol Head Neck Surg 115:830–833

Lawson W, Boek S, Loscalzo L et al (1982) Experience with immediate and delayed mandibular reconstruction. Laryngoscope 92:5–10

Lindqvist C, Soderholm AL, Hallikainen D, Sjovall L (1992a) Erosion and heterotopic bone formation after alloplastic TMJ reconstruction. J Oral Maxillofac Surg 50:560–561

Lindqvist C, Soderholm AL, Laine, Patsama J (1992b) Rigid reconstruction plates for immediate reconstruction following mandibular resection for malignant tumours. J Oral Maxillofac Surg 50:1032–1037

Lukash FN, Tenebaum NS, Moskowitz G (1990) Long-term fate of the vascularized iliac crest bone graft for mandibular reconstruction. Am J Surg 16:399–401

Moscoso JF, Urken ML (1994) The iliac crest composite flap for oromandibular reconstruction. Otolaryngol Clin North Am 27(6):1097–1117

Moscoso JF, Keller J, Genden E et al (1994) Vascularized bone flaps in oromandibular reconstruction. A comparative anatomic study of bone stock from various donor sites to assess suitability for enosseous dental implants. Arch Otolaryngol Head Neck Surg 120(1):36–43

Prein J (in press) Review of benign tumours of the maxillofacial region and considerations for bone invasion. In: Greenberg A, Prein J (eds) Craniomaxillofacial bone surgery. Springer, Berlin Heidelberg New York

Prein J (in press) Condylar prosthesis for the replacement of the mandibular condyle. In: Greenberg A, Prein J (eds) Craniomaxillofacial bone surgery. Springer, Berlin Heidelberg New York

Raveh J, Sutter F, Hellem S (1987) Surgical procedures for reconstruction of the lower jaw using the titanium coated screw reconstruction plate system: bridging defects. Otolaryngol Clin North Am 20:535–558

Sadove RC, Powell LA (1993) Simultaneous maxillary and mandibular reconstruction with one free osteocutaneous flap. Plast Reconstr Surg 92:141–146

Saunders JR, Hirata RM, Jaques DA (1990) Definitive mandibular replacement using reconstruction kplates. Am J Surg 160:387–389

Silverberg B, Banis JC, Acland RD (1985) Mandibular reconstruction with microvascular bone transfer: series of 10 patients. Am J Surg 150:440–446

Stoll P, Waechter R, Hodapp N, Schilli W (1990) Radiation and osteosynthesis. Dosimetry on an irradiation phantom. J Craniomaxofac Surg 18:361–366

Sullivan MJ, Baker SR, Crompton R, Smith-Wheelock M (1989) Free scapular osteocutaneous flap for mandibular reconstruction. Arch Otolaryngol Head Neck Surg 115:1134–1340

Tucker HM (1989) Nonrigid reconstruction of the mandible. Arch Otolaryngol Head Neck Surg 115:1190–1192

Urken ML, Buchbinder D, Weinberg H et al (1989) Primary placement of ossseointegrated implants in microvascular mandibular reconstruction. Otolaryngol Head Neck Surg 101:56–73

Urken ML, Weinberg H, Vickery C et al (1992) The combined sensate radical forearm and iliac crest free flaps for reconstruction of significant glossectomy-mandibulectomy defects. Laryngoscope 102(5):543–558

CHAPTER 6

Stable Internal Fixation of Osteotomies of the Facial Skeleton　　**6**

Chapter Author: Leon A. Assael
Contributors:　 Leon A. Assael
　　　　　　　　Joachim Prein

6.1 Introduction

Internal fixation of osteotomies of the facial skeleton ensures bone healing under stable conditions that permits immediate full function. Internal fixation also determines at the time of surgery the position of functional bony units of the face. Internal fixation provides fixation forces to counteract functional muscle forces on the facial skeleton and thereby helps to maintain the planned surgical position throughout the course of healing.

For surgery involving such precise fitting subunits as the maxilla and mandible, stable internal fixation requires careful planning and expert execution. Functional dental occlusion must be established with very low tolerance for error. While achieving stability is the greatest asset of internal fixation, it is also its greatest demand.

6.2 Treatment Planning for Internal Fixation of Osteotomies

Stable internal fixation demands that the final position in which bony segments are placed is determined at the time of surgery. Meaningful adjustments of bone position are not possible without a return to the operating room. Careful, systematic preoperative planning is necessary to achieve fixation in the correct position. The most important aspects of preoperative planning to emphasize with stable internal fixation are:

- Determining thoroughly the planned movements of bone in all dimensions
- Determining the movements based on a correct condylar position

After clinical, cephalometric, and model evaluation to design the main features of the planned surgery the final planning for internal fixation is made from the model surgery. Two sets of alginate casts are taken and poured in stone plaster. Only with a bite registration that reflects the desired postoperative condylar position can accu-

rate internal fixation at the time of surgery be achieved. Bite registration is taken in a comfortable neuromuscular centric position that reflects the desired condylar position. The use of a nondeformable silicone or aluminum wax bite registration is recommended. In order to confirm the accuracy of the bite registration temporomandibular joint laminograms can be taken with the bite registration in place. In cases where a centric slide is a potential problem preoperative laminograms taken in the planned centric position can be compared with postoperative laminograms in the planned final occlusion to assess the accuracy of condylar position. Confirmation of the bite with the mounted casts at the next patient visit can also ensure that there is no "slide" in the bite registration.

Dental casts are trimmed to closely resemble the bones to be moved. The maxillary cast is trimmed to the height of the palatal plane. It is trimmed back to show the location of the piriform rim, malar buttress, tuberosity, and posterior maxilla. The mandibular cast is trimmed to the height of the symphysis (incisal edge to gnathion). The cast height is trimmed to match the height of the horizontal ramus as determined by the cephalogram back to the gonial angle. The back of the cast is trimmed flat at the level of the gonial angles and mid ramus.

These two pairs of trimmed casts are then mounted on a semianatomic articulator with a face bow transfer (Fig. 6.1 a,b). Each cast is waxed to a plaster base. The two pairs of casts are mounted in sequence on the same articulator. Marks and measurements are made to assess movements at all critical sites, including the occlusal plane, Le Fort 1 osteotomy site, and chin. Marks on the external oblique ridge and inferior border in the third molar areas determine movement at those locations. Marks on the backs of the cast reflect the medial lateral rotation of the segments.

Model surgery is performed to reflect the correction of the occlusion and the planned movement of the bone as determined by the clinical and cephalometric assessment of the patient. In deciding on the final position of segments attention is given to tissue tolerances and the limitations of applying internal fixation. For example, in the ramus planned for sagittal split particular attention

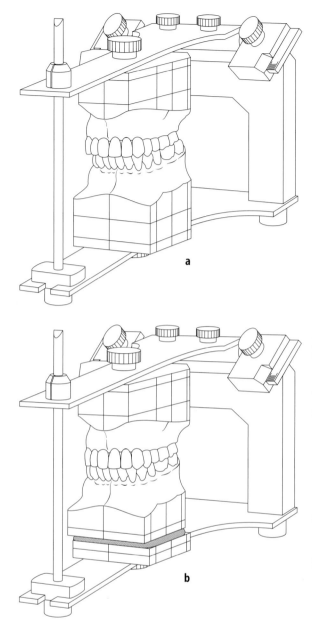

Fig. 6.1 a, b

a Trimmed mounted casts in a class 2 situation. The plaster has been trimmed to match the measurements to be taken for bony movements. The hinge axis is reflective of the face bow transfer.

b Movements on the articulator into class I situation. The anterior displacement of the mandible is visible through the marks on the cast.

is given to rotational movements, ramus lengthening movements, mandibular plane angle changes, and amount of anterior-posterior change at both the external oblique ridge and inferior borders. Records of these movements are made and are brought to the operating room for intraoperative confirmation of segment position (Fig. 6.2)

Occlusal wafer splints are constructed for all patients in order to accurately achieve the planned position of segments. When the surgery is in both jaws, an intermediate splint that reflects the maxillary movement is made. These splints are constructed as follows. After the planned movements are completed on the first set of casts, a final acrylic occlusal wafer is made by: (a) lubricating the final casts and eliminating undercuts, (b) applying cold cure acrylic wafer to the maxillary teeth first, and (c) when the acrylic is doughy, closing the mandible into occlusion leaving the bulk of acrylic attached to the maxillary dentition. The resulting shallow occlusal contacts in the mandible allow a path of closure in a natural hinge axis permitting immediate mobilization of the mandible and full function without intermaxillary fixation (Fig. 6.3).

Intermediate Splint. If the surgery is for movements in both jaws, an intermediate splint reflecting only the maxillary movement is then constructed as follows:

1. The mandibular cast showing surgical movement is removed and replaced with the uncut mandibular cast. (Alternatively, the surgical cast may be broken out and returned to its "preoperative" position using the line measurements).
2. With the final splint in place and attached to the maxillary casts that reflect the surgical movement of the maxilla, the casts and splint are greased.
3. Cold cure acrylic is applied to both the mandibular occlusion and the maxillary occlusal splint as the casts are closed to the first contact. The resulting splint reflects only the maxillary movement against the uncut mandible.

With the model surgery completed, the intermediate and final splints are brought to the operating room. These are accompanied by accurate three-dimensional measurements of movements at all critical sites. These measurements can be recorded on a form or reflected in constructed templates.

The critical sites for these measurements in maxillary surgery are:

- Central incisor midline at the occlusal plane
- Anterior nasal spine
- Piriform rims at the palatal plane
- Canine tips
- Mesiobuccal first molars occlusal plane
- Zygomatic buttresses at the palatal plane

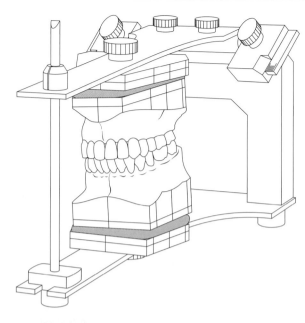

Fig. 6.2

Movements on the articulator for bimaxillary procedure. The complex asymmetrical movement in this patient demonstrates the changes at pogonion, anterior nasal spine and the mandibular rami. These are reflective of changes that are seen at the time of osteotomy fixation.

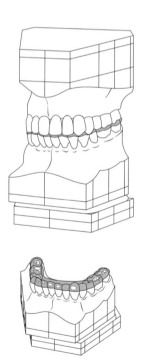

Fig. 6.3

The occlusal wafer on the casts. The final position of the planned osteotomies is determined by the occlusal wafer constructed on the mounted dental casts.
Inset: Occlusal cast visible from above on the mandibular teeth.

These measurements are essential to ensure good transverse and vertical symmetry of the face in the surgical plan. All movements are correlated with the clinical data base. For example, if the database indicates a left ramus that is 5 mm longer than the right with a deviation of pogonion 7 mm to the right, these measurements ensure that the surgical plan corrects not only the malocclusion but the asymmetry as well. The need to alter the surgical movements or incorporate adjunctive procedures such as genioplasty or bone grafting becomes apparent at this time.

It is essential that these exact measurements are reflected in the position of osseous segments when stable internal fixation is applied. This must incorporate the establishment of the preoperative condylar position and the reapplication of condylar position at the time of surgery. With the intermediate splint and final splints in place, movements of the jaws are compared with movements on the casts in the operating room to determine whether the proper position of segments and condylar position has been achieved.

6.3 Surgical Procedures

6.3.1 Mandibular Surgery

6.3.1.1 Sagittal Split Osteotomy

Since introduced by Spiessl, lag screw fixation has remained the most frequent means of stable internal fixation of sagittal split osteotomies of the mandible. Miniplate fixation and positional screw fixation are also used.

Several modifications of technique are helpful in achieving stable internal fixation of the sagittal split osteotomy. The Dalpont modification extends the buccal vertical cut down the anterior oblique ridge to the 2nd molar area where it is completed in the horizontal body of the mandible. This modification permits a greater surface area for screws, particularly in mandibular advancement surgery. In the Hunsuck modification the split is along the lingual surface of the ramus behind the nerve. This improves the ability to set back the mandible without impinging posteriorly. It also helps in procedures lengthening the ramus as the masticator sling is extended less as the distal segment moves inferiorly. The Hunsuck modification does not permit easy placement of screws at the inferior border however. With the Hunsuck modification it is often necessary to place all screws at the superior border (Fig. 6.4)

The technique for performing the sagittal split must also include careful attention to the mandibular nerve, which results in its placement in the distal segment without impingement. When the segments are placed, the position of the nerve must be confirmed. The place-

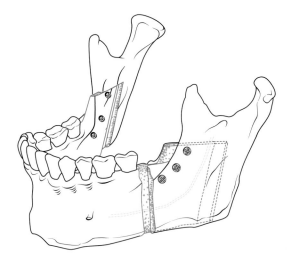

Fig. 6.4

Hunsuck modification. The sagittal split osteotomy is modified by incompletely performing the osteotomy to the posterior border above the lingula. This results in an osteotomy within the lingual cortical plate.

ment of screws only on the superior border or the use of monocortical plate fixation may result in less risk of neurotmesis and compression injury of the mandibular nerve.

The position of the distal segment of the sagittal split is determined when the patient is placed in occlusion in the final splint. Proximal segment position can be determined either by a condylar positioning device or manually. In either case the recorded movements of the model surgery are compared with those achieved in the operating room at the superior and inferior border. If manual positioning is performed, a Dingman bone holding forceps or other clamp on the anterior border is a useful device to maintain the segments since its paired beaks engage while they are still separated. This prevents overcompression of the proximal segment, which may result in lateral positioning of the condyle.

The surgeon may elect to position the proximal segment via direct measurements taken from the model surgery or through the use of a condylar positioning device. Condylar positioning devices are designed to reproduce the preoperative relationship between the

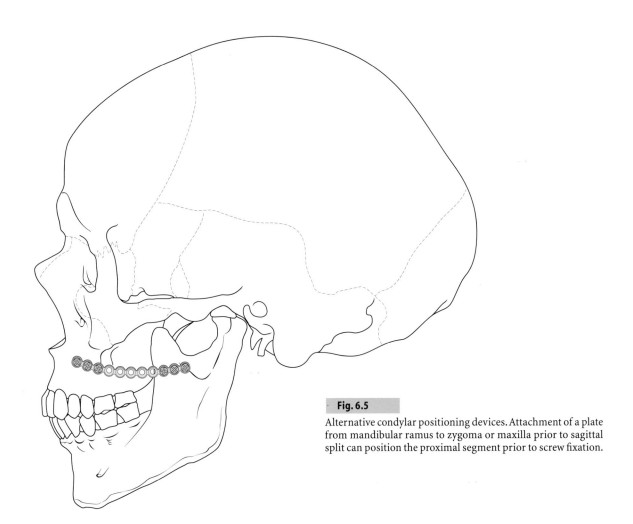

Fig. 6.5

Alternative condylar positioning devices. Attachment of a plate from mandibular ramus to zygoma or maxilla prior to sagittal split can position the proximal segment prior to screw fixation.

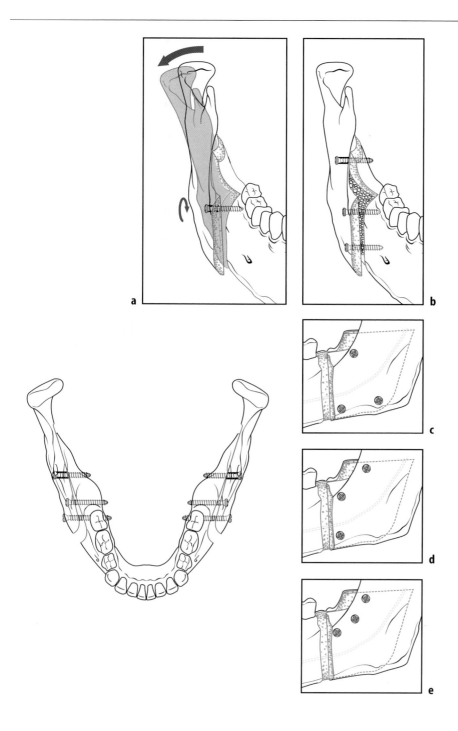

Fig. 6.6

Correct fixation of sagittal split osteotomy and anterior advancement of mandible. Anterior gaps are kept and stabilized with positioning screws. Posterior natural contact area is stabilized with a lag screw.

Inset a: Lateral condylar displacement due to lag screw fixation in natural gap area. Under these circumstances the distal aspect of the proximal segment is displaced medially.

Inset b: The use of a shim of bone to prevent lateral condylar displacement can be performed with a single lag screw in the most proximal position followed by positional screws placed through the sandwiched shim bone graft. A piece of the distal aspect of the proximal segment can be removed to serve as this graft.

Insets c, d, e: The various possible placements of either lag or positioning screws.

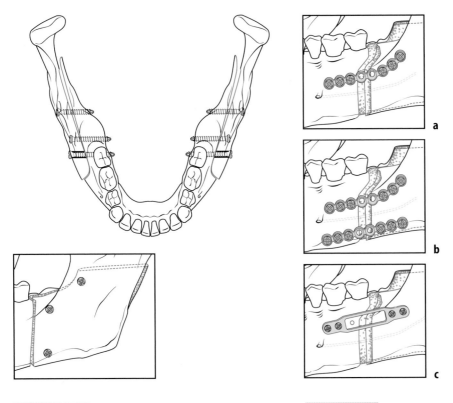

Fig. 6.7

Fixation of sagittal split osteotomy for class 3 occlusion. Natural contact area in distal aspect of proximal segment where a lag screw is used. The other screws are placed as position screws.

Fig. 6.8 a–c

Plate fixation of sagittal osteotomy. Monocortically applied plates provide accurate positioning but inferior fixation forces in the mandibular sagittal split osteotomy.
a One 2.0 miniplate.
b Two 2.0 miniplates.
c Split fix plate, or adjustable saggittal split plate.

proximal segment of the mandible and the maxillary base. In this case a plate is bent and fixed to the lateral border of the ramus and maxilla (cephelad to any maxillary osteotomy) before the osteotomy is completed. The plate is removed. Following the completion of the osteotomy the plate is replaced while the final ramus fixation is completed (Fig. 6.5).

Understanding the planned movements in three dimensions assists the surgeon in deciding what modifications in the osteotomy to perform, whether to use bone graft shims, and which method of internal fixation to employ. In mandibular advancement surgery tight clamping (or a lag screw at area of natural gap) of the ramus causes the condyle to position laterally (Fig. 6.6, inset a). In this instance positional screws or a single lag screw can be used at the point of natural contact followed by two positional screws (Fig. 6.6, inset b). Additionally, bone contact without condylar displacement can be assisted by placing a "shim" between the segments (Fig. 6.6, inset b) with lag screw fixation. Further examples of the geometry of screw fixation are shown in Fig. 6.6, insets c–e). Figure 6.7 shows the placement of lag

screws and positioning screws in retropositioning of the mandible.

Condylar position and stable internal fixation can also be achieved through the use of a monocortically fixed plate with 2.0-mm screws on the external oblique ridge. This permits fixation without condylar displacement. Mechanical load resistance with this technique is inferior to that with screw fixation of the ramus. For this reason two plates are used by some surgeons for each osteotomy (Fig. 6.8).

6.3.1.2 Other Ramus Osteotomies

The vertical ramus osteotomy is not commonly used with stable internal fixation because of the many problems in maintaining the preoperative condylar position and the risk to the mandibular nerve when transbuccal screws are applied. There have been reports of miniplate fixation of the proximal segment, but the ability to apply immediate full function has not been established. As a result most vertical ramus osteotomies are still per-

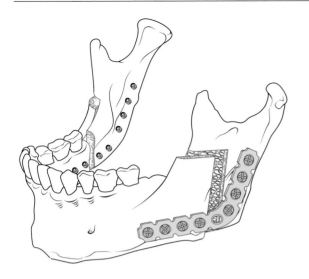

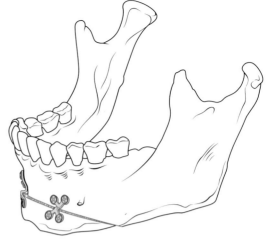

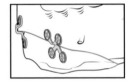

Fig. 6.9

Inverted L osteotomy. Fixation with a stabilization plate with four screws per segment is recommended since this osteotomy is the mechanical equivalent of a mandibular continuity defect.

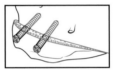

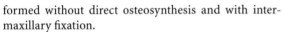

Fig. 6.10

Genioplasty fixation. Miniplate or lag screw fixation can be employed to fix the genioplasty osteotomy.

formed without direct osteosynthesis and with inter-maxillary fixation.

Inverted L osteotomies are used with stable internal fixation when the procedure is used for ramus lengthening and advancement with an interpositional bone graft. The inverted L is especially useful in a short ramus such as hemifacial microsomia when a large ramus lengthening and onlay bone grafting is planned.

This procedure is performed with a retromandibular transcervical incision. After intermaxillary fixation the proximal segment can be positioned with the AO bone holding forceps spread apart with the wing nut engaged. Movements at the inferior and superior borders are checked with the surgical plan to ensure condylar position. (Alternatively, a transoral condylar positioning device attached to the coronoid process may be used.) Fixation of the segments and graft are completed with a 2.4 reconstruction plate or a Universal Fracture plate. Four screws in both the proximal and distal segment are recommended to permit full function in this procedure. Onlay bone grafts, if indicated, can then be attached with lag screws (Fig. 6.9).

6.3.1.3 Genioplasty

Anterior mandibular horizontal osteotomy is performed with a power saw in the routine manner. For complex movements temporary fixation can be obtained with a transosseous wire or a single lag screw. Final three-dimensionally stable fixation of this osteotomy can be achieved with two or more lag screws, a pair

of straight plates, or a single T-, Y-, H-, or X-shaped 1.5- or 2.0-mm plate. When combined with a subapical osteotomy, a single H-shaped plate or straight plates can provide fixation to both osteotomies simultaneously. Screws are usually 4–6 mm long.

Lag screws may be placed transorally with genioplasty. The inferior border of the distal segment to the lingual plate of the superior segment provides the appropriate direction for many situations. The advantages of the 2.0 screw (16–22 mm long) are that mentalis muscle and muscle resuspension can be reattached more easily, and that no plate is palpable in the mental fold (Fig. 6.10).

6.3.1.4 Mandibular Segmental Surgery

Anterior mandibular subapical osteotomy is performed in the usual manner, with attention to making the inferior osteotomy at least 5 mm apical to the canine apex. The segment is positioned in its occlusal wafer with maxillomandibular fixation. A straight plate, T, L, H, or X plate can be employed to provide monocortical fixation with 2.0- or 1.5-mm screws. Lag screws are usually not practical due to the proximity of the tooth apices.

Fixation of subapical osteotomy can be combined with genioplasty fixation through the use of a variety of

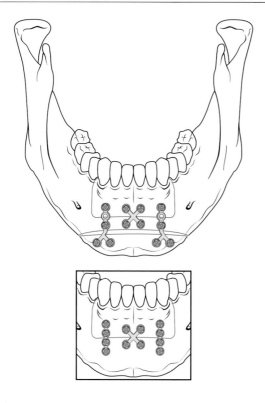

Fig. 6.11

Subapical osteotomy and genioplasty. Miniplate fixation is combined to support both osteotomies via the isthmus of bone between the segments.

plate combinations. Fixation of the isthmus of bone between the genioplasty should be part of the screw fixation scheme in order to prevent rotation of the segment (Fig. 6.11).

6.3.2 Midface Surgery: Le Fort I Osteotomy

The performance of the Le Fort I osteotomy is not substantially altered by the use of plate and screw fixation. The surgeon should give attention to recording the movements of the maxilla by making score lines or holes to measure maxillary movement. The location of the osteotomy in the piriform rim should allow the placement of screws apical to the teeth in the premaxilla. At least 5 mm of bone apical to the molars and premolars is helpful in permitting the safe placement of screws in these locations. Prior to the initiation of any fixation the closure of nasal mucosal rents, any necessary turbinectomy, septoplasty, and relief of the medial sinus wall should be completed. Hemostasis should be ensured prior to fixation with attention to impingement around the anterior palatine arteries.

The maxilla is positioned in all three dimenions for fixation by assuring the following components:

- The placement of the teeth into the final occlusal wafer
- The position of the condyles in centric relation
- The vertical position of the maxilla as measured at the osteotomy site

Teeth must rest passively in the occlusal wafer with the patient in maxillomandibular fixation. Wire fixation of the appliances is normally performed with a stiff arch wire and at least four maxillomandibular loops. Positioning of the condyle with the patient supine under general anesthesia is often problematic. The tendency is for the maxilla to come too far forward in superior autorotation due to the forward slide induced at the posterior medial sinus wall. This thick bone of the vertical process of the palatine bone must be relieved after the patient is in the splint, and interferences are identified. An additional site of interference for upward and backward movement of the maxilla is the pterygoid plates. Since the pterygoid plates project forward superiorly, relief of the tuberosity bone may be necessary to permit upward movement.

Forcing the condyle too far backward during maxillary positioning may result in a maxilla that is fixed too far posteriorly. The mandible is best rotated into the final maxillary position with upward manual movement of the angles of the patient's mandible. Backward pressure on the chin risks overseating the condyle.

The vertical position of the maxilla is determined from the model surgery. Measurements are easily taken at the piriform rim and zygomatic buttress. Measurements in the midline or incisor can be made only with a cranial positioning device. These devices are not necessary when maxillary movements are measured from models that are articulated via face bow transfer. For example, a 4-mm downward movement at the piriform rim accomplished by mandibular autorotation might result in 6 mm of movement at the incisor. Vertical positioning of the maxilla is also assisted by the placement of interpositional bone grafts when downward movement is planned. These grafts are placed in the piriform rim and zygomatic buttress regions.

Fixation of the Le Fort I osteotomy depends upon the direction of movement and the buttressing of the maxilla achieved by direct bone contact. If the patient is not in maxillomandibular fixation, the loads applied to the osteotomy site are predominantly compressive. For superior movement of the maxilla where bone contact is excellent, the use of two plates at the piriform rim with six screws per plate can be sufficient. The most widely used are 2.0- and 1.5-mm screws with L plates or arched plates. The bone of the lateral piriform rim and the bone

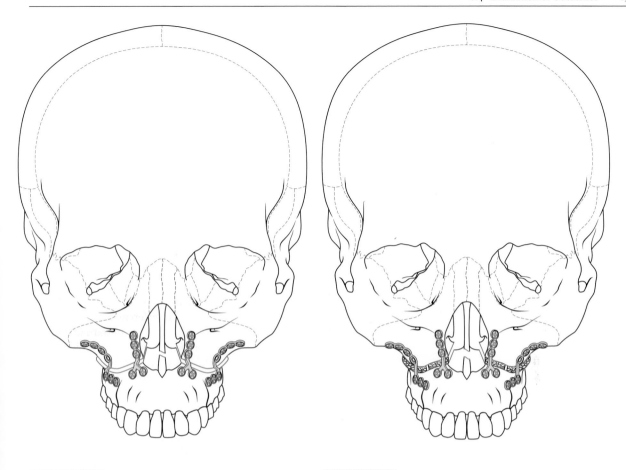

Fig. 6.12

Miniplate fixation of the Le Fort I osteotomy. Plates at the piriform rim and zygomatic buttress provide support in the thickest bone of the maxilla.

Fig. 6.13

Interpositional bone grafts. The Le Fort I osteotomy performed for downward movement can incorporate interpositional bone grafts wedged beneath the miniplates. This should be performed for gaps wider than 4 mm.

apical to the central and lateral incisor generally provide the best stability. Bicortical fixation of these screws can be achieved by passing the inferor screws as far as the nasal floor and the superior screws can engage both the piriform rim and the lateral nasal wall. Usually for all osteotomies where bone contact buttressing is incomplete, additional plates are subsequently placed at the zygomatic buttress (Fig. 6.12). For downward movement of the maxilla interpositional grafts can be wedged beneath the miniplates (Fig. 6.13).

If segmental maxillary surgery is performed, the occlusal splint creates a single unit of the maxilla. Four plates are generally used to provide maximum stability once the occlusal wafer is removed several weeks postoperatively. Cross-arch stability can be assisted by placing a plate across the midline on the facial aspect of the premaxilla. If the maxilla has been split for access as in a tumor case, transpalatine fixation is sometimes used (see Fig. 4.2.10, inset 3).

6.4 Evaluation of Outcomes

Patients are allowed full function after osteotomies performed with stable internal fixation. Initial postoperative clinical evaluation should ensure that the patient is closing into the splint perfectly. Postoperative radiographs assess jaw position, osteotomies and the position of plates and screws are taken with the patient closed into the splint (Fig. 6.14b). Lateral and posterior anterior cephalograms and orthopantomogram are normally taken (Fig. 6.14b–d).

Elastics are often used to guide the patients jaw function since proprioception of the postoperative jaw position is sometimes difficult. Elastics can manage only very small errors in jaw position and should not be used to provide orthopedic forces.

The use of stable internal fixation does not obviate the possibility of late surgical relapse. Careful assess-

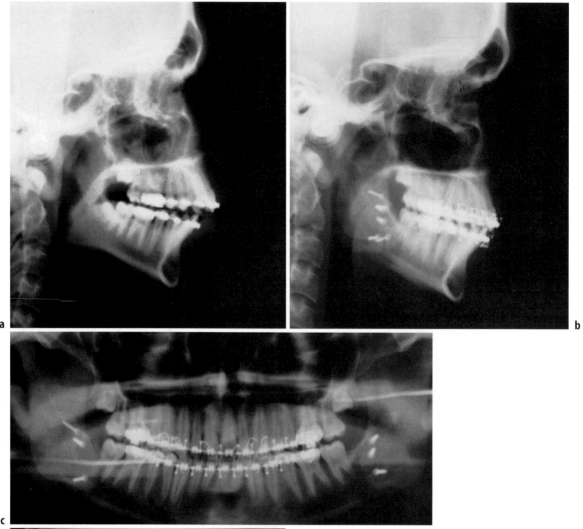

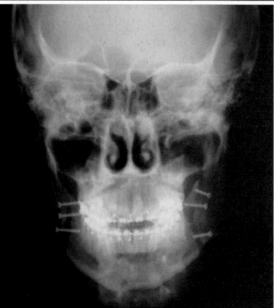

Fig. 6.14 a–d

Radiographic documentation. Comparison of the preoperative and postoperative cephalograms (**a, b**) along with orthopanto-mogram (**c**) and posterior anterior cephalogram (**d**) allows complete radiographic analysis of the surgical outcome.

ment of stability in the first 3 months is necessary to ensure uneventful initial healing phase.

Figures 6.15 and 6.16 show further clinical cases.

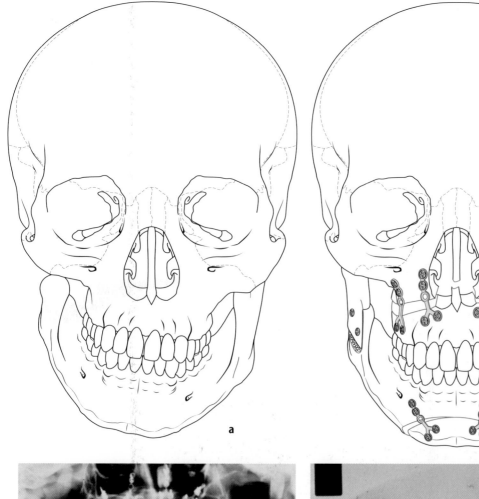

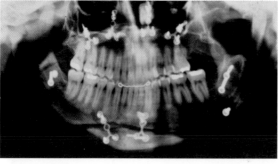

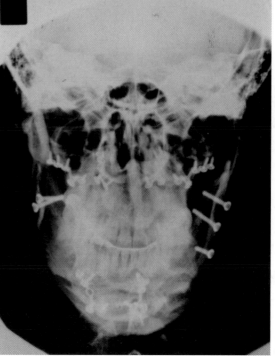

Fig.6.15 a–d

a Facial asymmetry due to loss of condylar area on the right side during childhood. The mandibular ramus on the right side is too short and in consequence the occlusal plane is deviated. The facial height on the right side is shorter than on the left. This facial asymmetry is comparable to hemifacial microsomia.

b Surgical correction of facial asymmetry described in **a**. The correction consists of a Le Fort I osteotomy, a sagittal split osteotomy on the left, a chin osteotomy and correction with a bone graft in the right mandibular area.

c Postoperative orthopantomogram of the situation shown in **b**.

d X-ray showing posterior-anterior view of the same operation as described in **b**.

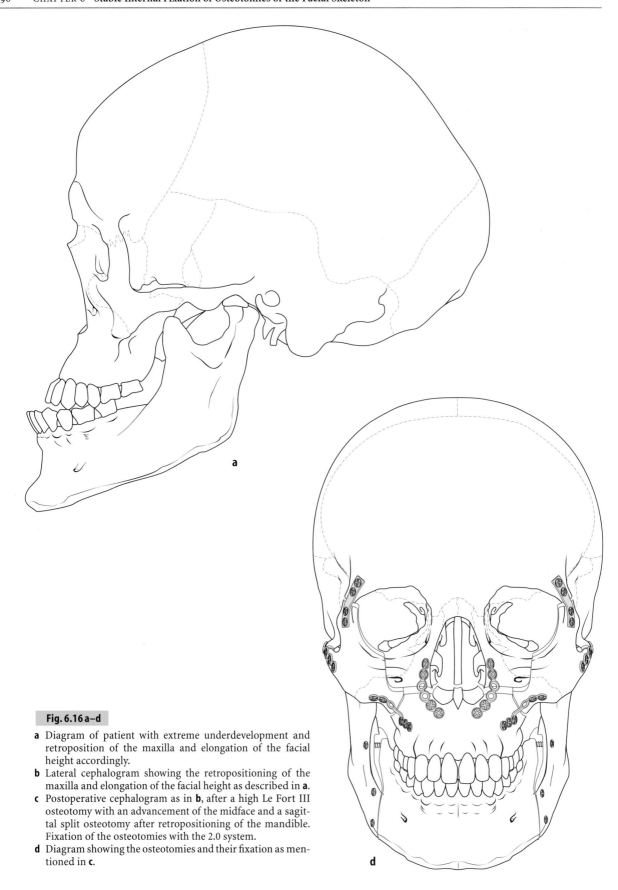

Fig. 6.16 a–d

a Diagram of patient with extreme underdevelopment and retroposition of the maxilla and elongation of the facial height accordingly.

b Lateral cephalogram showing the retropositioning of the maxilla and elongation of the facial height as described in **a**.

c Postoperative cephalogram as in **b**, after a high Le Fort III osteotomy with an advancement of the midface and a sagittal split osteotomy after retropositioning of the mandible. Fixation of the osteotomies with the 2.0 system.

d Diagram showing the osteotomies and their fixation as mentioned in **c**.

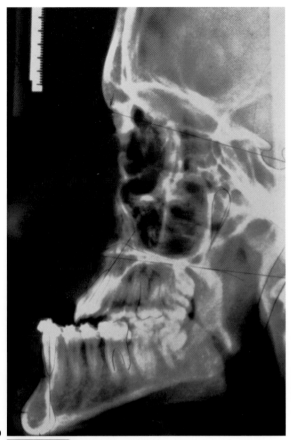

b

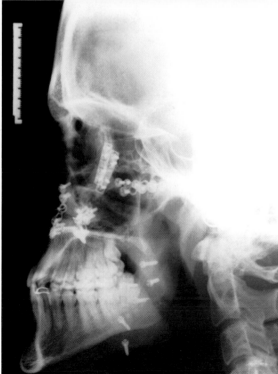

c

6.5 Complications

Comminuted osteotomies may occur during mobilization or during plate and screw fixation. This is most frequent during the sagittal split osteotomy. Care should be taken to identify weak areas for fixation and to avoid overtightening screws. The most frequent sites for comminution are the lingual plate at the angle region, particularly when a third molar is present, and the buccal plate in midramus. If comminution occurs, the comminuted segment can be built in larger subunits, permitting stable internal fixation in most cases (Fig. 6.17).

Palpable hardware is most often a factor at the piriform rim and nasomaxillary region. The use of 1.5-mm plates has not substantially reduced the palpability of this hardware. Due to the thinness of the cortical bone in the ramus osteotomy countersinking is seldom carried out. Symptomatic hardware is rare, but when it is a factor it may be due to muscle gliding over plates and screws during movement.

Malocclusion in stable fixation of osteotomies may be the result of malpositioned segments or problems in the splint, condylar position, temporomandibular joint disc position, path of closure, or neuromuscular guidance. Postoperative malocclusion calls for early analysis of the cause and appropriate intervention. This may include the use of temporomandibular joint imaging with the patient in correct maxillomandibular fixation. It may include removal of the splint, removal of the plates and screws and refixation in the corrected position, a new clinical data base, and diagnostic casts.

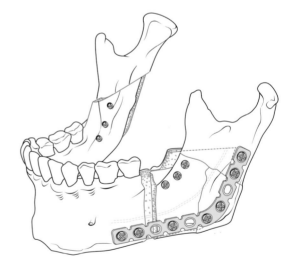

Fig. 6.17

Comminution of the sagittal osteotomy. Reconstituting major segments in the event of comminution usually produces stable internal fixation of the comminuted osteotomy.

6.6 Summary

Stable internal fixation of osteotomies of the jaws affords the opportunity for immediate function, assuring the planned surgical position, and less relapse for the orthognathic surgical patient. Successful application of this technique depends upon careful planning and achievement of the surgical treatment plan in the operative setting.

References and Suggested Reading

Ardary W, Tracy D, Brownridge G, Urata M (1989) Comparative evaluation of screw configuration on the stability of the sagittal split osteotomy. Oral Surg 68:125–129

Ellis E (1990) Accuracy of model surgery: Evaluation of an old technique and introduction of a new one. J Oral Maxillofac Surg 48:1161

Ellis E, Hinton RJ (1991) Histologic examination of the temporomandibular joint after mandibular advancement with and without rigid fixation: an experimental investigation in adult *Macaca mulatta*. J Oral Maxillofac Surg 49: 1316–1327

Ellis E, Tharanon W, Gambrell K (1992) Accuracy of face bow transfer. Effect on surgical prediction and postsurgical result. J Oral Maxillofac Surg 50:562–567

Foley W, Frost D, Paulin W, Tucker M (1989) Internal screw fixation: comparison of placement of pattern and rigidity. J Oral Maxillofac Surg 47:720–723

Franco J, Van Sickels J, Thrash W (1989) Factors contributing to relapse in rigidly fixed mandibular setbacks. J Oral Maxillofac Surg 47:451–456

Hackney F, Van Sickles J, Nummikoski P (1989) Condylar displacement and temporomandibular joint dysfunction following bilateral sagittal split osteotomy and rigid fixation. J Oral Maxillofac Surg 47:223–227

Harle W (1980) Le Fort I osteotomy using miniplates for correction of the long face. Int J Oral Surg 9:427

Harsha B, Terry B (1986) Stabilization of Le Fort I osteotomies utilizing small bone plates. Int J Adult Orthod Orthog Surg 1:69

Jeter T, Van Sickels J, Dolwick M (1984) Modified techniques for internal fixation of sagittal ramus osteotomies. J Oral Maxillofac Surg 42:270–272

Kent J, Craig M (1996) Secondary autogenous and alloplastic reshaping procedures for facial asymmetry. In: Atlas of oral and maxillofacial surgery clinics of North America, vol 4. pp 83

Kirkpatrick T, Woods M, Swift J, Markowitz M (1987) Skeletal stability following mandibular advancement and rigid fixation. J Oral Maxillofac Surg 45:572–576

Precious D, Armstrong J, Morais D (1992) Anatomic placement of fixation devices in genioplasty. Oral Surg 73:2–8

Shafer D, Assael L (1993) Rigid intrnal fixation of mandibular segmental osteotomies, vol 1. Atlas of oral and maxillofacial surgery clinics of North America. pp 41–53

Smith B (1993) Presurgical management. In: Atlas of the oral and maxillofacial surgery clinics of North America, vol 1. pp 1–15

Spiessl B (1976) Rigid internal fixation after sagittal split osteotomy of the ascending ramus. New concepts in maxillofacial bone surgery. Springer, Berlin Heidelberg New York

Spiessl B (1989) "Osteotomies" in internal fixation of the mandible. Springer, Berlin Heidelberg New York

Steinhäuser E (1982) Bone screws and plates in orthognathic surgery. Int J Oral Surg 11:209

Taylor T (1993) Complications of osteotomies with rigid fixation. In: Atlas of the oral and maxillofacial surgery clinics of North America, vol 1. pp 87

Tucker M (1988) Use of rigid internal fixation for management of intraoperative complications of mandibular sagittal split osteotomy. Int J Orthod Orthognath Surg 3:71

Van Sickels J, Tiner B (1993) Midface and periorbital osteotomies. In: Atlas of oral and maxillofacial surgery clinics of North America, vol 1. pp 71–86

Van Sickels J, Larsen A, Thrash W (1986) Relapse after rigid fixation of mandibular advancement. J Oral Maxillofac Surg 44:698

CHAPTER 7

Craniofacial Deformities

7

Chapter Author: Paul N. Manson
Contributors: Paul N. Manson
Craig A. Vander Kolk
Benjamin Carson

7.1 Introduction

The earliest craniofacial surgery began in the 1930s with Gillies' Le Fort III osteotomy in a patient with Crouzon's syndrome. In the 1950s and 1960s Tessier demonstrated that midface and intracranial approaches can be used for cranial vault and facial osteotomies for correction. The field rapidly expanded with complex craniofacial deformity correction: hypertelorism, frontal and facial retrusion, facial clefts, orbital dystopia, enophthalmos, Treacher Collins syndrome, and hemifacial microsomia were managed.

The early surgical techniques consisted of direct visualization of deformed segments, skeletal osteotomies, wire fixation, and the use of liberal amounts of bone graft to complete the reconstruction. Complex osteotomies were initially designed with "tongue in grove" and "Z-plasty" techniques to splint and reenforce the reconstruction. The current use of rigid fixation has made design of such complex osteotomies obsolete. Although craniofacial surgeons largely prefer fresh, autogenous bone for transplantation and reconstruction, the use of newer materials (such as bone forming materials, hydroxyapatite, Medpor, and bioceramics) offer promise for the future if their long-term safety and efficacy can be documented.

Craniofacial surgery has received a tremendous stimulus from the development of computed tomography, to include three-dimensional reconstructions. These reconstructions currently function to provide a detailed and composite picture of the deformity and its correction (Fig. 7.1). Surgical simulations may be performed with computer imaging, providing a standard for planning the reconstruction and assessing the postoperative result.

The main advantage of internal fixation is that it creates stability of osteotomized bone segments. It has been shown that bone survives better with stable fixation in most circumstances. In young infants the use and placement of stable fixation devices should be carefully determined to avoid problems with translocation of plates (intracranial or intracalvarial) which generally occurs in syndromal synostoses and in the temporal region. Since intracranial migration is especially prone to occur in those with syndromal craniosynostosis, some consideration for removing fixation materials, especially in the temporal region, should be given in these cases. The placement of fixation material can also contribute to palpable or visible plates. Craniofacial surgeons were initially concerned about growth restriction from fixation; however, it has been difficult to document that growth restriction exceeds 5%–8%. Currently its benefits therefore exceed its disadvantages by virtue of the increased stability created.

Reliable internal fixation stabilizes osteotomy segments and thus maintains their position. Often the expansions created in craniosynostosis correction are subject to considerable soft-tissue pressure. This pressure produces forces creating relapse which are effectively opposed only by strong fixation material. Internal fixation stabilizes the reconstruction for protection of patient positioning postoperatively, even on the osteotomized segment.

Stable fixation counteracts soft-tissue forces acting on the osteotomized segment in the early postoperative period. The patient can also be positioned on the reconstructed area. Stable fixation prevents relapse and collapse of the reconstruction, decreasing the potential for secondary revision.

Sufficient internal fixation also limits bone motion in the postoperative healing phase, thereby increasing bone survival. It produces less complicated bone wound healing, with progress toward primary bone healing. Stable fixation most probably decreases the tendency toward infection. The disadvantages of internal fixation include the cost and concerns about potential growth restriction, loosening, migration, and plate prominence. Loosening, plate prominence, and translocation are seen mostly in the temporal regions and in younger patients and those with syndromal synostoses.

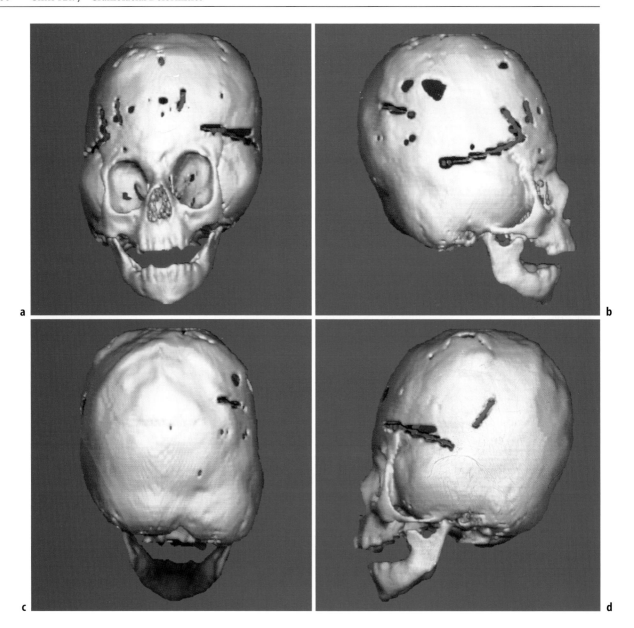

Fig. 7.1 a–d

Three-dimensional CT reconstructions provide a detailed and composite picture of the cranial deformity.

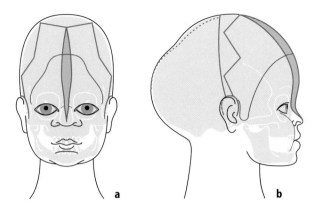

Fig. 7.2 a, b

Incisions used for cranial reconstruction include the coronal incision and extensions. This involves an incision from ear to ear which is generally carried out behind the ear if lower extension is required (dotted lines). It can be "zigzagged" for a less apparent incision (technique of Munro or "stealth" technique; see also Chap. 2).

The use of a posterior "T" incision extending from the coronal to allow for improved exposure for posterior reconstruction.

When hypertelorism with a bifid nose is present requiring resection of anterior skin and correction of the bifid nose, an anterior T can be extended to the nasal tip which allows direct exposure and excision of excess tissue.

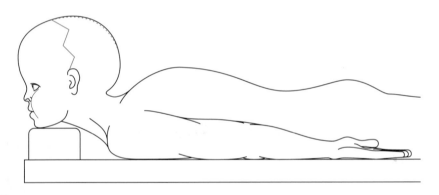

Fig. 7.3

The sphinx position.

7.2 Incisions for Craniofacial Reconstruction and Patient Positioning

The coronal incision is the most common incision used for craniofacial reconstruction (Fig. 7.2). When the full cranium is reconstructed (Fig. 7.2b), a "T" is developed from the coronal incision which extends posteriorly to allow for reconstruction. When hypertelorism with bifid nose is present, an anterior "T" (see Fig. 7.2b) allows exposure and permits excision of excess tissue. The positioning for a full cranial reconstruction in older children can be the "sphinx" position (Fig. 7.3). When the reconstruction is staged, the anterior and posterior coronal or "T" incisions are used, and the patient is positioned prone for the posterior and supine for the anterior.

7.3 Craniosynostosis

Craniosynostosis, or premature fusion, can involve any cranial suture. Early fusion of the suture limits cranial growth. There are eight identifiable cranial sutures. Three sets are paired: right and left coronal, right and left lambdoid, and right and left squamosal (Fig. 7.4). The two midline sutures include the sagittal suture and the metopic suture (Fig. 7.5a). One should also be aware that there is a nasal frontal suture (Fig. 7.5a) anteriorly and cranial base suture extensions (Fig. 7.5b).

When sutures undergo premature fusion or have a growth restriction, they decrease the ability of the skull to adapt to the growing brain. It is now known that the size of the brain in patients with craniosynostosis is generally normal or increased. The complex relationship between the dura, brain, and signals providing suture

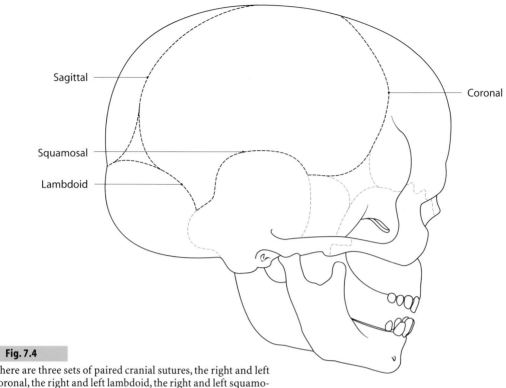

Fig. 7.4

There are three sets of paired cranial sutures, the right and left coronal, the right and left lambdoid, the right and left squamosal.

closure are not presently known. Several general theories have been formulated to predict the etiology. Virchow stated that the deformity is related to the fusion of the suture itself. Moss' theory was related to the postulate that the abnormality begins in the cranial base in the synchondroses and secondarily affects the cranial vault. Other investigators have suggested that the abnormality begins in the mesenchymal blastema and is related to the dura where tensile forces of the growing brain are not adequately transmitted in signal fashion to the suture, providing an inadequate stimulus to grow.

Recent reports suggest that abnormalities of growth factors occur within the suture. It is known that some of the syndromal synostoses, such as Crouzon's syndrome, have a mutation in the *FGFR-2* gene. Fibroblast growth factor is one of the growth factors. In the Boston craniosynostosis syndrome there is a mutation of a Homeobox gene, *MSX-2*, which is thought to control the growth and expression of other genes that control differentiation and growth. As craniosynostosis develops, the growth of the skull is limited in a direction perpendicular to the suture. A flattening in the region around the suture results in cranial deformity. There is usually compensatory overgrowth on the contralateral side. When multiple sutures are fused, the tendency to develop increased intracranial pressure increases as the ability to compensate with compensatory overgrowth decreases.

The term "plagiocephaly" is derived from the Greek and means literally "twisted skull." It is used to describe the syndrome in which a coronal or lambdoidal suture fuses prematurely and results in lack of growth. The term "anterior plagiocephaly" refers to involvement of the coronal suture and "posterior plagiocephaly" to that of the lambdoidal suture. Coronal suture synostoses cause ipsilateral or bilateral frontal flattening. In unilateral deformities one finds a decrease in the transverse diameter of the ipsilateral orbit, anterior placement of the ear, deviation of the chin point to the opposite side, deviation of the nose to the ipsilateral side, contralateral frontal "bossing," and contralateral occipital flattening (Fig. 7.6).

True lambdoidal synostosis is rare; many posterior postural or positional deformities can be mistaken for synostosis; three-dimensional computed tomography is necessary to document fusion of the suture to confirm partial or complete synostosis (Fig. 7.7). Positional deformities are generally managed by the use of a helmet or positioning techniques for infant sleeping which molds or relieves sleeping pressure on the skull. When both coronal and lambdoidal sutures are involved, anterior or posterior brachycephaly occurs. The deformity consists of anterior-posterior flattening, increased vertical height of the skull and shortening of the cranial base (Fig. 7.8).

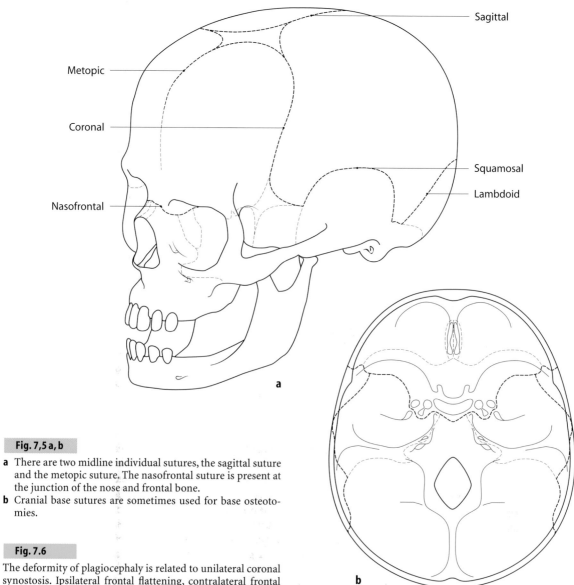

Sagittal

Metopic

Coronal

Squamosal

Lambdoid

Nasofrontal

a

b

Fig. 7,5 a, b

a There are two midline individual sutures, the sagittal suture and the metopic suture. The nasofrontal suture is present at the junction of the nose and frontal bone.
b Cranial base sutures are sometimes used for base osteotomies.

Fig. 7.6

The deformity of plagiocephaly is related to unilateral coronal synostosis. Ipsilateral frontal flattening, contralateral frontal bossing, ipsilateral occipital flattening, deviation of the chin point to the opposite side, deviation of the nose to the ipsilateral side and movement of the ear position anteriorly are characteristic of the deformity.

▼

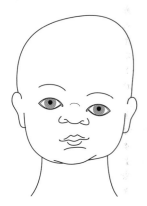
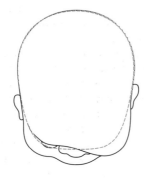
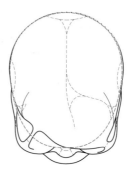

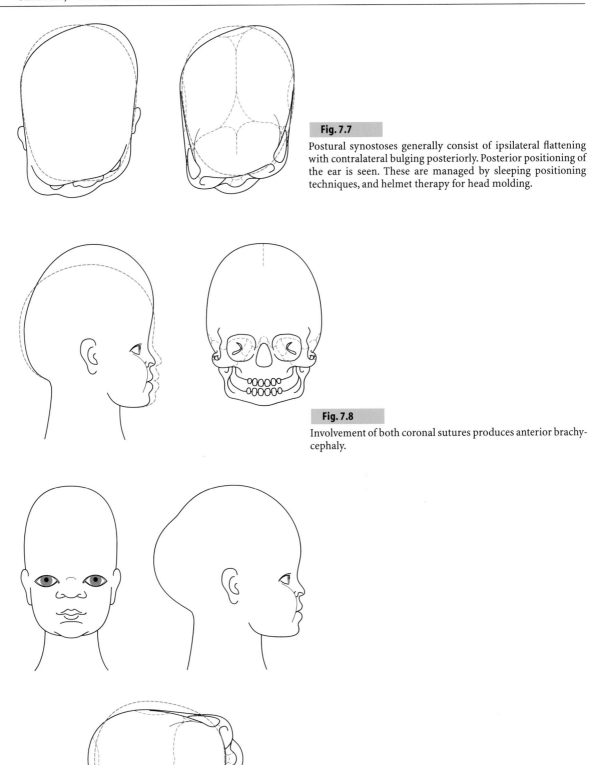

Fig. 7.7

Postural synostoses generally consist of ipsilateral flattening with contralateral bulging posteriorly. Posterior positioning of the ear is seen. These are managed by sleeping positioning techniques, and helmet therapy for head molding.

Fig. 7.8

Involvement of both coronal sutures produces anterior brachycephaly.

Fig. 7.9

Sagittal synostosis produces scaphocephaly.

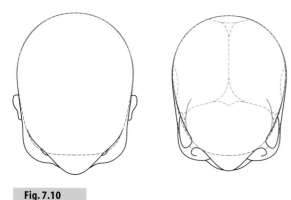

Fig. 7.10

Trigonocephaly is produced by premature closure of the metopic suture. It is often accompanied by hypotelorism.

Isolated sagittal suture synostosis is one of the most common synostoses. Skull growth is restricted laterally, causing an increased anterior-posterior length of the skull. Sagittal synostosis in infants under 4 months of age is managed initially by resection of the involved suture. Thereafter sutural resection and osteotomies are required to expand the cranial vault. Sagittal synostosis demonstrates impaired growth in an elongated skull with increased anterior-posterior length. This produces dolichocephaly or scaphocephaly (Fig. 7.9). When the metopic suture undergoes premature fusion, there is diminished growth in the right and left sides of the forehead, with a prominent ridge anteriorly. The triangular skull shape produced is known as trigonocephaly (Fig. 7.10). Hypertelorism is also frequently noted in these patients. Bilateral coronal synostosis produces brachycephaly, a tower skull with reduced anterior-posterior growth.

The deformities resulting from synostosis are always more complex than those seen in the local area around the involved suture. Compensatory changes are seen at a distance in the skull. Delashaw has postulated that other sutures of the cranium try to compensate for the synostosis. The variable effects produced require consideration not only of the area of major growth restriction but contralateral areas as well. Therefore in treating a plagiocephaly there are techniques for both unilateral and bilateral forehead osteotomies. Most surgeons generally prefer a bilateral osteotomy because the compensatory changes on the noninvolved side are addressed better by the bilateral osteotomy, permitting increased symmetry to be achieved.

Three types of reconstruction are commonly performed in craniofacial reconstruction: anterior cranial expansion, posterior cranial expansion, and total cranial expansion. There are two varieties of hypertelorism procedures, the "box" orbital osteotomy and the "V" excision bipartition or facial split osteotomies of Vander Muellen, Monasterio, and Tessier, which are used in

Apert's syndrome. Anterior cranial expansions include procedures performed for either right or left isolated coronal synostosis, right and left bilateral coronal synostosis, and metopic synostosis. Posterior cranial expansion is used for the right or left isolated and bilateral lambdoid deformities. Subtotal or total calvarial expansion is used for sagittal synostosis if it does not respond early to osteotomy. Le Fort III, frontal cranial advancement, and monoblock procedures correct the midface and frontal bone deformities singularly or simultaneously (monoblock).

7.4 Planning and Reconstruction

The planning for reconstruction is based on a physical examination and an initial diagnosis which is supported by data obtained from axial and three-dimensional computed tomography (see Fig. 7.1). This scan can be placed in a data base for archival data collection and retrieval. Both bone and brain windows should be collected to provide maximal information. Brain windows evaluate the amount of compression of the brain and the restriction of the fluid spaces or ventricles secondary to the growth restriction. Redistribution of the subarachnoid fluid with brain compression directly below the area of synostosis often occurs with digital impressions in the bone. Cerebral circulation may be decreased in the scan. Compensatory changes are sometimes seen on the contralateral side in unilateral deformities.

7.5 Surgical Technique: Anterior Cranial Expansion and Reconstruction

Anterior cranial expansion begins with a coronal incision. The frontal and temporal areas are exposed subperiosteally, leaving the temporalis muscles attached to the subcutaneous tissue. This provides a generous exposure to the entire frontal and both temporal regions (see Fig. 7.2).

An anterior bone flap (Fig. 7.11) is developed which permits dissection along the anterior cranial base to expose the orbital rooves and crista gali. The olfactory nerves are not disturbed.

The orbits are dissected medially, superiorly, and laterally down to the body of the zygoma. Osteotomies are performed (Fig. 7.12) across the roof of the orbits; the sphenoid and frontal process of the zygoma are sectioned at the malar eminence on the involved side and at the zygomaticofrontal suture on the uninvolved side (Fig. 7.12a). If the deformity is bilateral (Fig. 7.12b), such as in metopic synostosis, the osteotomies are performed at the junction at the malar eminence and the frontal process of the zygoma. This allows a complete "lateral canthal advancement" with anterior rotation. Osteoto-

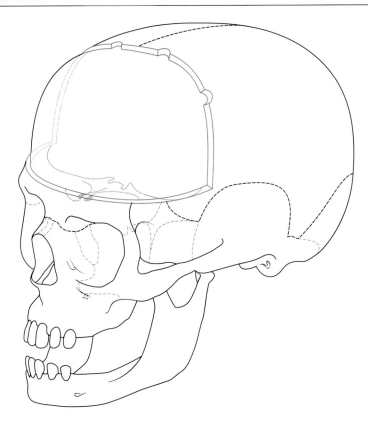

Fig. 7.11

The anterior frontal bone flap can be removed following its dissection by peripheral or central burrholes. Its removal permits dissection along the anterior cranial base, roof of the orbits and exposure of central structures such as the cribriform plate and crista gali. The olfactory nerves are not disturbed.

Fig. 7.12 a, b

After dissecting the orbits medially, superiorly and laterally ▶ down to the body of the zygoma, osteotomies may be performed on the involved side at the malar eminence and at the zygomaticofrontal suture on the uninvolved side. Advancement of the frontal process of the zygoma produces a complete lateral canthal advancement by anterior rotation of the lateral orbit. Frontal bar advancement may be unilateral (**a**) or bilateral (**b**).

mies are made across the nasofrontal suture. This exposure allows the entire area of the deformity to be accessed, osteotomized, and repositioned.

When a temporal region is recessed, the temporal bone can be removed and replaced in an improved position (Fig. 7.13). The temporal regions were formerly used for a "tongue in groove" articulation of bone for stabilization (Fig. 7.14). Now, however, temporal bones can be widely exposed, removed, recontoured, and repositioned without compromising stability because of stable fixation techniques, correcting the temporal contour. If the orbit is constricted in a mediolateral direction, it can be osteotomized and an interpositional bone graft placed (Fig. 7.15). Otherwise, the frontal bar is bent to conform to a normal, bilateral symmetric configuration and plated into position at the lateral temporal and nasofrontal junctions. It is generally plated and posi-

tioned by plates placed in the temporal hollow region (Fig. 7.16).

Finally, the frontal bone is contoured by bending barrel stave or partial or complete peripheral osteotomies. The frontal bone is then plated into position (Fig. 7.17; junctional stable fixation). The bone dust saved from the osteotomies and burrholes is then placed on the areas of the osteotomies. An anterior osteotomy is generally performed at the nasofrontal region, which avoids dissection of the insertion of the medial canthal ligament. In younger infants the segments of bone can be bent with finger manipulation or a Tessier bone-bending forceps. After the age of 1 year, the bone is too brittle for bending; inner table scoring is then used to allow for bending, as are greenstick fractures. Sometimes greenstick fractures or partial osteotomies need to be supported by plate and screw fixation to maintain position. The orbi-

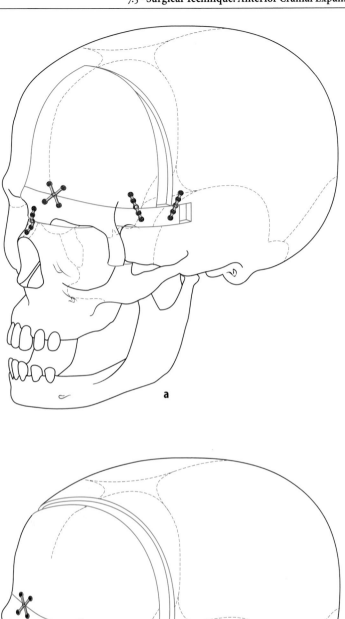

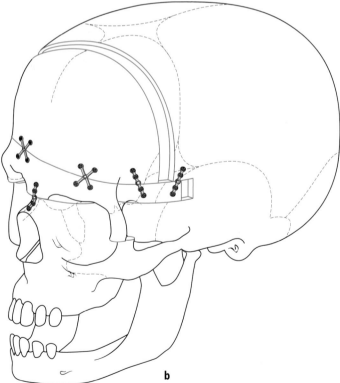

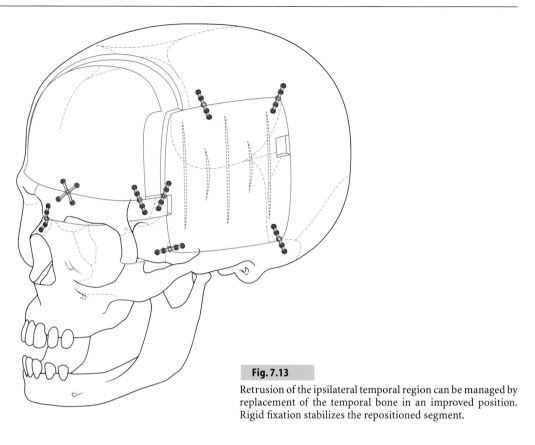

Fig. 7.13

Retrusion of the ipsilateral temporal region can be managed by replacement of the temporal bone in an improved position. Rigid fixation stabilizes the repositioned segment.

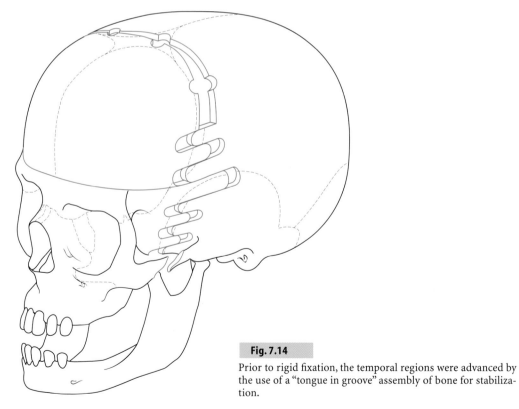

Fig. 7.14

Prior to rigid fixation, the temporal regions were advanced by the use of a "tongue in groove" assembly of bone for stabilization.

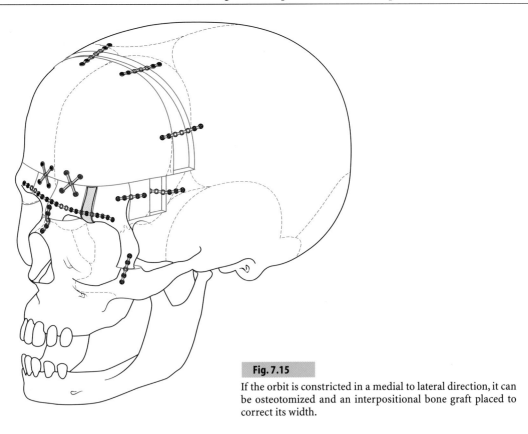

Fig. 7.15

If the orbit is constricted in a medial to lateral direction, it can be osteotomized and an interpositional bone graft placed to correct its width.

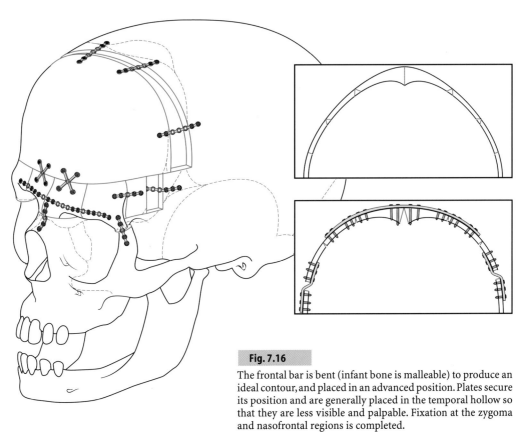

Fig. 7.16

The frontal bar is bent (infant bone is malleable) to produce an ideal contour, and placed in an advanced position. Plates secure its position and are generally placed in the temporal hollow so that they are less visible and palpable. Fixation at the zygoma and nasofrontal regions is completed.

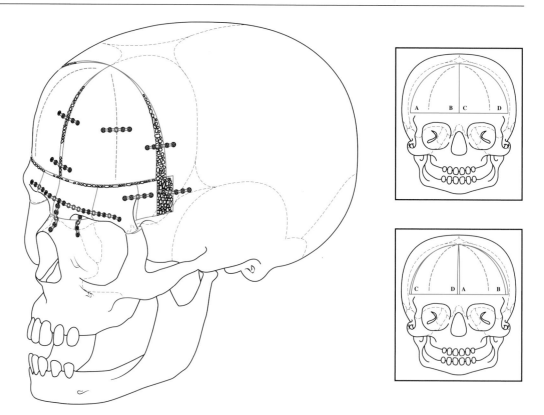

Fig. 7.17

The frontal bone flap may be reversed 180° in plagiocephaly correction. It can be further contoured by peripheral, "barrel stave" or sectional osteotomies which can be stabilized with small internal fixation devices. The frontal bone flap is stabilized by marginal rigid fixation. Bone dust saved from the osteotomies and burrholes is placed into areas of osteotomy gap.

tal segments are advanced into a slightly overcorrected position and held in place with microreconstruction plates or 1.3 plates. In children 3-mm screws should be used since these have not been shown to cause dural penetration if intracranial migration occurs. Bone grafts can also be used in contour modes and lag screwed into position. Some fixation is usually necessary at the nasofrontal junction.

7.6 Posterior Cranial Expansion

Isolated posterior cranial expansion is carried out through a biparietal incision (see Fig. 7.2). Subperiosteal dissection is used to expose the occiput and lambdoid areas down to the occipital region, in the junction of the posterior neck muscles. A two-piece parietal-occipital craniotomy is usually performed in a transverse fashion, completely encompassing the skull deformity. The oste-

otomy begins 5–8 cm above the junction of the left lambdoidal sutures and along the sagittal suture. It then extends in a curvalinear fashion to involve the asterion region. The inferior osteotomy is performed below the transverse sinus. A central transverse osteotomy below the junction of the lambdoidal sutures divides a posterior craniotomy into two segments (Fig. 7.18). The segments are elevated, and a lower "occipital bar" can be harvested which allows the same facility of reconstruction as anterior by moving and positioning the "frontal bar."

For right or left isolated lambdoid suture synostosis, the bone segments may be rotated 190°. This allows the expanded bone from the contralateral (compensatory) area to be placed on the ipsilateral or flattened side. The flattened ipsilateral bone can be placed loosely on top of the bulging dura and the contour deformity corrected. Extending the rotation a little bit beyond 180° assists in providing adequate expansion and fixation.

If an occipital bar is not required, the advanced segment is held in place with "stepped" reconstruction plates bent to allow the appropriate advancement. "Barrel stave" peripheral osteotomies are sometimes performed in the bone flap to increase the contour. The barrel staving allows contouring to be performed. This same technique can be used in the frontal bone.

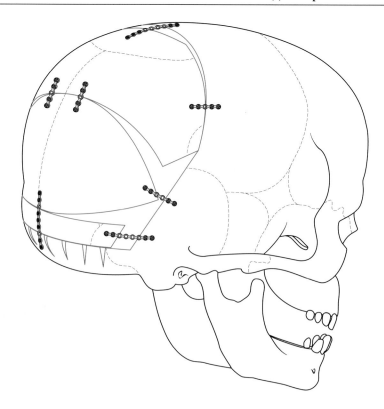

Fig. 7.18

The posterior cranial expansion involves removal of the posterior skull and vertex with creation of a one of two segments and posterior expansion and vertical height reduction. A lower occipital bar can be harvested, which allows advancement and repositioning.

The occipital bar has been advanced strongly posteriorly.

7.7 Complete or Subtotal Calvarial Expansion

Full cranial expansion is an extensive operation reserved only for those patients with total calvarial deformities which cannot be corrected by simpler procedures. One-stage full cranial expansion procedures are generally avoided in those under 2 years of age, due to blood replacement and monitoring difficulties and the potential for significant complications related to the sphinx position, such as air embolism. Two-stage anterior and posterior cranial expansions are sometimes performed to permit correction of the deformities with less complicated operations (Fig. 7.19). Older individuals, however, can have a full cranial expansion with or without a frontal bar in one stage. The use of the frontal bar depends upon the deformity observed.

A full cranial expansion allows all of the bone segments of the frontal, parietal, and occipital areas to be

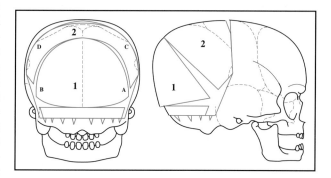

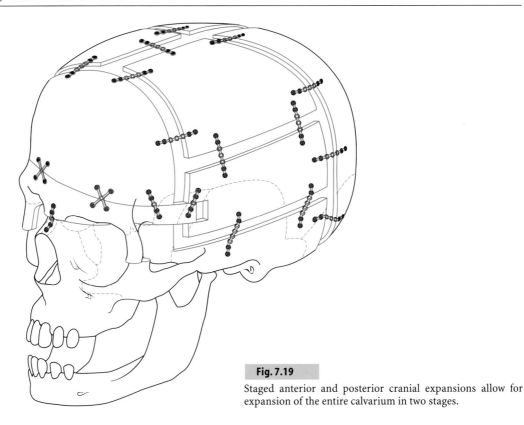

Fig. 7.19

Staged anterior and posterior cranial expansions allow for expansion of the entire calvarium in two stages.

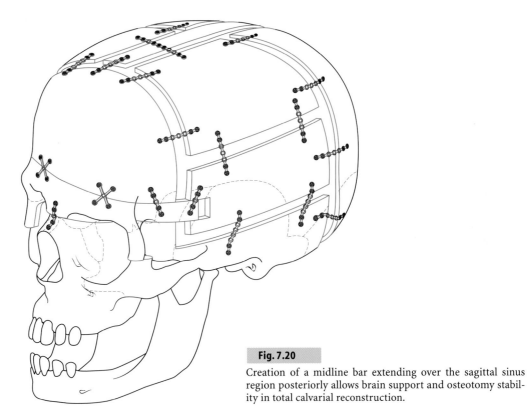

Fig. 7.20

Creation of a midline bar extending over the sagittal sinus region posteriorly allows brain support and osteotomy stability in total calvarial reconstruction.

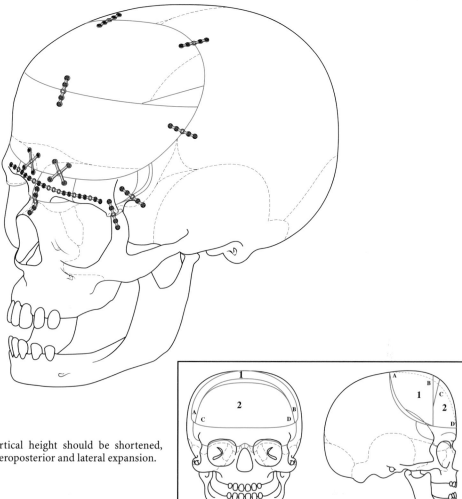

Fig. 7.21

In brachycephaly the vertical height should be shortened, which is permitted by anteroposterior and lateral expansion.

removed, appropriately contoured, and repositioned. A bar is usually left either in the center or posteriorly to provide brain support (Fig. 7.20). Subtotal cranial expansions are generally performed in patients with recurrent or severe deformities who have not achieved significant correction with simpler procedures. These patients usually demonstrate delayed growth, and some have microcephaly resulting in "secondary synostosis." In some cases a frontal bar advancement is required along with a posterior expansion which is a full cranial expansion. One must tailor the expansion to the amount of stretch that the scalp can tolerate and still be able to close the incision. In almost all cases this requires mobilization of the scalp and galeal scoring.

The reconstruction proceeds with the placement of the frontal bar in an appropriate position. The two wings of the frontal bar and frontal bone are then "fanned" laterally to increase the frontal width. The temporal and parietal segments, usually separated in individual segments, are then advanced laterally and "step-plated" to the basal skull. This allows for lateral expansion of significance. These bone segments sometimes require contouring, barrel staving, or shortening superiorly to allow

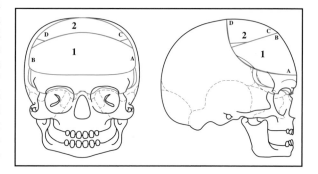

the bone to be rotated laterally and inferiorly and maintain the proper height. The possibility of too much vertical expansion is managed by superior osteotomies; a decision needs to be made as to how much superior volume increase is required.

Finally, the occipital and lambdoid segments are advanced anteriorly into position and rotated laterally to decrease the anterior-posterior skull length which improves the transverse diameter. If decrease in the anterior-posterior length of the skull is desired, the frontal and occipital bones are moved posteriorly and anteriorly, respectively, so that the skull length is decreased. The brain is compressed in the anterior-posteror dimension and moves laterally to occupy the expanded lateral bone framework. In patients who demonstrate brachycephaly, the expansion should occur anteriorly and posteriorly, and the vertical height should be reduced (Fig. 7.21).

Bone defects cannot be expected to heal by spontaneous osteogenesis in patients who are over 2 years of age. Therefore bone is split from the inner tables of the skull so that a full bone reconstruction can be completed. Bone defects should be filled with grafts in anyone over 3 years of age. The grafts are positioned to provide stability of expansion. Occasionally there is so much expansion that scalp closure is not possible even with "criss-cross" galeotomies. This situation must be corrected by decreasing the amount of interpositional bone graft in the expansion and replating the segments in a less expanded position.

7.8 Hypertelorism

The correction of hypertelorism classically involves "box" osteotomies performed around the orbital region (Fig. 7.22). Complex osteotomies, or facial bipartitions (Fig. 7.23), are designed to reduce the transverse diameter of the upper face and improve the width of the maxillary arch and the entire maxilla, creating a "V" excision where the orbits are rotated into position. The path of these osteotomies must be guided to avoid teeth. The presence of the slanted orbit (inferior displacement of the lateral orbit) requires correction by orbital rotation. The osteotomy cuts are visualized in Fig. 7.22 and 7.23. The use of 1.3 plates and screws is ideal for these osteotomized segments.

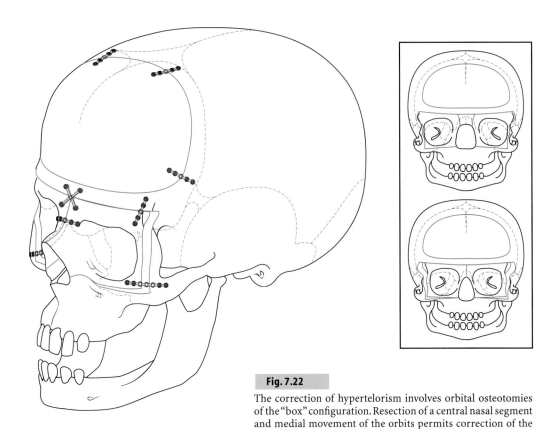

Fig. 7.22

The correction of hypertelorism involves orbital osteotomies of the "box" configuration. Resection of a central nasal segment and medial movement of the orbits permits correction of the hypertelorism.

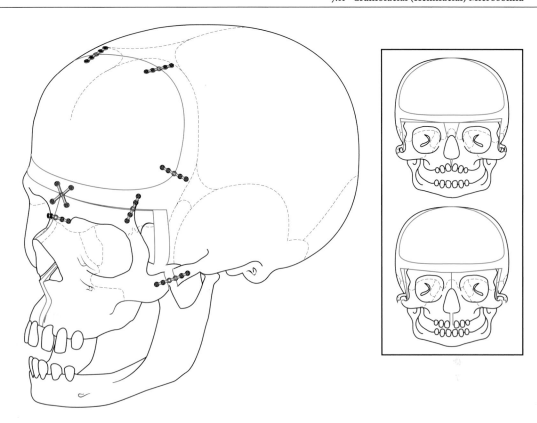

Facial bipartition osteotomies involve rotation of the entire maxilla and frontal bone as a single unit. A central "V" is excised permitting the orbits to rotate into position. This is especially useful in correction of the inferior rotation of the lateral orbit. Additionally, the width of the maxillary dental arch is improved by lateral rotation. The use of this osteotomy avoids the inferior orbital osteotomy illustrated in Fig. 7.22 which would impair developing teeth.

7.9 Monoblock Osteotomies

In monoblock osteotomies the use of a simultaneous advancement of the midface and frontal bone allows correction of the exorbitism and midface retrusion in a single operation (Fig. 7.24). The operation has been plagued by a 10% incidence of infection which occurs from nasal-subcranial communications and contamination in "dead space" behind the advanced frontal bone. Most patients benefit from the use of stable fixation as opposed to wires.

7.10 Orbital Dystopia

Simultaneous orbital osteotomies are used for the vertical correction of cranial-orbital deformities, such as ver-

tical correction in orbital dystopia. A single orbit can be moved up or down (Fig. 7.25). A minicraniotomy or a standard frontal craniotomy provides the exposure. Some overcorrection (4 mm) is suggested. The judicious use of plate and screw fixation in cranial osteotomies allows the surgeon to obtain consistently good results while minimizing complications.

7.11 Craniofacial (Hemifacial) Microsomia

The syndrome of craniofacial (hemifacial) microsomia involves malar hypoplasia, the possibility of facial weakness, paralysis, underdevelopment, or absence of the zygoma, lateral and inferior orbit, and temporal mandibular joint (Fig. 7.26). In its complete form the cleft is a Tessier #7 cleft with macrostomia, microtic external ear and underdeveloped ipsilateral tongue, soft palate, and muscles of mastication. The parotid gland and duct can be absent. The seventh cranial nerve may have absent, partial, or complete function, hypoplasia, or aplasia. When the external and the middle ear are affected, conductive hearing loss is present.

The osseous manifestations involve mandibular deficiency, which can vary from minor flattening of the condylar head to complete absence of the entire mandibular ramus, with deviation of the mandible and the lower face toward the affected side. The maxilla is tilted, and

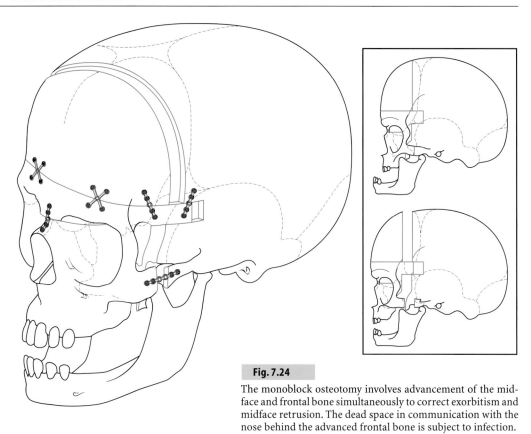

Fig. 7.24

The monoblock osteotomy involves advancement of the midface and frontal bone simultaneously to correct exorbitism and midface retrusion. The dead space in communication with the nose behind the advanced frontal bone is subject to infection.

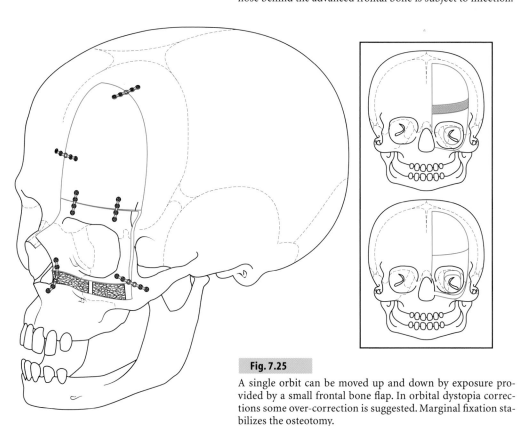

Fig. 7.25

A single orbit can be moved up and down by exposure provided by a small frontal bone flap. In orbital dystopia corrections some over-correction is suggested. Marginal fixation stabilizes the osteotomy.

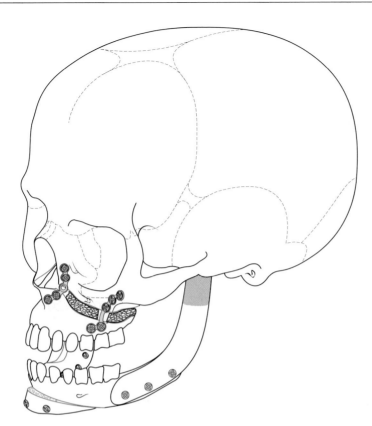

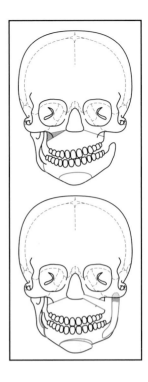

Fig. 7.26

In hemifacial microsomia a short mandible and maxilla are found on the ipsilateral side. The syndrome is classified by the amount of mandibular hypoplasia and development of the condyle.

therefore the occlusal plane is canted superiorly. Various degrees of zygomatic hypoplasia are seen with absence of the zygomatic arch and condylar fossa in severe cases. The orbit may be inferiorly dystopic, and cranial asymmetry may be present. The surgical procedures involved in correction use mandibular osteotomies, and recently also bone lengthening, costal chondral bone grafting, and bimaxillary osteotomies with genioplasty (Fig. 7.26).

7.12 The Treacher Collins Malformation

The malformation in Treacher Collins syndrome is thought to be a combination of the Tessier #6, #7, and #8 clefts. Absence of the zygoma, coloboma of the lateral lower eyelid, antimongoloid slant of the palpebral fissure, deformity of the orbit, and absence of the eyelashes, hypoplasia of the mandibular ramus, anterior open bite, severe retrusion of the chin and an absence of the zygomatic arches, fusion of the temporalis and the masseter, macrostomia, palatal clefts, choanal atresia, and absence of the malar prominence characterize the deformity.

Skeletal correction involves soft-tissue transfer from the upper to the lower eyelids, osteotomies or bone grafting of the mandible, maxillary osteotomy (Fig. 7.27), genioplasty and reconstruction of the zygomas with calvarial bone grafts. Lateral canthopexies improve the lateral position of the eyelids, and generally a soft-tissue flap must be added to the lateral portion of the lower lid.

7.13 Encephaloceles

Encephaloceles are bone defects in the cranial vault or base which allow prolapse of meninges and brain tissue into the nose, orbit, or temporal region. These are approached by frontal bone flap and repositioning of the prolapsed meninges and brain tissue. A bone graft (Fig. 7.28) can be placed over the defect. Excess skin is resected.

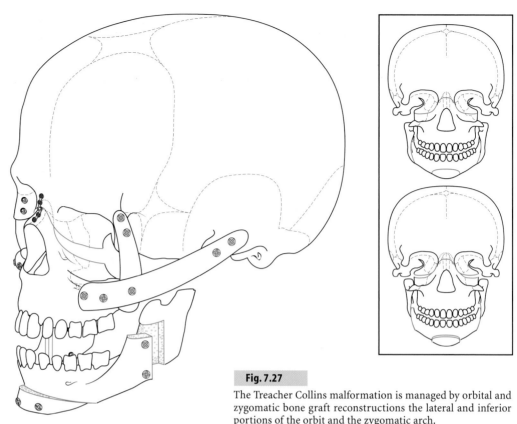

Fig. 7.27

The Treacher Collins malformation is managed by orbital and zygomatic bone graft reconstructions the lateral and inferior portions of the orbit and the zygomatic arch.

The mandible is advanced with bilateral interpositional bone graft, and osteotomies. The maxilla must be rotated as well.

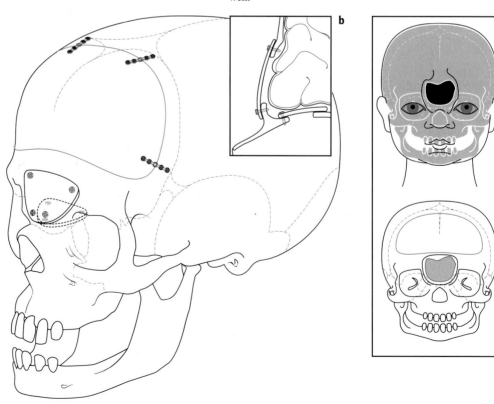

7.14 Bone Lenghthening by Continuous Distraction

In recent years Ilizarov's idea of bone lengthening via distraction after osteotomies has been introduced into craniomaxillofacial surgery.

7.14.1 Distraction for Mandibular Deformities

In the past many deformities of the mandible required complex reconstruction. The reconstruction either took the form of the bone graft being plated in a mandibular defect followed by stable fixation, or, occasionally, the tissues required vascularized bone to optimize the final results.

Distraction osteogenesis has the advantage of allowing reconstruction of mandibular deformities in a controlled fashion with the native bone. In mandibular defects from either trauma or tumor this can be accomplished by performing an osteotomy of the bone on either side of the defect, transporting this bone across the defect to reach ultimately the other side of the defect, creating bone as the segment is moved into position. In congenital defects in which the mandible is smaller on a unilateral or bilateral basis (hemifacial microsomia, or Treacher Collins syndrome) the mandible can be increased in size by, again, creating an osteotomy and lengthening the bone in the direction in which normal growth should occur.

Patients with congenital deformities are those most commonly undergoing distraction at this time. Patients with asymmetries of the mandible in moderate deformities are the best candidates. Mild deformities require a choice between a scar versus improved bone symmetry. In severe deformities the mandible may be too small to perform an adequate osteotomy. Bilateral deformities frequently have a significant esthetic deformity, but are of more concern for functional problems with the airway and sleep apnea. Distraction can open the airway and decrease the need for tracheostomy by bringing the mandible forward.

Evaluation prior to the procedure usually requires orthodontic assistance, as do regular osteotomies and the traditional advancement techniques. The records include cephalometric, panorex, and computed tomog-

raphy examinations for more complex deformities. The orthodontist may have to play an important role, assisting the surgeon in planning the movement and position of the osteotomy. Patients frequently require functional orthodontic treatment following the procedure in order to maintain or improve the occlusion. The orthodontist can assist the surgeon in monitoring the process of the distraction to obtain the ideal functional occlusal and esthetic results.

The procedure begins by placing a nasal airway for bilateral and, to a lesser extent, unilateral procedures. Appropriate antibiotics are usually given. A buccal incision is performed near the site of the proposed mandibular osteotomy. A subperiosteal dissection is then performed. The location of the osteotomy is planned with consideration of the position of the inferior alveolar nerve and tooth follicles. The osteotomy should ideally be perpendicular to the plane of the movement that is desired. A burr can be used to mark the position of this osteotomy. The position of the pin placement is then determined. The ideal condition of the pin should be parallel to the direction of the movement and perpendicular to the osteotomy (Fig. 7.29 a).

A trocar is used to place the pins after a small incision is made in the skin. A drill guide is used to protect the soft tissues. Once the drill hole has been completed, pins are placed. Some distraction devices require placement of plate and screws, which are then the focus of the distraction. An osteotomy is then performed along the buccal surface with a Lindeman round burr or a reciprocating saw. The completion of the osteotomy along the lingual cortex is performed with an osteotome. The completion of the osteotomy is then confirmed. The device is then placed and activated to determine whether the segments can move (Fig. 7.29 b).

Standard postoperative care includes pin tract cleaning for an external device, thorough cleaning for internal devices, and probably liquid, progressing to soft diet depending on the amount of stability. Distraction begins in the early postoperative period. Some physicians allow a latency period of 5 days, and some begin distraction immediately. Distraction should be initiated within 5 days. It begins with 1 mm distance per day, using a cycle of at least two times or preferably four times a day. Follow-up is on every 3rd day to assess the device position and care, making sure that distraction is occurring. Obviously, if the device is activated in the wrong direction, compression occurs, and the result is compromised. Cephalometrics and panorex records are obtained after 1 week, 2 weeks, 1 month, and 2 months.

The device is activated until the desired skeletal reconstruction is achieved. Visual confirmation of this reconstructive result should be obtained. The device is left in place until there is evidence of further consolidation on the X-ray.

Fig. 7.28 a, b

◄ Encephaloceles involve defects in the cranial base with prolapse of the meninges and brain tissue. Correction involves exposure with a frontal bone flap (**a**), retraction or resection of the prolapsed tissue and bone graft obliteration of the defect (**b**).

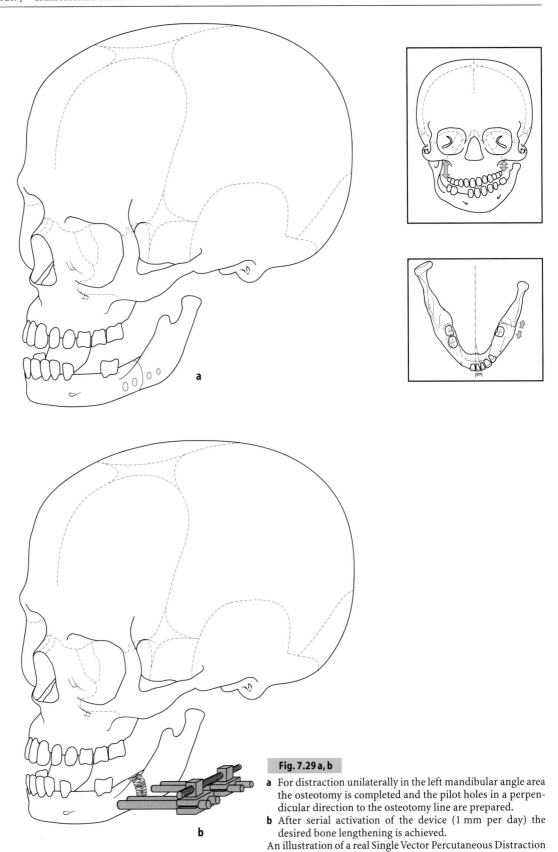

Fig. 7.29 a, b

a For distraction unilaterally in the left mandibular angle area the osteotomy is completed and the pilot holes in a perpendicular direction to the osteotomy line are prepared.

b After serial activation of the device (1 mm per day) the desired bone lengthening is achieved.

An illustration of a real Single Vector Percutaneous Distraction Device is shown in Fig. 1.29 a–d.

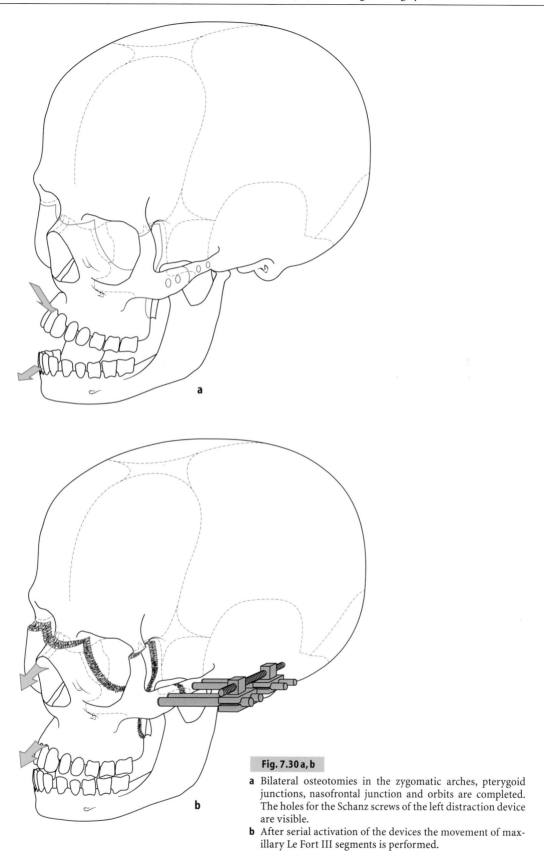

Fig. 7.30 a, b

a Bilateral osteotomies in the zygomatic arches, pterygoid junctions, nasofrontal junction and orbits are completed. The holes for the Schanz screws of the left distraction device are visible.

b After serial activation of the devices the movement of maxillary Le Fort III segments is performed.

7.14.2 Midface Distraction

Midface distraction is potentially a new area for investigation and clinical application. This would be appropriate for patients such as clefts and Binder's syndrome, along with Crouzon's and Apert's syndromes (Fig. 7.30a). Preoperative evaluations and consultation are performed similar to the mandible. The device for distraction by nature has fewer degrees of freedom since the devices are typically not worn on the middle portion of the face. Typically they utilize the zygomatic arch as the point of force application. Clinical experience of the future will indicate the most appropriate distraction devices for this purpose. At present posterior-anterior advancement is possible with a slight rotation side to side. Other options for midface distractions can occur with orthodontic manipulation using rubber bands and a fixed orthodontic appliance after osteotomy in the area planned for advancement. A maxillary tuberosity-pterygoid dysjunction is usually required. Follow-up and techniques of distraction are similar to those described for the mandible (Fig. 7.30b).

References and Suggested Reading

Argenta L, David LR, Wilson JA, Bell WO (1996) An increase in infant cranial deformity with supine sleeping position. J Craniofac Surg 7:5–11

Arnaud E, Renier D, Marchac D (1994) Development of the frontal sinus and glabellar morphology after frontocranial remodeling for craniosynostosis in infancy. J Craniofac Surg 5:81–94

Bruneteau RJ, Mulliken JB (1992) Frontal plagiocephaly: synostotic, compensational or deformational. Plast Reconstr Surg 89:21–31

Chadduck WM, Chadduck JD, Boop FA (1992) The subarachnoid spaces in craniosynostosis. Neurosurg 30:867–871

Cohen MM (1991) Etiopathogenesis of craniosynostosis. Neurosurg Clin North Am 2:507

Cohen SR et al (1993) Surgical techniques of cranial vault expansion for increases in intracranial pressure in older children. J Craniofac Surg 4:167–173

David LR, Wilson JA, Watson NE, Argenta LC (1996) Cerebral perfusion defects secondary to simple craniosynostosis. J Craniofac Surg 7:177–185

Eppley BL, Sadove AM (1994) Effects of resorbable fixation on craniofacial skeletal growth: modifications in plate size. J Craniofac Surg 5:110–114

Gault DT et al (1990) Intracranial volume in children with craniosynostosis. J Craniofac Surg 1:1

Jabs EW et al (1993) A mutation in the homeodomain of the human MSX2 gene in a family affected with autosomal dominant craniosynostosis. Cell 75:443

LeBourq N et al (1992) Value of 3D imaging for a study of craniofacial malformations in children. J Neuroradiol 18:225

Lo LJ, Marsh JL et al (1996) Plagiocephaly: differential diagnosis based on endocranial morphology. Plast Reconstr Surg 97:282–291

McCarthy JG, Glasberg SB et al (1995) Twenty-year experience with early surgery for craniosynostosis. I. Isolated craniofacial synostosis – results and unsolved problems. Plast Reconstr Surg 96:272–283

McCarthy, Glasberg SB et al (1995) Twenty-year experience with early surgery for craniosynostosis. II. The craniofacial synostosis syndromes and pansynostosis – results and unsolved problems. Plast Reconstr Surg 96:284–298

Munro IR (1993) Rigid fixation, skull reconstruction, and fiscal responsibility (editorial)

Ohman J, Richtsmeier J (1994) Perspectives on craniofacial growth. Clin Plast Surg 21:489–499

Persing JA, Posnick J et al (1996) Cranial plate and screw fixation in infancy. An assessment of risk. J Craniofac Surg 7:267–270

Posnick JC (1996) Monobloc and facial bipartition osteotomies: a step-by step description of the surgical technique. J Craniofac Surg 3:229–250

Posnick JC et al (1992) Indirect intracranial volume measurement using CT scans: clinic applications for craniosynostosis. Plast Reconstr Surg 89:34–45

Posnick JC, Armstrong D, Bit U (1995) Metopic and sagittal synostosis: intracranial volume measurements prior to and after cranio-orbital reshaping in childhood. Plast Reconstr Surg 96:299–315

Posnick JC, Goldstein JA, Saitzman AA (1993a) Surgical correction of the Treacher Collins malar deficiency: quantitative CT scan analysis of long term results. Plast Reconstr Surg 92:12–22

Posnick JC, Kin KY, Jhawar BJ, Armstrong D (1993b) Crouzon syndrome: quantitative assessment of presenting deformity and surgical results based on CT scans. Plast Reconstr Surg 92:1015–1024

Posnick JC, Lin KY, Chen P, Armstrong D (1992) Sagittal synostosis: quantitative assessment of presenting deformity and surgical results based on CT scans. Plast Reconstr Surg 92:1015

Posnick JC, Lin Ky, Chen P, Armstrong D (1994) Metopic synostosis. Quantitative assessment of presenting deformity and surgical results based on CT scans. Plast Reconstr Surg 93:16–23

Prevot M, Renier D, Marchac D (1993) Lack of ossification after cranioplasty for craniosynostosis: a review of relevant factors in 592 consecutive patients. J Craniofac Surg 4:247–254

Ripley CE, Pomatto J et al (1994) Treatment of positional plagiocephaly with dynamic orthotic cranioplasty. J Craniofac Surg 5:150–159

Sadove AM, Eppley BL (1991) Microfixation techniques in pediatric craniomaxillofacial surgery. Ann Plast Surg 27:36–43

Turk AE, McCarthy JG, Thorne CH, Wisoff JH (1996) The "back to sleep campaign" and deformational plagiocephaly: is there cause for concern? J Craniofac Surg 7:12–18

Waitzman AA, Posnick JC, Armstrong DC, Pron GE (1992) Craniofacial skeletal measurements based on computed tomography. II. Normal values and growth trends. Cleft Palate Craniofac J 29:118–128

Williams JK, Cohen SR et al (1995) Outcome assessment in craniosynostosis: a longitudinal, statistical study of reoperation rates. Presented at the VI International Symposium of Craniofacial Surgeons, St. Tropez, France

Wolfe SA, Morison G, Page KL, Berkowitz S (1993) The monobloc frontofacial advancement: do the pluses outweigh the minuses? Plast Reconstr Surg 91:977–987

Yaremchuk MJ (1993) Commentary on craniofacial growth following rigid fixation. J Craniofac Surg 4:245–246

Yaremchuk MJ, Thomas GS et al (1994) The effects of rigid fixaiton on craniofacial growth of rhesus monkeys. Plast Reconstr Surg 93:11–15

Subject Index